REVISED AND UPDATED

THE ASTHMA HANDBOOK

A Complete Guide for Patients and Their Families

REVISED AND UPDATED

THE ASTHMA HANDBOOK

A Complete Guide for Patients and Their Families

Stuart H. Young, M.D.,
with Susan A. Shulman and
Martin D. Shulman, Ph.D.

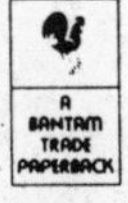

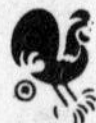

BANTAM BOOKS

NEW YORK • TORONTO • LONDON • SYDNEY • AUCKLAND

To my mother and father—Sylvia and John,
my brother Jonathan and my wife, Marcia.
Stuart H. Young, M.D.

To our sons, Lawrence and Andrew, who all too often had to hear
"we'll be with you as soon as we're finished writing,"
thanks for being patient with us.
We give you our infinite love.
Susan A. Shulman and
Martin D. Shulman

The authors have written a comprehensive book on asthma and its treatment which should provide you with solid information and guidance in coping with this serious condition. Asthma, however, like other diseases, requires formal medical attention and, therefore, we advise that you use this book only as a secondary source of medical advice in conjunction with your physician's primary treatment.

THE ASTHMA HANDBOOK:
A COMPLETE GUIDE FOR PATIENTS AND THEIR FAMILIES
A Bantam Book / February 1985

PRINTING HISTORY
Revised Bantam trade edition / August 1989

Illustrations for Breathing Exercises and Directions for Postural Drainage were reproduced with the permission of Merrell Dow Pharmaceuticals, Inc., Subsidiary of the Dow Chemical Company, Cincinnati, Ohio 45215.

Illustrations by Patricia Tobin.

Library of Congress Cataloging-in-Publication Data

Young, Stuart H.
The asthma handbook : a complete guide for patients and their families / Stuart H. Young, with Susan A. Shulman and Martin D. Shulman.
p. cm.
Includes index.
ISBN 0-553-34712-8
1. Asthma—Popular works. 2. Asthma in children—Popular works.
I. Shulman, Susan A. II. Shulman, Martin D. III. Title.
RC591.Y68 1989
616.2'38—dc20 89-6589
CIP

Published simultaneously in the United States and Canada

Bantam Books are published by Bantam Books, a division of Bantam Doubleday Dell Publishing Group, Inc. Its trademark, consisting of the words "Bantam Books" and the portrayal of a rooster, is Registered in U.S. Patent and Trademark Office and in other countries. Marca Registrada. Bantam Books, 666 Fifth Avenue, New York, New York 10103.

PRINTED IN THE UNITED STATES OF AMERICA

S 0 9 8 7 6 5 4 3

ACKNOWLEDGMENTS

I realize that writing a book is never an individual effort. Even if one were to utilize no other resource than one's own imagination, there are many influences filtering in through the eye of that imagination. There are many people from whom I have received contributions because of their association with me.

I would like to express my gratitude to my many teachers who over the years have inculcated in me knowledge, judgment, and above all, a love and respect for medicine.

I would like to specially thank five mentors and friends, each of whom was extremely helpful to me at some point in my career: the late Jonathan Trumball Lanman, M.D.; also Edwin Bronsky, M.D., Elliot Ellis, M.D., Richard Farr, M.D., and David Pearlman, M.D.

I am appreciative of the knowledge and satisfaction gained from my patients during the course of my treatment of them. In addition, I am happy to thank Patricia Burbage, R.N., Karen Rubenstein, and Leon Zacharowitz, patients who were kind enough to read this book and offer me advice and encouragement.

I would like to thank my wife, Marcia, for her forbearance and encouragement while I prepared this book and for her help in formulating its concepts and principles.

My gratitude also goes to Edith Frank who very carefully reviewed this book and offered me advice and encouragement.

I received valuable comments from my colleagues, several of whom carefully read sections of this book. The contributions they made to this book, I gratefully acknowledge. I accept full responsibility for any oversights or errors. The physicians are: James Rubin, M.D., Katherine Teets Grimm, M.D., Lois Stark, M.D., Joseph Nieder, M.D., Alan Fay, M.D., and Bernard Adelsberg, M.D.

I would like to especially thank my associate Bruce Dobozin, M.D., who extensively and methodically reviewed this book and offered constructive criticism and support in its preparation.

Special thanks to my loyal hardworking staff, especially Charmaine Murphy. Also thanks to Jean Laird, Jeanette Mendez, Andrea Reid, and Ruby Vasquez.

Special thanks to Ronnian Feintuch who extensively reviewed the manuscript and offered much helpful advice, criticism, and encouragement.

And finally, there are many others, too numerous to mention, to whom I am grateful and whom I have already thanked personally.

SPECIAL ACKNOWLEDGMENT

I owe a special debt of gratitude to Harlan Daman, M.D., my close friend and colleague with whom I have collaborated on many books and scientific articles. Dr. Daman has carefully read every section in the book. He has made invaluable suggestions and checked everything from concepts to drug dosage. I gratefully acknowledge his very valuable assistance in the preparation of this book.

Stuart Young, M.D.

We welcome this opportunity to acknowledge the people who offered their consistent support and constructive criticism during the years of writing this book.

Thank you to all of our friends who couldn't wait to see this book in print so that they finally could stop hearing about it. You all know who you are and we thank you most sincerely.

Susan's parents, Shirley and Marvin Krumholz, deserve our deepest thanks for their daily words of encouragement and confidence. Ellen and David Mandel, sister and brother-in-law, have been our constant cheerleaders. Thanks also to Aunt Cele and to our cousin Bud for his guidance right from the start. Special thanks to Marty's family, Hy, Fay, Julie, Shelli, Howie, and Marlene Shulman for sharing our excitement and believing in us.

We would like to thank our agents, John Boswell and Pat Brown of John Boswell Associates, for their continuous support, expert guidance, and involvement in the publishing of this book.

We would also like to express our appreciation to our editor, Linda Loewenthal of Bantam Books, for her expert editorial guidance, always cheerfully offered to us in the preparation of the second edition of this book.

Thanks to New Dawn Health Food Shoppe for allowing us to peruse their shelves and barrage them with questions.

Susan and Martin Shulman

CONTENTS

Foreword by Stuart H. Young, M.D. xiii

Preface by Susan A. Shulman xv

1. The Facts About Asthma 1
2. How to Know If You Have Asthma and How to Get Help 14
3. Asthma and the Environment 38
4. Food Allergy and Asthma 67
5. Immunotherapy 134
6. Pharmacological Management of Asthma 143
7. Case Studies: Basic Therapy Approaches in Action 202
8. Psychological Aspects of Asthma and Stress-Reduction Therapies 219
9. A Physical Therapy Approach to Asthma 232
10. Asthma and Pregnancy 248
11. Asthma in Children 265
12. The Acute Attack 285
13. Surgery 304
14. Asthma Centers and Clinics 309
15. Daily Dos and Don'ts 318
16. The Future 327

Appendix 1: Pollination Time of Trees, Grasses, and Weeds 332

Glossary 349

Index 359

FOREWORD

I have been a practicing allergist for twenty years. Of the many types of allergic diseases that I treat, none is more challenging than asthma. Asthma is a capricious illness that can inflict a lifetime of misery on one person, while another may wheeze just once in his entire life. Asthma's capriciousness is often seen in the same individual who may be deathly ill for three weeks, and who then suddenly, and for no apparent reason, is perfectly well. Asthma is an illness the cause of which is so profound that not until we completely untangle the genetic code will we truly unravel its mystery or find a cure. Asthma is not curable now because we cannot change one's genes. However, with the knowledge that is available today it is usually controllable, and most asthmatics can function in a normal or near-normal fashion. Asthma's causes are so variable and its treatments so diverse that it takes a great deal of education for both the patient and the physician to understand and control it. It is the purpose of this book to educate you, the patient, so that you are prepared in concert with your physician to deal with asthma using all of the tools that are presently available.

I wrote this book because it is my belief that the treatment of any illness is facilitated by both an educated physician and layman. I have been, and I am presently, involved in writing scientific articles to educate physicians in their understanding of asthma. I also attend many courses and conferences where many of my colleagues educate me. The treatment of asthma changes and improves every year, and it is important for a physician to keep abreast of any innovations. Thus an educated, knowledgeable, and compassionate physician is a very important member of the team. The other member of the team—equally important, if not more so—

is you, the patient. One of the primary responsibilities of the physician is to train his patient. In my opinion this is an extremely important task, and one that I have taken very seriously. However, I have found that very often the task is easier said than done!

There have been countless times when I have been in the position of having to explain the underlying mechanisms of asthma, available medications, and general management procedures. While most of these times have been with an individual patient, I have also experimented with group discussions and lectures to patient groups. Despite slow, clear, and logical explanations, I have been generally disappointed that intelligent, motivated patients have not gained a clear understanding of what was being said. While they try very hard, their intense involvement and high anxiety seems to preclude a thorough comprehension. Something I say sounds familiar, and soon the patient is lost in a string of associations of past experiences and stops listening objectively to the whole story. They are frustrated and I am frustrated. They want to learn, but they would really prefer to take me home with them and digest the information I am offering, slowly, at their own pace, delving into issues that are relevant to them at a certain time.

Knowing this, I have often suggested that my patients read literature on asthma, allergy, and environmental control. However, the material is scattered in sundry books, magazines, journals, and pamphlets that are often not clear, concise, well organized, or helpful.

This all culminated in my motivation and desire to write this book. Susan Shulman, one of my patients, suggested that she also had a message to pass on to other asthmatics. She felt that I had the knowledge and dedication to write this book, and she had the skill, empathy, and firsthand experiences to enhance and translate the basic, factual information into a highly readable, informative, and usable book. We have catalogued all the current, relevant information into a book that is written on a level that is sophisticated enough to impart the necessary knowledge to the patient, but with a minimum of "scientificese" so that the lay person can understand what is being presented.

Stuart H. Young, M.D.

PREFACE

Can you imagine being frightened of the wind, perfume, laughter, trees, colds, smoke, dogs, or chalk? Are there really people who have all of these fears? If so, how can they possibly expect to live through the day?

Such people do exist. They are among the more than ten million Americans who suffer from a devastating and sometimes life-threatening disease known as asthma. Their fears are unfortunately justified because they have learned through painful experiences that, due to certain variables, their air passages may clog and create difficulty in breathing. They know what it's like to be in the midst of an asthma attack. Fearing for their lives, they may swallow a few pills and hope they work quickly, or use an asthma spray and pray it will end the choking sensation, or rush to an emergency room and demand Adrenalin immediately.

Statistics say they will probably survive the ordeal, but it will leave them exhausted, weak, depressed, frightened, and angry. Attack after attack will make them unsure of their own body's ability to function.

This disease will change their life-styles and their expectations. They may have to change jobs, leave social gatherings and leave theaters until they can stop coughing. They may have to avoid smoking and people who smoke; perfume; walking against the wind or walking too far; laughing too much; getting too fatigued; eating too much; climbing too many stairs; using powdered cleansers; dusting furniture or shaking out sheets; visiting friends who have pets; going to the zoo or to the circus; or anyone, anything, or anyplace that may create a vulnerability to an asthma attack.

Life becomes much less spontaneous since the asthmatic is always on guard.

I know because I have been an asthma sufferer for twenty-three years. Indeed, asthma has made its indelible mark on me. It has intruded when it was not wanted.

For twelve of the twenty-three years when I suffered with severe asthma, I searched for anything that would allow me to function normally and to breathe more easily. I sampled a smorgasbord of medications, experimented with several diets, attempted to control my environment, and benefited from the advice of several very well intentioned doctors. Eleven years ago, I decided that my situation was no longer bearable. I couldn't sleep at night. I couldn't keep up with my children without wheezing. I would spend an hour each morning waiting until I could breath normally. In short, I was miserable and desperate.

One afternoon I decided to call the National Jewish Center in Denver and see if they could help me. I was prepared to pack my bags and check into this hospital, which is dedicated to the treatment of this "pain in the neck disease." I tried to find out what they had to offer so that I wouldn't make a dramatic exodus to a fool's errand. After all, I was a wife, mother, and teacher, and leaving would not be so easy. The person I spoke with suggested that I first see a Dr. Stuart H. Young, a Manhattan allergist who had trained at the center and was a renowned asthma specialist. This sounded reasonable to me, so I decided to give the East Coast one more try.

I vividly remember my first meeting with Dr. Young. I began to cry as I recounted my history and explained my present treatment program. Dr. Young realized that I had not neglected my asthma as some patients tend to and that helping me would be a challenge; but he did indicate that he couldn't offer an immediate cure, although he had some new ideas. His straightforward attitude was refreshing, and I was convinced that he would try to get an overview of my situation. After an initial diagnostic workup, we experimented with a basic drug program enhanced by diet therapy. This was a constructive process, and we were continuously evaluating my progress. The result has been rewarding and I can breathe normally again.

During one of our first sessions, I asked Dr. Young if he could recommend a good book on asthma. There were so many times, especially during my pregnancies, that I could have used some suggestions on dealing with asthma. I had not been able to find any source that had everything I needed. Dr. Young agreed that there was very little to be found. He himself was looking for a book that he could recommend to his asthma patients, to their parents and relatives, to his colleagues less directly involved in treating asthma who needed a reference at times, to other professionals who come in contact with asthmatics, and to training institutions. We both saw the serious need for such a handbook to serve the ten million Americans who are asthmatic, and the additional numbers of significant others in the lives of asthmatics, since they know too little about their condition or are misinformed. Before long we pledged that we would get the job done. We both knew that there were many people like me with many, many questions about asthma who would be desperately and passionately awaiting our book.

As we began to formalize our plans, I became more and more convinced that Dr. Young and I were a perfect team. Dr. Young is an expert in asthma care, having treated hundreds of asthmatics in his practice while incorporating the most modern methods into his treatment approaches.

While Dr. Young was the expert in the treatment of asthma symptoms, I was also an expert since I was the patient and had intimate knowledge of what it's like to be asthmatic. My experience has created in me a moral obligation to help other asthmatics. I have made certain that the facts and suggestions presented in our book are not only sound, but realistic and usable.

Between Dr. Young's expertise and my experience, we have a great deal to offer you, whether you are an asthma sufferer or someone who cares about an asthmatic. We have compiled all the available information that we feel is important and relevant to you into a guidebook that is comprehensive, up-to-date, and readable.

There has been a tremendous change in the treatment of asthma during the last ten years. Research has led to a better understanding of the disease, to new medication, and to new treatment approaches. We can now be optimistic; no asthmatic is beyond help. I vividly remember hearing my grandmother's constant wheezing as she climbed the stairs in the home we shared. She seemed to passively accept that asthma was her ''lot in life''; that she would be burdened with wheezing, coughing, sudden and frequent asthma attacks followed by hospital stays, and a restricted life-style.

Years later when I became asthmatic, while I strived to emulate my grandmother's intelligence, good nature, and courage, I did not want to inherit her fate. In her time, when the disease was often shrouded in misconceptions and prejudices, she may have had to settle for suffering. I do not, and neither do you. We know more. We can do more, and you can and must expect more.

It is this optimism and determination that compelled us to write this book. The best thing that you can do in your quest to conquer asthma is to become a well-informed and involved participant in your own treatment program, in cooperation with your doctor. Use this handbook, then, to give you this knowledge so that you can work toward better breathing and happier living.

Susan A. Shulman

1

THE FACTS ABOUT ASTHMA

The first and most obvious thing to say about asthma is that it is a serious and often devastating disease, affecting almost eleven million Americans (and perhaps millions more "closet" asthmatics). It appears to affect more males than females. While asthma can begin at any age, its onset is most common before the age of fifteen and after the age of forty-five, and it is among the leading causes of absenteeism in schools and in industry.

According to the most recent task force report of the National Institute of Allergy and Infectious Diseases

1. One billion dollars is spent each year on asthma medication.
2. Another billion dollars is paid each year in disability benefits for asthma, emphysema, and chronic respiratory diseases.
3. More than 125 million school days are lost each year by asthmatic children six to fifteen years old—61.3 percent of total school days lost.
4. A recent study found that in one year more than twenty-five thousand people missed more than six million workdays because of chronic allergic conditions.
5. Some studies have shown that as much as 18 percent of a family's income may go toward an asthma sufferer's treatment.
6. There are twenty-seven million patient visits each year for the treatment of asthma.

7. In one study of 134,000 hospital cases of asthma and hay fever, the average hospitalization was more than eight days long and the total cost exceeded $62 million.
8. There are as many as five thousand documented deaths from asthma each year, and worse, despite better medication and increased understanding of asthma, the death rate rises each year.

These are startling statistics about respiratory disorders that remain shrouded in myths and misconceptions.

WHAT IS ASTHMA?

In my practice, I see hundreds of asthmatics every year. It is easy to recognize asthma but not easy to define it. It is a disease with many causes and symptoms and with widely varying degrees of severity.

Although no single definition of asthma is possible, all asthma sufferers have one thing in common: they have trouble breathing. Most patients experience a tightening in the chest accompanied by a choking sensation and the inability to take in enough air. There is often coughing and wheezing and almost always a feeling of panic. My patients tell me of the discomfort and exhaustion and finally, the anger and fear that follow an asthma attack. They feel betrayed by their own bodies.

What makes it even worse is that asthma is often unpredictable. The asthmatic is really at the mercy of the disease. When the asthmatic is not in a symptomatic state, everything is just fine. In fact, one of the most distinguishing features that separates asthma from other seemingly similar diseases is its episodic nature. Difficulty breathing, as well as wheezing and coughing are also symptomatic of other disorders, such as cystic fibrosis, emphysema, chronic bronchitis, heart failure, and lung cancer. In these, however, the difficulty is more or less permanent, while in asthma it is not.

To many asthmatics, asthma can mean any or all of the following:

- They cannot exercise freely.
- They cannot mow the lawn.
- They cannot smoke or be near people who do.
- They cannot dust furniture.
- They cannot take the kids to the zoo or circus.
- They cannot rely on feeling well enough to go to work every day.
- They cannot make long-range plans.
- They cannot even laugh too much.

No wonder my more symptomatic patients tell me they long to regain control over their lives! As we shall see, the happy answer is that they can.

WHAT THE ASTHMA ATTACK IS LIKE

In simple terms, an asthma sufferer's lungs do not work properly. The airways of the lungs (large airways are called bronchi, small ones are bronchioles) are constricted by certain abnormalities. For reasons I'll discuss later, the asthmatic's lungs are supersensitive and easily provoked into constriction.

The constriction begins as a bronchial spasm. This is often followed by a swelling of the lining of the airways and the production of excess sticky mucus. The mucus may form plugs and block (occlude) the air passages completely. Usually, there is a combination of the three: spasm, swelling, and excess mucus.

Since the airways have narrowed, it takes more effort to force air through them; this makes breathing very hard work for the asthmatic. During severe attacks, the sufferer may be exhausted, sweating, and speechless.

Forcing air through constricted airways is what causes wheezing (high-pitched rattling noises). During the onset of an attack, the problem is getting air out of the lungs, and wheezing is heard during exhalation. As the attack progresses, the wheezing can be heard during inhalation as well.

Wheezing may be loud enough to hear across the room or, if the air passages are seriously constricted, almost no sound may be heard.

Coughing is another common feature of asthma. It happens when the air passages are irritated by excessive mucus.

When the asthmatic has trouble breathing, most people would assume it is because he is unable to take in enough air. In fact, it is initially easier for asthmatics to inhale than to exhale.

Too much air remains in the lungs after inefficient asthmatic exhalation. This increased amount of stale air (residual volume) left in the lungs decreases the vital capacity, which is the amount of fresh air used by the lungs. The less fresh air available, the poorer the oxygenation of the whole body, not just the lungs. This is why asthma attacks are more dangerous the longer they persist.

CAUSES OF ASTHMA

While the description of the symptoms of asthma and the possible limitations that result from these symptoms are clear, such clarity cannot be found when discussing the underlying causes of the disease. The patients I see come to me with a wide variety of theories about what they think causes their asthma. These theories are often based on their own beliefs or those of their family, friends, or well-intentioned neighbors.

Some of their hunches are quite accurate. Patients may stress family history, blaming genetics for their asthma. Some patients may list environmental factors such as grass, trees, pollen, and pets. Some feel that their asthma is provoked by a variety of foods. Some attacks occur only after an infection. Others feel that their asthma is caused by physical exertion. All of these factors can indeed play a role in causing asthma symptoms, and I will elaborate later.

Although some patients' theories are accurate, some of their hunches are not. The cause of asthma is surrounded by several myths. Let us dispel them now.

MYTHS

Some patients believe that their asthma is psychosomatic. This is just not true. As a matter of fact, the report of a purely psychosomatic case of asthma is so rare that it would be a case for the medical journals!

The myth that stress causes asthma is a tough one to dissipate. It is reinforced on television, in books, and in movies. When the parents argue, the child suddenly begins to wheeze. It seems that when the character needs to be portrayed as emotionally weak or traumatized, he becomes asthmatic. The myth lives on!

The fact is, however, that for the vast majority of us, no matter how nervous we get, or how traumatized we are, we will not become asthmatic. If you do not have the underlying respiratory disease (which I will describe later), you cannot become asthmatic. Stress does not cause asthma.

However, in an already established asthmatic, stress can sometimes make things worse. More often than not, stress does not act alone, but is just one of many factors triggering the symptoms. Thinking of asthma as a psychosomatic disorder, present only in high-strung, neurotic people, is just plain wrong.

There is a classic story told by a psychiatrist that depicts the error of viewing asthma as a purely psychological problem. A young woman in the 1940s broke away from her family to live with her boyfriend. Since the 1940s were definitely not the 1980s in terms of morality, moving in with her boyfriend was greatly frowned upon, to say the least. Therefore, when the young woman developed asthma symptoms, it was obvious to all of the disapproving, condemning relatives and "friends" that the asthma was a direct result of the great guilt she must have suffered. This was confirmed by the psychiatrists she visited who compared her wheezing to a "crying" out of her innermost emotion. The clincher was that she was only symptomatic at her boyfriend's apartment. What a perfect example of psychosomatic asthma!

She finally made her way to an astute allergist who did not take very long to uncover the truth. The fact that she was symptom-free at home and not at her boyfriend's was the clue he needed.

He found the true culprit. It was not guilt, but feathers! The young woman had a severe allergy to feathers. She had been sleeping with a feather pillow at her boyfriend's apartment, but at home, she slept on foam. Removing the feathers removed the symptoms. It is easy to get carried away by myths.

Another myth about asthma that I hear from my patients all the time is that asthma is caused by the geographic locations of their homes. Like hundreds of other asthmatics who have done so, these asthmatics truly believe that they should move to Arizona. They should not! Airborne irritants or certain weather patterns may affect individual asthmatics. As a group, asthmatics appear to have a respiratory system that is "programmed" to react abnormally to certain environmental stimuli. It may take some time, but you will begin to react wherever you are, since you are programmed to react.

The Arizona desert, by the way, has plenty of vegetation and some of the highest pollen counts in the world! The basic problem is that asthma is not precipitated by external factors only. You need not pack your bags!

CLOSER TO THE TRUTH

We have some theories that are accurate and some that are not. Let us try to get closer to the truth. We know that the lungs of the asthmatic function differently from normal lungs, but what are the underlying causes?

Allergens were suspected of being the sole culprits, or "triggers" in the asthmatic condition until approximately twenty years ago. Although allergies play a definite role for some asthmatics, they are not the underlying cause we are searching for.

In the asthmatic, there is an imbalance in several of the biochemical systems involved in proper lung functioning.. This stems from a dysfunction of the autonomic nervous system. All asthmatics have this dysfunction that is the basis for their programmed abnormal lung reaction. This chemical malfunction then sets up the lungs for cellular-level interactions that are also abnormal and that interrupt smooth muscle functioning.

So, the asthmatic individual appears to be programmed to react abnormally to certain stimuli. These stimuli serve as "triggers." A trigger is anything that initiates the production of mediators that, in turn, results in abnormal, harmful reactions (spasms, swelling, and mucus production). Francis Rackermann, a prominent pioneer in allergy research in the 1920s, was instrumental in discovering the various triggers that precipitate an asthma attack. Rackermann used the term trigger, and elaborated on the analogy to a gun. He felt that while it is very important to know what pulls the trigger in an asthma reaction, to really understand the disease you also needed to know how the gun is loaded. This eluded him and has been unclear until recently.

We now know that the ammunition appears to come from a biochemical imbalance in the autonomic nervous system, of genetic origin, that affects proper lung functioning. Once the gun is loaded, it can go off as soon as one pulls the trigger. The lungs of the asthmatic are like the fingers of a trigger-happy gunfighter. They are very vulnerable, sensitive, and quick to react in an exaggerated way. Let us discuss the triggers.

THE TRIGGERS OF ASTHMA

1. Allergies

Many people can have allergies and not have the underlying dysfunction of the autonomic nervous system. Their allergy may manifest itself in nasal congestion, hay fever, and skin problems, but not as asthma. On the other hand, the allergic reactions of an individual with the underlying lung disorder can lead to asthma symptoms.

If an allergy is the critical trigger for a particular individual's asthma, the asthma is generally known as extrinsic asthma. If the trigger is not allergy related, the asthma is referred to as intrinsic. It is most common to have a combination of both intrinsic and extrinsic asthma. The reactions that produce asthma appear to result from abnormal reactions to stimuli, both internal and external.

Even though this gets a bit technical, let me explain how the allergens play a role in provoking asthma symptoms. We all produce antibodies that help us prevent and fight disease, specifically, immunoglobulin-E or IgE, which wards off parasites, worms, or even cancer. However, IgE can also initiate harmful allergic reactions. The IgE will attack a pollen granule with the same gusto as if it were attacking a parasite. This only occurs in some people—allergic people—and, in effect, is a mistake on the part of the body. The scenario is as follows: IgE molecules are fixed on mast cells that line the respiratory tract like sentinels guarding the passageway to the lungs. When a parasite enters the respiratory tract, the mast cell-IgE complex attacks it and removes the parasite; when a pollen grain enters the respiratory tract, the same thing happens. "Killing" the pollen is useless and harmful, whereas killing the parasite is beneficial. When the IgE combines with specific allergens, the mast cells release mediators. These mediators are also basically helpful, except in the case of asthma. They send out messages to the nervous system and to the immediate environment that result in abnormal biochemical reactions. For example, one mediator, histamine, causes an inflammation of the air passages in the lungs as well as increased mucus and mucus plug production. Although not generally viewed as a significant culprit, histamines can work against the asthmatic.

Other mediators are very important in our asthma story, and I will just mention them in passing. Leukotriene LTE_4, a chemical formerly known as SRS-A, interferes with smooth muscle functioning and causes the air passages to go into spasm. Certainly, you can see that the combination of IgE and LTE_4 can give an individual a great deal of trouble. Many other mediators are being investigated to determine their role in asthma; for example eosinophil chemotatic factor of anaphylaxis (ECF-A), platelet-aggregating factor of anaphylaxis (PAF-A), basophil chemotatic factor of anaphylaxis (BCF-A), arachidonic acid, and the prostaglandins.

The most common allergens include pollens, mold, food additives (for instance, monosodium glutamate, or MSG), animal dander, house dust, dust mites, feathers, insect particles, kapok, cottonseed, chemicals used in industry, and certain medications such as aspirin. Because each person is programmed with his own sensitivities, the list can go on and on. Allergic sensitivities appear to be programmed genetically. The person who tells me that he has never had any allergic reactions before his current bout with asthma is the person who has been lucky enough not to have had enough exposure to his particular trigger to spark the abnormal reactions.

2. Exercise

Another trigger is exercise. Exercise forces the lungs to work more quickly and to exchange air more rapidly. When one exercises, dry air is inhaled which is disruptive to the lungs and causes the release of mediators just as if an allergic reaction has occurred. The asthmatic's lungs can tolerate this for only a short period of time, and then the hyperactive mast cell-IgE complex breaks down and the now familiar chain of events begins. A hallmark of asthma is that these symptoms begin six or seven minutes after he starts exercising or even shortly afterward. When a new patient tells me that he wheezes or in some way demonstrates breathing difficulty after a short period of exercise, I suspect asthma.

Because the asthmatic can exercise for some time without symptoms, some sports are better than others. For example, baseball, doubles in tennis, and golf do not require constant physical activity. Any sport that requires short spurts of activity followed by some rest (even if it is not a very long rest) is suitable for the asthmatic. The asthmatic might be an excellent sprinter but not a long-distance runner. Swimming is an appropriate sport for asthmatics, for although it requires fine breath control and constant movement, it is done in a very moist environment.

3. Infections

Asthmatics and nonasthmatics alike can develop respiratory infections in which the bronchial passages become inflamed, reducing their size. Mucus production is increased when there are infections resulting in mucus that is thicker than usual. The asthmatic's respiratory system is working at a handicap, by definition. The added constriction and possible mucus plugging caused by infections further complicates the situation. Asthmatics should take every possible measure to prevent getting colds and other infections. Symptoms can change from controlled and tolerable to uncontrolled and intolerable.

4. Airborne Irritants

Asthmatics often become symptomatic when they come in contact with some airborne irritants. These irritants may be allergens for the allergically based asthmatic, and they may serve to provoke the irritable lungs in the nonallergic asthmatic. There are many such irritants that impose themselves upon us in our daily lives. Some of the more common irritants are cigarette smoke, dust, odors, perfumes, sprays, and air pollution. A sudden change in air temperature or pressure may also serve as an irritant. Some individuals, because of their occupations, are exposed on a daily basis to large quantities of some specific irritant. For example, it is not uncommon for a baker to develop asthmatic symptoms from the constant inhalation of flour. A toll collector, spending his day among cars that are stopping and going, may react to the exhaust fumes. While many of the irritants are mere annoyances to the nonasthmatic, to the asthmatic individual, they can mean big trouble!

5. Emotions

My inclusion of emotions as one of the triggers of asthma must not lead you to think that I view asthma as a psychosomatic disease. I do not! As I have already stated, you do not become asthmatic unless you have a dysfunction of the autonomic nervous system. Without this underlying disorder, emotions cannot cause asthma. In the asthmatic, however, it is conceivable that a great deal of psychological stress can trigger symptoms. Tension and anger in anyone can result in rapid and shallow breathing. The asthmatic depends upon smooth and relaxed lung functioning. When there is tension, the asthmatic is at a disadvantage.

6. Gastroesophageal Reflux

Gastroesophageal reflux can also trigger asthma symptoms. Reflux, the regurgitation of digestive fluid upward through the cardiac orifice (opening) between the stomach and the esophagus, occurs commonly with hiatus hernia, usually in older people. We have all experienced reflux, that acid aftertaste after belching that is so unpleasant. When the highly acidic, regurgitated contents of the stomach get into the esophagus, a slight short-lived indigestion results. To most of us that means an unpleasant sensation and perhaps a bit of heartburn. But to the susceptible asthmatic it may mean a severe attack of asthma or an incapacitating coughing spasm.

This is a new syndrome. It was always believed that the contents of an acidic stomach would become problematic only when they hit the surface of the lung. Doctors did not realize that when these contents were in the esophagus, a reflex action could trigger severe asthma. (What is happening is that the reflux is causing a reflex.) In adults, reflux has also been associated with recurrent bronchitis, pneumonia, and fibrosis.

Although reflux can occur during the day, it happens more frequently at night when one is lying down. This is because when we are upright, gravity helps the cardiac orifice stay closed. But when we lie down, the cardiac orifice must stay closed without the help of gravity, and if it is the least bit incompetent, acid fluid will leak through into the esophagus. The syndrome is also more common in adults than in children because, sad but true, as we age, all of the body's valves get a little leaky. Other factors (progesterone, theophylline, isoproterenol, anticholinergic agents such as Atrovent, meperidine, morphine, calcium channel blockers, nicotine, coffee, caffeine, fatty foods, alcohol, chocolate, peppermint, tomato, and citrus fruits) may play a role in this situation because they reduce the effectiveness of the cardiac orifice.

The above factors must be reduced so that the asthma symptoms that reflux causes may also be reduced. Patients are encouraged to eat three or more small meals a day, not to lie down after eating, and to eat the last meal several hours before retiring. Since the more you eat, the higher your probability of reflux, the overweight patient is encouraged to reduce food intake and lose weight. Frequent feedings are recommended. The head of the bed should be elevated six inches to reduce reflux and all of the above mentioned foods and medications should be avoided. Two medications, cimetidine (Tagamet) and Ranitidine (Zantac) are helpful.

The bottom line is this: Gastroesophageal reflux can cause in susceptible individuals an asthmatic attack that may occur more often at night. If you suspect that this condition exists for you, talk to your doctor about it. It can be diagnosed and treated. There are simple tests such as an upper GI (gastrointestinal) series that can identify it, or if the GI series does not prove helpful, more sophisticated tests can be done. The treatment is simple and many cases respond favorably.

By now, I hope that I have given you a clear idea of what asthma is, what it means to both patient and doctor, and what its possible causes are. To review, it is a respiratory disorder that results in shortness of breath, wheezing, and coughing. It reflects underlying lung dysfunction and is "triggered" by many things, including allergies, exercise, infections, airborne irritants, emotions, and reflux. The lungs react by airway constriction, swelling, and excess mucus production. These symptoms may come and go, making the disease unpredictable by nature. Depending upon the severity of their symptoms, asthmatics describe their asthma as anywhere from being a mild inconvenience all the way to being a devastating and debilitating burden for themselves and their families.

Asthma needs to be managed appropriately and quickly. The decision whether or not to seek medical intervention is a crucial one—one that I will discuss in detail in Chapter 2.

2

HOW TO KNOW IF YOU HAVE ASTHMA AND HOW TO GET HELP

THE SIGNS AND SYMPTOMS OF ASTHMA

Do you have asthma? You probably do if

1. After running to catch a bus, you are wheezing, coughing, and you can't catch your breath.
2. You wake up in the middle of the night and you find yourself opening the window to let in more fresh air because you can't breathe very well.
3. You have been telling your friends that you have a cold, but it's been lingering for three months; you tell them that the wheezing and the coughing will eventually stop.
4. You visit a friend who has three cats and your chest tightens, your breathing becomes shallow, and your constant coughing is not bringing much relief.
5. When you breathe deeply, you sound like an orchestra tuning up.
6. You go to see a play and during intermission the smoke in the lobby forces you to leave and you miss the second act.
7. You are laughing at a good joke, but after the laughter has died down your coughing has not.

8. You are dusting your furniture and you feel as if your air passages are narrowing; someone else has to finish dusting.
9. You step out into the cold winter air and you feel as if your breath has been taken away from you.
10. You get into an elevator with a colleague who has doused herself with perfume and even after the elevator ride, you are still not breathing well.
11. One day you can beat your four-year-old in a running race and the next day your child wins, leaving you huffing and puffing.
12. You are sitting and doing nothing and all of a sudden you are gasping for air.
13. A bad coughing spell doesn't end until you have been able to "clear the passage" by coughing up some mucus.
14. You choose to go to the movies instead of playing tennis, when you have always preferred tennis.
15. You have started to join in on conversations pertaining to asthma; glance at the over-the-counter asthma medications; make the TV louder when commercials for asthma drugs are being shown; and you are starting to sound and maybe feel like your friend's grandmother who's been asthmatic for years!

The Symptoms of Asthma

SHORTNESS OF BREATH

There are countless other situations that I can use to depict asthma. Nevertheless, the most common denominator is reduced efficiency of breathing. It does not matter whether impaired breathing results from physical exertion (running a race or dancing), eating certain foods, ingesting airborne irritants (smoke, dust, or pollen), infection, or a sudden change in air flow (laughing or walking against the wind).

Some deny the possibility of asthma just because their breathing difficulty comes and goes. Don't do this. As a matter of fact, this on-again, off-again pattern is a trademark of asthma. This type of reversibility helps me to differentiate asthma from other respiratory problems. I always make a point of finding out if my patient's symptoms are sporadic or continuous.

If I've described how you are feeling, or if you know someone who fits the description, a diagnosis of asthma is a good guess.

WHEEZING

Almost all asthmatics wheeze, whereby there are audible vibrations caused by air being forced through constricted air passages. It occurs during inhalation or exhalation and may be relatively faint or quite loud. In addition to reflecting breathing difficulty, the sound itself may be annoying and anxiety producing. One patient reported that her own wheezing often woke her up. Another patient reported that she had become accustomed to her wheezing except during physical exertion or during lovemaking. Then it was a depressing interruption. Some patients report that they get so accustomed to their wheezing that they don't even hear it. One couple that I treated reported that they often had lighthearted arguments as to which one of them was wheezing. Whenever it occurs, however, it is a sign that breathing is not efficient.

While wheezing frequently accompanies asthma, it is symptomatic of other conditions as well. In fact, there is a popular expression that says, "All that wheezes is not asthma." Here is a good example. One of my patients was a thirty-five-year-old woman with asthma; under my treatment she had become virtually symptom-free. She called me to report that her mother had recently developed asthma. She was hoping that I would be able to help her mother as I had helped her. I told her I would try, and we set up another appointment. When the woman brought her mother in for an evaluation, I immediately realized that she was acutely uncomfortable. I did not bother finishing the case history before I examined her. Her heart was racing and had an extra sound, her liver and ankles were swollen and her chest noises sounded like pulmonary edema. The patient was in acute heart failure, or cardiac asthma. She eventually did very well under the care of an excellent cardiologist. In this case, her wheezing was not attributable to asthma.

Another story, on a sadder note, involved a male patient who had been smoking for many years and who just recently had begun to wheeze and cough up blood-streaked sputum. Immediately after I examined him, I sent him to a radiologist for a chest X ray. He had a small coin lesion on his lung and he, in fact, had lung cancer.

Wheezing must always be taken seriously since it could be a danger sign indicating a number of different diseases. Two such syndromes will be discussed at the end of this section.

COUGHING

It is also true that most asthmatics cough, especially children. The cough may be a full, loose cough. This kind of cough often is caused by mucus secretion in the passageways. The cough might be a dry, hacking cough, reflecting tight, spastic air passages. Of course, coughing is a natural accompaniment to an upper respiratory infection. But in the nonasthmatic, the cough should lessen in severity and frequency over a relatively short period of time. If the cough becomes persistent and remains constant, and if it occurs during any of the situations I have described at the beginning of this chapter, one should suspect asthma.

EXCESS MUCUS

Asthmatics often have to put up with excessive mucus production; the normal person, however, rarely brings up mucus while coughing. Some asthmatics bring up crystallinelike spirals of mucus (Kirschman spirals) that have plugged up and taken the shape of the small air passages; these are known as mucus plugs. Excessive mucus production is very irritating; that's why most of my patients tell me that they are relieved once they are able to cough up trapped mucus.

SYNDROMES THAT MIMIC ASTHMA

Recently several new syndromes that mimic asthma have been identified. Although much less common than asthma, the symptoms must be differentiated from asthma so that appropriate treatment can be given. I shall describe each of these syndromes, comparing and contrasting them to asthma, thus enabling you to analyze your symptoms, and if anything seems familiar, by all means discuss it with your physician.

Glottic Dysfunction refers to a problem with vocal cord behavior. Almost everyone has heard and seen a child with croup (a loud barking cough with labored breathing). It has been known that if the area in the larynx at the level of the vocal cords is narrowed, or if the vocal cords are swollen, difficulty in inhaling and croup will ensue. Only recently has it been discovered that when the vocal cords are swollen or not working properly, there can be severe problems both inhaling and exhaling, producing asthmalike symptoms. As of May 1987, only thirty-one cases of this rare syndrome have been reported.

Twenty were misdiagnosed as having bronchial asthma. It is imperative that this syndrome be differentiated from true upper airway closure and asthma.

Glottic dysfunction manifests itself with alarming symptoms of upper airway closure. The patient appears to be asphyxiating. When individuals present themselves to the emergency room or to a physician unfamiliar with this syndrome, they are often intubated or tracheotomized. If the differences between glottic dysfunction and true upper airway distress and asthma were known, such extreme procedures could be prevented.

In an asthma attack, patients are short of breath (dyspnea), breathing quickly (tachypnea), unable to hold their breath, speaking with great difficulty. Although patients with glottic dysfunction appear to be in distress, they can speak and hold their breath. Coughing or panting makes an asthmatic worse, while a cough may actually stop the spasm in a patient afflicted with glottic dysfunction. It is also true that glottic dysfunction patients feel better when they are distracted, and their symptoms disappear when they fall asleep. This is not usually true of the asthmatic. (If an asthmatic is symptomatic before he falls asleep, symptoms usually do not disappear.) Pulmonary function studies *during the acute attack* will show inspiratory problems in the patient with asthma. After an attack, pulmonary functions will be abnormal in the asthmatic, but not in the individual with "only" glottic dysfunction. During an attack, the doctor is able, with proper instruments, to see that the vocal cords are moving improperly in glottic dysfunction patients.

A mecholyl challenge test can also be used to distinguish between the asthmatic and the patient with glottic dysfunction. This test uses methacholine, a substance that will not induce wheezing in a nonasthmatic subject, even in high doses. An asthmatic will wheeze when he inhales even a small dose of mecholyl. Under controlled circumstances, monitored by pulmonary functions, an individual is given mecholyl in increasing doses to measure when he wheezes. If he wheezes before a certain critical concentration, this suggests the diagnosis of asthma. This test is used only when the diagnosis of asthma is in question or in research situations. It is generally agreed that glottic dysfunction is a psychosomatic disorder and treatment is primarily psychological. Speech therapy to train the correct vocal cord action can also be of supplemental help.

Alpha one antitrypsin defect, a defect in which a lung-protecting substance is missing, also results in asthmalike symptoms. Trypsin is a natural substance which slowly dissolves lung cells, but fortunately the body maintains a proper balance with antitrypsin, preventing this from happening. A deficit in antitrypsin is rare and can be detected by a simple blood test. The syndrome simulates asthma, but it may appear later in life and leads to severe emphysema if not treated. When identified early, it is possible to replace the alpha one antitrypsin substance, thus avoiding the problem.

If you do have symptoms of asthma, you should see a doctor. However, we all know people who prefer to try to treat themselves or who just refuse to seek medical help. Let's consider, then, the question of when to see a doctor.

Should You Wait to See a Doctor?

Almost always the answer is no! The waiting game that many patients play is often responsible for the trouble that they are in when they finally come to see me. Every day I speak with new patients who say

1. I waited because I was sure that my cold would eventually go away.
2. I waited because my spouse told me that the wheezing was "all in my mind."
3. I waited because I wanted the allergy season to pass.
4. I waited because I did not want you to tell me I had asthma.

As a general rule of thumb, waiting can be dangerous. Breathing problems, even if they are not asthma, can be serious. Early diagnosis and treatment are crucial.

If you are still hemming and hawing about going to see a doctor, several factors may help you make up your mind.

SEVERITY

If you are wheezing all day or can't get rid of a monthlong cold or can't get through a night's sleep without a coughing spell, your symptoms are severe. What are you waiting for?

AGE

If your baby is wheezing, run (do not walk) to your doctor. Breathing problems in an infant can become critical in a matter of hours. While the wheezing may signal asthma, it may signify heart failure or acute epiglottitis, in which the tissue hovering over the larynx and trachea begins to swell, closing the air passages and thus mimicking asthma. Foreign matter might be lodged in the respiratory passages as well. For more information see Chapter 11, Asthma in Children. In the elderly, asthma symptoms may mean heart failure and should receive immediate medical attention.

YOUR GENERAL PHYSICAL CONDITION

If the asthma symptoms that you are trying to ignore occur when you also have a general feeling of malaise, you should seek attention. Your body has a good signal system that warns of malfunction. Listen to it! If you tire more easily than you used to, if you are more susceptible to viruses and infections than previously, or if you have become a "party pooper," see a doctor.

YOUR ATTITUDE

Even if your symptoms don't seem all that severe, if you're worried, see a doctor. Symptoms do not have to reach a certain level of severity before it is legitimate to seek medical help.

YOUR FAMILY'S FRIEND'S ATTITUDE

We all have people who love us and care about us. It's very difficult for them to watch us suffer. As my patients explain their symptoms and frustrations, they often speak about a loved one or a friend who is more worried than they are. It is often significant others who have to coax us to make an appointment to see the doctor. If your family or friends have been after you to do something about your present health, then do it. We can't always see the obvious as well as others can. Get on the phone and make your appointment.

YOUR FAMILY'S MEDICAL HISTORY

If there is a history of respiratory problems in your family, your symptoms should be considered a warning sign that you may be carrying on the family tradition. Consider them an unlucky legacy and see a doctor.

PREGNANCY

As you will see later, pregnancy is a special case in asthma. The typical pregnant woman may put up with a headache so as to avoid taking aspirin, and she might tolerate nausea without taking any medication. There is a compulsion to avoid medication. Most often this is valid. However, when asthma symptoms occur, the pregnant woman should not just tolerate them. If the mother is not breathing well, the fetus is not breathing well. The pregnant woman with asthma symptoms should see a doctor! Her fear that the doctor might prescribe medication that might harm the baby should not keep her away. Untreated asthma may hurt the baby more than the medications.

Choosing a Doctor

Now that the decision to seek medical assistance has been made, your next step is to choose the appropriate type of doctor.

FAMILY PHYSICIAN/INTERNIST

In my opinion, you should start with your primary physician who is usually a family physician, general practitioner, or internist. It is possible that your doctor can decide upon the best course of treatment (seeking a specialist's consultation or trying some medications). Hopefully, you have a good working relationship with this doctor. If not, perhaps it would be a good idea to go directly to a specialist.

PEDIATRICIAN

With a child, the pediatrician plays a major role since he is in charge of, and is most familiar with, your child's health. As in the case of the family physician, you and the pediatrician will decide if he can handle the child's asthma, or if a referral is necessary.

ALLERGIST

If it becomes obvious that your asthma symptoms are in response to allergic reactions, or if you have a family history of allergies, consult an allergist. If the disease is not easily controllable, your physician will usually refer you to an allergist who will evaluate and treat both the allergic and nonallergic aspects of asthma.

OTHER SPECIALISTS

Symptoms that mimic asthma may not be asthma. If your child suffers from difficulty in breathing and is also not thriving or growing well, there is reason to suspect heart defects or cystic fibrosis. Your child's pediatrician will probably suggest a consultation with a pediatric pulmonologist. Any adult with breathing problems who has been spitting blood, experiencing chest pains, or who has been exposed to tuberculosis should also see a pulmonologist. Symptoms of chest pain, swollen ankles, gurgling sounds during breathing, and foamy mucus warrant the attention of a cardiologist.

The First Visit to the Doctor

Make an appointment. If your symptoms are acute and need immediate attention, you should tell this to the receptionist. I always set aside time to see such patients. If your symptoms are not acute, a three- or four-week wait for your first appointment is not unreasonable. The first visit to the doctor who will be treating your asthma is extremely important. Since asthma often requires long-term care, initiate the patient/doctor relationship so it can grow to be smooth, honest, productive, and helpful. This first visit may also be somewhat anxiety producing if you don't know what to expect. You can help to make the first meeting between doctor and patient more productive if you are prepared. Let me describe a typical first visit.

HISTORY

Expect the doctor to gather relevant information on your background. Although each doctor's approach will differ, having a general idea of what kinds of questions you will be asked can be beneficial. It is sometimes difficult to think on the spot. Here, then, is a list of those questions I usually ask when I take a case history.

I. Background information
   A. When did your symptoms begin?
      1. Did your symptoms begin suddenly or gradually?
      2. How long have you been symptomatic?
      3. Has the severity of your symptoms been changing?
   B. What are your symptoms?
      1. Do you wheeze? Cough?
      2. Do you cough up a great deal of mucus? What color? What consistency? How often? How much?
      3. How often are your attacks?
      4. When was your first attack?
      5. What are your attacks like?
      6. What were your worst attacks like?
   C. Have you ever been treated for these symptoms?
      1. What type of treatment (allergy shots, medications, diets, environmental control, or psychoanalysis)?
      2. By whom?
      3. When and for how long?
      4. What were the results (successes and failures)?
   D. Do any other family member(s) have similar symptoms?
   E. Have you ever been hospitalized for asthma?
      1. What caused the hospitalization?
      2. When were you hospitalized?
      3. For how long?
      4. What was done?
      5. How effective was the treatment?
   F. Do you know the results of any previous laboratory tests (chest X rays, sinus X rays, pulmonary function study)? If you have them, bring them.

G. How are you now treating your symptoms?
H. How are the symptoms affecting your life?

II. Possible triggers
A. Do you have any ideas about what makes your symptoms noticeably worse (for instance, dust, weather, food, stress, smoke, or infection)?
B. Are your symptoms worse at any particular time or are they constant?
C. What is your general environment like?
1. Do you have any pets?
2. Do you smoke? Does anyone in your home smoke?
3. What is your heating/air-conditioning system like?
4. Can you describe the makeup of your furniture (for instance, mattress, pillows, or carpets)?
5. What kind of work do you do? Where? Describe the setting?
6. Are you worse at home or at work or anywhere else?
D. Can you describe a typical week's menu? What are your favorite foods? Do your symptoms worsen after meals? How long after?
E. Are your symptoms influenced by physical activity?
1. Do you become symptomatic during or after physical activity?
2. Which activities are most problematic?
F. Do your symptoms get worse with laughter, crying, or walking against the wind?

III. General health
A. Are there any other health problems that you have?
B. Are there any other health problems in your family (for instance, heart disease, diabetes, or cancer)?

This list can go on and on. If there is relevant information about your particular situation, supply it, even if the doctor does not ask about it. Again, I'm including these typical questions to make you aware of the kind of information you will be asked to supply.

Some patients change their daily routines in order to cope with their asthma symptoms. At times, these people do not even realize how they have altered their life-styles to minimize their symptoms. One situation comes to mind. I was taking background information from an eighteen-year-old boy. I asked if he had any difficulty in keeping up with his friends. He said that he had no problems. From past experience, I decided to continue with further questioning. I asked whether he got short of breath when he ran and he replied, "Oh, I never run." When I pointed out that he had just told me that he had no trouble keeping up with his friends and that this seemed incongruous, he replied, "My friends and I play chess." He had limited himself to the activities that did not make him short of breath and had become so accustomed to this life-style restriction that he no longer realized it was a restriction.

Although the doctor is responsible for asking thorough questions, the patient is responsible for supplying answers. Patients should reflect upon their symptoms because sometimes they are too close to the situation to describe it objectively and completely. Think about the questions that you will be asked, and give some thought to the real facts.

EXAMINATION

After taking a case history, I usually examine my patient. While the extent of my examination may vary depending on his or her background, I almost always do the following: First I take a good look at the patient and get a general impression as to what shape he's in; then I take his pulse and blood pressure; note his skin color; and examine his ears, nose, throat, sinuses, heart, lungs, and abdomen. In this way, I can determine the extent of the asthma symptoms, look for a possible allergic component, assess the patient's general health, gather information for a total medical evaluation and for the differential diagnosis of his respiratory problem, and make certain that his wheezing and shortness of breath are really manifestations of asthma.

The information that I have gathered from the case history and from the physical examination usually leads me to some educated guesses regarding underlying causes. These need to be corroborated through further testing. Be prepared, then, for some laboratory tests to be done (or requested) during the first visit to the doctor. I may request any of the following:

1. Chest X ray. This helps me determine whether or not you really have asthma. Other conditions often mimic asthma. In children these include cystic fibrosis and foreign body ingestion. In adults, the main considerations are heart disease, malignancies of the chest (rare), and various forms of chronic lung disease, especially emphysema. A chest X ray is crucial in the differential diagnosis of asthma. Its results also give me a baseline from which to evaluate later progress.
2. Sinus X ray. This is extremely important when I feel that there may be a chronic focus of infection in the patient's sinuses. This may be important both for nasal disease and for chest disease. Sinuses very often can be a hidden focus for asthma. While this is not a routine test, it is very important that this be done if your asthma is relatively severe.
3. Blood Test. This is administered to evaluate your general state of health and includes a complete blood count and the determination of a minimum blood sugar measure to make certain that you do not have diabetes. Diabetes interferes with certain medication that I might prescribe. In addition, a blood test called a multiphasic blood scan is done that evaluates your general health. It is very important for me to have your entire health picture clearly in mind when I prescribe a treatment course for you.
4. Immunoglobulin Test. This test is given to determine the level of certain proteins in the blood that fight infection.
5. Sweat Test. This test measures the amount of sodium ions and chloride ions in sweat. (See glossary for further details.) It is usually given to children younger than ten years of age who have significant asthma symptoms. It helps to differentiate between asthma and cystic fibrosis.

6. EKG. An electrocardiogram will help me evaluate your heart. Sometimes heart failure will mimic asthma. In addition, some asthma drugs can irritate the heart and should be avoided when the EKG is not normal. An EKG is usually done in patients forty years or older.
7. Spirometry (Pulmonary Function Test). This test is used to evaluate the dynamics of breathing and is usually performed in a doctor's office and measures two major functions: the total amount of air that you can move out of your lungs and the speed at which you can do it. In addition, we measure these two factors before and after a bronchodilator (a drug that relaxes bronchial muscles resulting in expansion of the bronchial air passages) is administered to see if there is any improvement. This is called reversibility. The hallmark of asthma is that it reverses or improves with medication. Both the degree of impairment and the degree of reversibility help guide me in my choice of medication for my patients.

   The amount and speed of forceful exhalation is crucial in evaluating asthma. Several different measurements are used to evaluate this maneuver. One measurement that you should know is called "one second forced expiratory volume" (FEV_1). It is the greatest amount of air that you can force out of your lungs in one second. It is matched to your age and height. You should be able to exhale approximately 82 percent of all of the exhalable air in your lungs in one second. This is measured by spirometry, whereby you are instructed, usually wearing nose clips, to fill your lungs completely and blow out into the spirometer (an instrument for measuring the air entering and leaving the lungs) as hard and as fast as possible until the lungs are empty. This test may be performed three times and the best curve is the one that is used. If you cannot do this within the normal range, you have some degree of bronchospasm. The lower the percentage, the greater the degree of bronchospasm.

   Another measure of how fast you can expel air is called

the peak flow. This measures the maximum velocity of air going out of your lungs in one tenth of a second. It is measured by a little tubelike device called a peak flow meter. You blow into the mouthpiece of the tube as hard and as fast as you can. An indicator dial on the scale measures the velocity of your expiration. This is a very simple device and can be kept at home. It can be very useful in predicting asthma attacks. Your peak flow level very often will drop before you begin to feel ill. I use this device in my office when a patient is having an attack and it is used in emergency rooms to closely monitor a patient. There are other devices such as a peak flow whistle that will also measure your peak flow. My main experience is with the peak flow meter.

Phethysmography, using the body box, is a test in which you actually enter a box and are closed off from the outside air. Phethysmography utilizes very sophisticated equipment to evaluate severe asthmatics. It can measure many other factors about your lungs aside from the speed with which you can exhale. This is not a routine test.

8. Skin Test. This test is utilized to determine what you are allergic to and the degree of severity of your allergy. There are three types of skin tests, and they have been used since the nineteenth century.
   a. A scratch test in which multiple ⅜ inch (1 centimeter) superficial scratches that do not draw blood are made on the surface of the skin. The extract of the material in question is then rubbed in and the results are read in twenty minutes. If a wheal (an itchy red swelling of the skin that looks like a mosquito bite) of greater than 5 millimeters (⅕ inch) appears, it means that you have reacted to that material. It does not always mean that you are allergic to it.
   b. A puncture test; this is very similar to the scratch test except here the test material is placed on the skin and a needle punctures through it, not deep enough to draw blood. The same criteria of reactions are used.

c. An intradermal test in which the solution to be tested is injected directly into the skin producing a small ⅛ inch wheal. If the test is positive, the wheal will grow in size to equal or exceed 7 millimeters (⅓ inch).

If any of these tests are positive, this means that you have reacted to that substance; it does not necessarily mean that you are allergic to this substance at the present time nor does it mean that this substance is necessarily causing your asthma. It requires a great deal of judgment on the part of the doctor to determine which of these substances, if any, should be used in your treatment program.

9. In Vitro Test. This test represents a major recent advance in the diagnosis of allergies. Until recently, it has been impossible to make a diagnostic test of the blood in order to determine allergic reaction to a specific substance because the quantities involved were too small. With the recent advent of radio labeling (a space age bonus), it has become possible to do this. One such test that has become increasingly popular is the RAST (Radioallergosorbent test). This is a sophisticated blood test that measures the quantity of IgE in specific allergens. One blood sample can be substituted for numerous skin tests. The RAST is more convenient and comfortable for the patient than skin tests and there are no adverse reactions. However, the RAST is slightly less sensitive than skin tests. Therefore, in some cases, after the RAST, a few skin tests may still be necessary. When the RAST results are positive, as is usually the case, no further testing will be necessary.
10. ELISA (Enzyme-linked Immuno-Assay). This test uses an enzyme marker to measure the amount of IgE in specific allergens. This is detected by a sensitive instrument, called a spectrophotometer Phadezym. FAST and MAST are examples of this type of test and are comparable to RAST.
11. PRIST (Paper Radioimmunosorbent Test). This test measures the total IgE in your serum. Patients who have high levels tend to be allergic whereas those who have low

levels are usually nonallergic. This can be a very useful guide as to whether or not your physician should pursue an extensive allergic evaluation in your case.

These laboratory tests are very important. They help me to make a diagnosis, determine specific triggers, determine the effects of your problem on your respiratory system, plan an appropriate treatment program, and arrive at a baseline against which to measure and compare progress.

The preceding tests, just described, are used by many physicians in the evaluation of patients with asthma. All of these tests have been proven scientifically to be helpful. However, there is another group of tests that have never been proven scientifically to be of any help. The American Academy of Allergy and Immunology has evaluated these procedures and their opinion is that there is no evidence that the following tests are of any benefit in the evaluation of a patient with asthma. If your doctor suggests that any of the following procedures be utilized in your diagnostic evaluation, be very suspicious of the evaluation!

The first two are tests that focus on vitamin and mineral deficiencies. They are Hair Analysis and Vitamin Screening Panel.

Hair Analysis, when done with extremely careful collection techniques (which is rarely the case), can be useful in the diagnosis of certain vitamin and mineral deficiencies. However, it has not been shown that supplementing your diet to compensate for or eliminate these vitamin and mineral deficiencies will be useful in helping to control your asthma symptoms. I cannot envision any situation in which this test will be helpful in the diagnosis or treatment of asthma.

Vitamin Screening Panels, while very useful in determining suspected vitamin deficiencies, is of no value in diagnosing or treating asthma. If your physician begins to talk about hidden vitamin deficiencies, question the physician very closely!

Since some of the asthmatic population is allergic to some foods, it would certainly be helpful to be able to identify individual food allergens. Currently, skin tests, RAST, and diet experimentation are used to help discover food allergies. These are the only reliable tests available to us now. Two tests currently used that are not valuable are cytotoxic testing and provocative neutralization challenges.

The *Cytotoxic Test* is based on the premise that if the antigenic extract of a food to which you are possibly allergic is mixed with a drop of your blood, certain cells in your blood will attack the food if you are allergic or intolerant to that food. When this reaction occurs, the appearance of the cells in your blood will be altered, enabling a good microscopist to establish the relationship, thus determining which foods are the culprits. This test has been studied carefully by the Academy of Allergy and Immunology, and as intriguing as the theory is, it unfortunately does not work. The problem is that when several of the world's best microscopists were employed, they all came up with different results. If three different microscopists were given your blood, they would come up with three totally different lists of foods to which you were allergic. This test is not reliable and therefore it is worthless!

Provocative neutralization challenges (not to be confused with food challenges which are valuable) are also very questionable. The method is as follows: Assume you are allergic to milk. The proponents of this theory inject increasing quantities of milk subcutaneously, or place it under your tongue. When the correct dose is reached, you will wheeze. Then the doctor injects or places under your tongue decreasing amounts of milk, until the wheezing stops. This is the "magic neutralizing" dose. Once he has established this dose, you will be given the same dose by injection or have it placed under your tongue *ad infinitum*. This is supposed to stop your problems with milk. In my opinion and that of the Academy of Allergy and Immunology, this method is absolutely unproven. I will add that in my experience, it is of no help.

FIRST-VISIT HELPFUL HINTS FOR THE PATIENT

Now that you know what is going to happen to you during your first visit to the doctor, let me provide a list of guidelines to ensure a smoother, more productive session. The doctor is engaged in problem solving and needs all the pieces of the puzzle to be in the best position to solve the problem. Through years of experience with all kinds of patients, I have found the following to be helpful:

1. Plan the day. Eliminate any possible pressuring factors. I've had patients who bring their nine-month-old infant and spend more time worrying about the baby than listening and cooperating with me. Get a baby-sitter. Other patients schedule other appointments (social or business) after the one with me and are preoccupied with time. One patient left her husband double-parked outside and was unable to concentrate since she was anticipating what his reaction might be if our visit took a long time. First visits take quite a while. Allow time and plan appropriately.
2. Present the true you. Some patients exaggerate their symptoms, while others minimize their symptoms. Both tendencies are counterproductive. Accuracy is vital. If you are already taking some medications, don't undermedicate (so that your symptoms become so full-blown as to create an emergency situation) or overmedicate (so that your symptoms are masked or eliminated). Present the facts as they are!
3. Know your history. Your history should be familiar to you. Try to organize it. It is best, I have learned, to present it in chronological order. If you have been ill for a long time, it is best to briefly summarize "ancient" history and stress "recent" history. Salience is the key; highlight the important features. It is especially helpful if you bring reports from previous consultations. Any previous X rays are very helpful too. There is no such thing as too much information.
4. Know your medications. If you are presently taking medications, know their names and the dosages you are taking. If necessary, call your pharmacist. It always surprises me that so many people are unaware of what they are swallowing. Do not describe a small, round, chartreuse pill. Find out the name!

5. Speak clearly and precisely. I am aware of the fact that many patients are anxious during our first visit. This is understandable. The purpose of this chapter is to lessen these anxieties because they can create an obstacle that works against the success of this information-exchanging meeting. If you can, speak to the point and avoid rambling. Hard as I try, it is often impossible to gain an overview when one of my new patients goes on and on endlessly, with no particular direction discernible. Avoid vague descriptions. The patient who comes with a written list of facts and/or questions is indeed a joy.
6. Be straightforward and honest. I can only work with the information that is provided. There are times when I know that the patient is not telling me the whole story. This is a waste of time and furthermore, it will make it difficult for us to create a working relationship based on mutual respect. Be direct. After taking countless case histories, there is almost nothing that will surprise me. If it is relevant, be specific and supply the facts. It is not particularly rewarding to try to help someone who is not being helpful.
7. Be involved. Too many patients convey the feeling that their responsibility in their own care has ended when they come to see me. This is not so. Aggressive involvement in your own treatment is crucial. Patients who sit passively are doing themselves (and me) a disservice. It is human nature to want to be met halfway in any mutual endeavor and asthma care is a mutual endeavor. Ask questions. Seek clarification. Be responsive and involved!
8. Don't expect too much. Be patient and do not expect an instant cause/cure statement. Too many patients appear disappointed, even angry, when I tell them that some tests need to be done. Unless I am as certain as possible about the nature of the patient's illness, I am ill-equipped to prescribe treatment. Don't set yourself up for disappointment.
9. Demonstrate a commitment. The patients who clearly convey to me their commitment to the diagnostic and treatment processes are the most satisfying and, most often, the most

successful. Often my recommendations may be quite demanding. I might insist that a patient convince the spouse to stop smoking. I might stipulate that the family cat be removed from the patient's environment. I might have to recommend a change in jobs or job setting. Sometimes the patient agrees, but I know, for example, that the cat is still at home. Those patients who rise to the occasion and meet the challenge are demonstrating the commitment needed in asthma care. You must wait, experiment, report successes and failures, and monitor your body's reactions. I feel strongly that this commitment is a prerequisite for success. When it is demonstrated during the first visit, I know that the patient and I will work well together.

PATIENT'S BILL OF RIGHTS

In presenting a total view of the first visit, it is necessary to add a section on "consumer rights," in this case, the rights of the patient. Just as I hope that my new patients will be able to demonstrate honesty, clarity, involvement, and a sense of commitment, the patient has expectations that must also be met in order to make the first visit (and subsequent visits) successful and productive. The patient has the right to expect me, or any colleague to be

1. a good listener, able to integrate the information provided, without placing the patient in preconceived categories
2. patient, allowing the asthmatic time to present the information in his style, at his own pace, without the impression that the doctor is in a rush
3. responsive to the patient's questions about symptoms
4. easily understandable, using language that is appropriate for the patient
5. considerate of the patient's feelings, what he has gone through, and what was done to him
6. competent and knowledgeable, demonstrating familiarity with the patient's symptoms and the ramifications and possible treatment alternatives available to him

7. operating in facilities that are up-to-date, clean, and run by a staff that is polite, considerate, efficient, and helpful
8. able to offer a "game plan" with short- and long-range goals, thus providing the patient with stopgap measures if he is severely symptomatic, as well as an idea of the overall treatment program planned for him
9. reachable and flexible, demonstrating an open-minded willingness to maintain a relationship based on mutual respect, credibility, and cooperation

The first visit sets the stage for an effective asthma treatment program. If this visit goes smoothly, a significant first step has been taken. A typical first visit provides me with the raw data upon which to base a plan for reducing or eliminating the asthma symptoms in my patient. Some patients will have to alter their diet or their environment. Some will best be treated with medications. Finally, some patients may have to avoid certain substances and may be good candidates for allergy shots (immunotherapy). Most will have to monitor a combination of these factors.

Whichever route I take, I will continue to rely upon my patient to provide the data upon which to judge the success or failure of our treatment choices. The patient and I will continue to exchange information throughout the treatment. Master the skill of providing such information, for it will play an important role in your relationship with your doctor.

LUNG-LINE

An excellent, free service, which is available through the National Jewish Center for Immunology and Respiratory Medicine in Denver, Colorado, is Lung-Line. A staff of trained registered nurses answer your general questions about asthma, allergy, and lung diseases. They can provide you with names of hospitals and specialists in your area as well as the titles of helpful books and other literature. Their knowledge ranges from information about air-purifying systems to facts about special diets. Although the service is not intended to answer specific questions about your medication or your unique situation, there is a physician who will get back to you if the phone staff thinks it is appropriate. The Lung-Line is open from Monday through Friday, 8:30 A.M. to 5:00 P.M. Calls received after hours will be returned as soon as possible. The toll-free telephone number for all areas outside of Colorado is (800) 222-LUNG. For residents of Colorado the number is (303) 398-1477. More information about the National Jewish Center for Immunology and Respiratory Medicine is found in Chapter 14.

3

ASTHMA AND THE ENVIRONMENT

INTRODUCTION

Because of the supersensitivity created by the autonomic nervous system, the asthmatic is always in a vulnerable state. He walks a tightrope much of the time, trying to avoid the various stimuli that could throw him off balance and into an asthmatic attack. The troublemakers are everywhere, from the air that he breathes to the food that he eats. The asthmatic needs to be familiar with all of the environmental stimuli that can cause his asthma to flare up.

What are these troublemakers? Allergens are the most common triggers. Because they are usually a prime suspect and are quite controllable, I will devote most of this chapter to discussing them. An allergen is anything that causes an allergic reaction. Allergens come in different forms. There are aero-allergens that are found in the air that we breathe and there are food allergens.

Aero-allergens are the more common culprits. Some airborne allergens can be managed through environmental control. For example, eliminating animal dander from the environment will reduce your chances of developing an adverse allergic-asthmatic reaction to an animal. You may have to give up horseback riding and stick to the merry-go-round.

But, some airborne allergens are not so easy to get rid of because they are everywhere, almost all of the time. For example, eliminating household dust or mold is very difficult, often impossible. When total removal of the allergen is not possible, a combination of environmental control and immunotherapy can be used. If we cannot eliminate exposure to the allergen, we can at least attempt to minimize its effects. Allergy injections can be very effective in diminishing or preventing reactions to some specific allergens.

Food allergens are a less common cause of asthma than airborne allergens. They require a very individualized approach and may be controlled through diet.

Nonallergic environmental stimuli such as atmosphere pollutants and even extremes in weather can also produce asthmatic symptoms. The exact mechanisms by which smoke, a potent irritant; auto fumes; smog, a form of pollution; or high or low humidity precipitate asthma symptoms are not always clear. Nevertheless, these factors can cause serious problems.

Many of these environmental stimuli are controllable. You should be aware of them. This chapter will describe how allergens cause an allergic reaction, and I will describe in detail the environmental troublemakers. This chapter on asthma and the environment deals with the first of four basic ingredients in asthma treatment. Chapter 4 deals with asthma and food allergy in which I discuss diets designed to reduce the ingestion of food allergens. Chapter 5 deals with immunotherapy in which I discuss allergy shots as a means to reduce the asthmatic's reaction to troublemakers. Chapter 6 deals with drug therapy and discusses a variety of medications used to establish and maintain control over asthma symptoms.

Environmental Stimuli in Asthma

How does an allergen provoke an allergic reaction? To answer this, recall the discussion in Chapter 1, regarding allergic triggers. The following chain of events takes place:

- The allergen is inhaled or ingested.
- Specific antibodies (IgE) are produced by the asthmatic's white blood cells. Their function is to protect the body against various

particulate invaders such as parasites. Unfortunately, in the allergic asthmatic, such elements as pollen, dust, mold, and parasites (all of which are particulate) are mistakenly viewed by the body as invaders.

- Mast cells line the entire respiratory and gastrointestinal tract or other places that are in contact with external substances.
- The IgE molecules are in pairs and are fixed on the membrane of the mast cell. These IgE molecules are specifically programmed to recognize certain molecules from particulate matter (pollen, parasites, and dust) when the IgE molecules have been exposed to the particulates several times.
- After exposure to the appropriate allergen, the allergen will combine with the IgE antibody on the mast cell.
- The union of allergen and IgE on the mast cell is disruptive, causing the secretion of various chemical mediators.
- These mediators cause physiological changes that, in turn, cause asthmatic symptoms.

Thus, there is an interaction between an inhaled allergen and an IgE antibody bound to the mast cell surface that triggers a series of steps that lead to the generation and release of mediators. A very important mediator in general (but not always the most important one in asthmatics) is histamine. Histamine causes swelling, irritation, and inflammation of the lining of the bronchi (mucous membrane). It also produces increased mucus production and temporary or transient bronchospasm.

Another mediator, Leukotriene (LTE_4), plays an important role. It has a very slow onset, but its action is very prolonged. This is why the bronchi stay contracted or constricted hours after the initial allergen attacks them.

Brief mention should be made of the prostaglandins, important mediators in proper lung functioning. There are many prostaglandins. Some produce relaxation of the bronchi, while some are potentially harmful, producing constriction. It is not clear how the prostaglandins work, but it appears that they will eventually become very important agents in helping to control asthma. More about that later.

As you can see, medical science has become very aware that mediators play a very important role in the changes in both maintaining the normal state of the lungs and in producing asthma.

THE VULNERABLE ASTHMATIC

There are several characteristics of an asthmatic that put him at a disadvantage by facilitating the unfortunate chain of events just described. The asthmatic has as many mast cells as a nonasthmatic. He also has as many receptor sites on the mast cells as the nonasthmatic. He may have more IgE than the nonasthmatic patient, but not always. However, as we discussed before, he has an enzyme deficiency that makes him more vulnerable; he will react to allergens and any other stimuli to which the nonasthmatic will not.

In the asthmatic, you have a situation in which the mast cells are more vulnerable and sensitive, more available and possibly more easily penetrated than they should be. People with asthma have more porous mucus membranes than the nonasthmatic person. The basement membrane of the respiratory tract leaks. The spaces between the cells are not as tight as in nonasthmatic people and therefore antigens can leak down from the respiratory tract into the rest of the cells, increasing the asthmatic's exposure to antigens. All these are troublesome. If the asthmatic is exposed to some of his triggering allergens, his immune system is easily provoked into defensive reactions.

Knowing that allergens mean trouble, the asthmatic must be aware of his reactive allergens. He must be on the lookout! Our next question is: What are the allergens one should guard against?

Aero-allergens: The Space Invaders

An aero-allergen is any substance that is particulate in nature, capable of producing an allergic reaction, present in the atmosphere, and inhaled. All aero-allergens are naturally substances as opposed to aero-irritants, which are man-made. Both can cause problems and are often unavoidable. For an aero-allergen to be a problem, there must be both a plentiful source of it and a sufficient transport system to bring it to its victims. For example, airborne pollen fills all of these criteria, as it is produced in massive quantities. It is capable of producing an allergic reaction, and the wind is an excellent transport system to bring it to its victims. The following section will discuss various types of troublemaking aero-allergens.

1. POLLEN (NOTHING TO SNEEZE AT)

Pollen is a small grain produced by flowering plants, grasses, ragweed and other weeds, plantain, and trees. Those plants that are pollinated by the wind have been found to be much more of an allergic problem than those plants that are insect pollinated. The wind-pollinated plants are usually less attractive than the prettier insect-pollinated plants: a rose is insect-pollinated, whereas a ragweed is pollinated by the wind. The only time an insect-pollinated plant is a problem to an allergic person is when that individual sniffs the attractive flower.

Almost all grass pollens, with the exception of Bermuda grass, are very similar as far as an allergic person is concerned. Therefore, if you are allergic to grass, whether you breathe in timothy grass, ryegrass, or redtop grass, you will have problems. This is also true for ragweed. Tall ragweed and short ragweed are almost the same allergen. However, tree pollens are quite different. Red oak and white oak are the same, but sycamore pollen is quite different than birch pollen. If you are allergic to birch pollen, and you breathe in sycamore pollen, you will not experience any allergic reaction. However, if you are allergic to red maple, you will also have problems with silver maple. Therefore, knowing that you're allergic to trees is not enough. If trees are a source of trouble, you will have to investigate further to find out which trees cause you to react.

Weather Conditions and Pollen

The weather is a very important factor in determining the length and severity of a pollination season. If rain precedes the pollination season of a particular plant, it will produce and release much greater quantities of pollen during its pollination season. The converse is also true: If it is very dry prior to the pollination season of a plant, then lesser quantities of pollen will be produced and released by that plant. But if it is clear, dry, and windy during the pollination seasons of a particular plant, that season will be quite bad. The best possible combination is if it is dry prior to the pollination season and rains during the pollination season. Thus, rain before the pollination season and wind during means disaster.

Seasons of Pollination

It is important to know when various pollens are in the air; that is, when the plants are pollinating. Since this varies in different parts of the country, I will only give you a general guide (see Appendix 1). In the Northeast, trees pollinate in late March, April, and May. Elm, birch, and maple tend to pollinate earlier, in March and April. Oak, hickory, and sycamore pollinate later, in May. Grass starts to pollinate at the end of May just around Memorial Day and continues through June, July, and into early August. Very often oak trees and grass overlap around Memorial Day, making it all too "memorable" for those people who are allergic to both. Plantain tends to pollinate at the same time grass does. Ragweed starts in early August (although the official day is August 15) and tends to peak around Labor Day, making this holiday "hard labor" for people who are allergic to ragweed. Ragweed then tails off in mid-September. The farther south you go and the warmer the climate is, the earlier the trees start and the longer the grass season is. In southern California, grass and trees pollinate from February to December. So if you are allergic to grass and trees, do not go to southern California. Northern California is almost as bad. The trees do not really pollinate until the beginning of April. But grass continues into September, and trees do not stop until the middle of the summer. Weeds probably start in mid-July and pollinate well into October and November.

Arizona, where we are all told to rush to, has weeds and grass pollinating practically all year. So this is not exactly an allergy haven.

Northern Michigan, the Adirondacks, the White Mountains, and northern Maine have very little ragweed, an excellent environment for those who are ragweed sensitive. West of the Rocky Mountains, you will also find very little ragweed, although other irritating allergens occur west of the Rocky Mountains, as previously mentioned. Europe is also free of ragweed, except for the beaches of Normandy where there is a small amount of ragweed that was probably dropped there during the invasion of World War II.

Finally, if you think that December and January are good months for allergy sufferers, in the Texas Panhandle and in New Mexico mountain cedar pollinates from mid-December through January. This is a horrible season for those people who suffer from this allergy.

Do pollen counts count? We've all heard the local meteorologist quote a pollen count. This is a measure of the density of pollen in an air sample. To the extent that the air the meteorologist sampled is the same air that you will breathe, the pollen count is meaningful to you. However, pollen density varies greatly. If Long Island Hospital reports a high pollen count, don't cancel your New Jersey picnic. I tend to use a pollen count only as a very rough guide. However, when the overall trend of the pollen count is scrutinized carefully for several years, it is very helpful in predicting the future pollination pattern for a particular plant in a geographical area. Thus, we know from previous pollen counts that oak trees always pollinate in May in New York. I also know that grass pollinates in May in Los Angeles. Therefore, I can advise a severely grass-sensitive allergic patient to stay away from Los Angeles in May. Thus, the long-term trend of a pollen count is very meaningful, whereas the short-term trend is much less so.

2. FUNGUS (IT GROWS ON YOU)

A fungus is a parasite that can grow on organic matter either living or nonliving, is found everywhere, especially in humid places, and comes in many forms such as mold, dry rot, and downy mildew. Fungi are very hardy and are resistant to many environmental conditions. They may be a problem when they are ingested or inhaled.

Fungi reproduce by producing spores that are tiny little particles approximately one fifteenth to one tenth of the size of a red blood cell. The fungi produce copious amounts of these spores which are very light and buoyant and zoom through the air. There may be millions and millions of spores of mold in every breath we take. Thus, it is not the fungi itself that is the problem, but the spores that it produces to reproduce itself that cause us such woe.

Outdoor Sources of Fungi

Fungi can grow in the soil and on plants, hay, mulches, commercial peat moss, compost piles, leaf litter, and commercial crops. When a lawn is mowed or grain is harvested, the spores of the fungi become airborne. A humid climate is certainly more of a problem for a fungus-sensitive patient than a dry one.

Indoor Sources of Fungi

While outdoor sources of fungi are seasonal, indoor sources can be perennial. There are many potential troublemakers in one's home for the fungi-sensitive individual. Mold can grow in water vaporizers, humidifiers, air conditioners, especially central air conditioner systems with humidifiers and hot air systems. Pets and small children who leave food around can create a source of fungus. Houseplants are a source of fungus, but if they are not agitated, they may not be a severe problem. Indoors or out, moist conditions facilitate growth. Whenever there is water seepage that creates moist materials, there are breeding grounds for fungi. Beware of shower curtains, refrigerator drip trays, window moldings, and cold and moist basements.

Fungus in Foods

The fungi in the foods we eat are usually not severe troublemakers to asthmatics. Highly allergic patients, especially children, might react to ingested fungi. Yeast and other fungi are used to prepare a variety of foods such as baked goods, beer, wine, vinegar, processed meats, cheese, soy sauce, and even chocolate. Certain fungi can even grow in the refrigerator and may affect food stored after as little as seventy-two hours. Fungi come in many different forms and are often difficult to pinpoint.

Seasons for Fungi

Outdoor fungi (mainly alternaria and hormodendrum) have very clear-cut seasons. Starting in the Northeast, mold begins to become a problem as soon as the temperature exceeds fifty-five degrees. From April on, we see an increase in the mold population reaching a crescendo in July and August, when it begins to slowly fall off. However, we are then exposed to many other molds. I will not trouble you with their names. They are all very long and who wants to be on a first-name basis with a fungus?

When the first frost occurs in the Northeast or in any temperature area, it is not a continuous hard freeze. As soon as it warms up a little bit, the fungi grow again and a second blast of spores occurs producing a marked increase in symptoms. So the first frost is not the respite that you might expect it to be if you are mold-sensitive.

As we go south, mold is even more of a problem. In North Carolina, South Carolina, Florida, and Georgia, it is almost a year-round problem. In the West, where there are many more problems with weeds, grasses, and trees, mold is less of a problem until you go to the Pacific Northwest where it rains almost all of the time and mold grows constantly.

3. DUST (THE ENEMY OF THE WHITE GLOVE)

Even the "white glove" cannot win the fight against dust. It is everywhere and poses a problem on many levels. Even people who have never shown any allergic symptoms might sneeze and cough a little after cleaning out their dusty old shelves or attic. You could probably guess that dust would present an even greater problem for the twitchy-lunged asthma sufferer.

Dust can be seen as an irritant, an allergen, or a transport system for other allergens. It is a complex mixture of organic and inorganic substances. It can contain pollen, fungi spores (which we know as common allergens), animal dander, mites, insect debris, bacteria, human skin particles, plant particles, food remnants, and inorganic substances. In fact, dust can contain breakdown products of many things in and around the home. In essence, dust is a smorgasbord of allergens that is unfortunately force-fed to the asthmatic.

You might ask if dust is an allergen by itself or if the ill effects from house dust are caused by the allergenic components of the dust. People who are allergic to pollen or fungi or animal dander will certainly react to dust since it carries these substances. In this way, dust is a transport system. However, there are other individuals who have allergic reactions to dust, but do not show any allergic reactions to the common allergic culprits in dust. In this way, dust can be viewed as an aero-allergen in its own right. Any way you slice it, dust is an ever-present nuisance for the asthmatic.

4. MITES (STRANGE BEDFELLOWS)

Even though mites are a component of dust, they should be singled out because of their importance in asthma. Mites are minuscule living organisms that feed on human skin particles that have been shed. As far as mites are concerned, you're the "hostess with the mostest," no matter how disturbing that might sound. Wherever a person rests for a while, mites collect. Mites become a part of household dust and are found in great density in mattresses and carpets. They also thrive in warm, humid environments and are abundant in damp houses.

In studies done with patients sensitive to household dust, exposure to the isolated mite extract from the dust induced asthma symptoms much more readily than exposure to common dust. This tells us that mites are potent aero-allergens. We'll see later how you can minimize the accumulation of mites.

5. ANIMAL EPIDERMIS (DON'T MEANDER IN THE DANDER)

Almost everyone has seen or heard about allergic reactions to pets. They are very common. Reactions to cats, dogs, and horses (in that order) are the most frequent. It is a misconception that it is the hair of the animal that causes the problem. The troublemakers are animal dander (the dry dead skin that flakes off the animal just like human dandruff) and saliva of cats and dogs. It probably follows that there are more allergic reactions to cats, since they lick themselves all the time. Animal epidermis, as an aero-allergen, is found in house dust. Removing the pet for the day does not remove the aero-allergen.

6. FEATHERS (A TICKLISH SUBJECT)

For feather-sensitive asthmatics, problems can be year-round rather than seasonal. Feathers are found in pillows, quilts, jackets, sleeping bags, and beds. If you're not careful, your entire night may be spent surrounded by feathers.

Since feathers may come from chickens, and chickens lay eggs, some people believe that those who are allergic to feathers are also sensitive to eggs; however, there is no connection.

7. KAPOK (A STUFFY SUBJECT)

Like feathers, kapok (seed hair from the kapok tree) is used as a stuffing in pillows, furniture, sleeping bags, stuffed animals, life preservers, and mattresses. Kapok is another aero-allergen that can cause perennial asthma.

8. COTTONSEED (THAT'S NOT JUST "OIL," FOLKS)

Cottonseed is used as a stuffing, as a constituent of animal feed, and in cooking. You are probably more familiar with cottonseed oil. In this ingestible form, it rarely triggers asthma symptoms. But, when used as a stuffing, it becomes an aero-allergen. When inhaled, it has been associated with severe reactions. In fact, challenge testing with cottonseed should be done with extreme caution.

9. FLAXSEED (CAN GIVE YOU FLACK)

Flaxseed (linseed) is inhaled from a variety of sources: cattle and poultry feed, dog food, wave-setting lotion, shampoos, some brands of depilatories, insulating materials, and some rugs. Like cottonseed, ingested flaxseed (found in Roman Meal Bread, some cough medicines, and laxatives) is not usually a problem. Inhaled flaxseed, also following the pattern of cottonseed, has been known to cause severe asthma symptoms. Testing must be done cautiously.

10. PYRETHRUM (COULD BUG YOU)

Pyrethrum is an insecticide. It comes from pyrethrum flowers and is similar to the ragweed plant. Asthma symptoms are often reported after an area has been sprayed with pyrethrum.

Irritants in Asthma

There are certain substances whose presence in the air causes an irritation that, in turn, provokes asthma symptoms. These are not aero-allergens, as they cannot be separated out and tested individually, but they also provoke bronchospasm and/or mucus buildup. These factors are common irritants for most people, but the asthmatic's supersensitivity exaggerates the problem.

SMOKING

Smoke is by far the most common airborne irritant. Smoking effectively reduces one's immune defense system: this may lead an asthmatic to be more susceptible to upper respiratory infection, something that he can ill afford to get! Smoking also paralyzes the tiny hairlike structures (cilia) which are part of the filtering system along the mucus membrane lining of our respiratory passageways. The asthmatic cannot allow his internal filtering system to be inefficient, permitting airborne particles to accumulate, enter, and clog his respiratory passageways. Smoking must be avoided. But this is just half of the job.

Even the nonsmoker has a great deal to cope with regarding smoke. The asthmatic who is passively exposed to smoke at home, at work, or at a social function, will often become more symptomatic. What about the nonasthmatic? What effect will exposure to smoke have on the pulmonary function? The research is clear that young infants who live with a parent or parents who smoke demonstrate increased frequency of respiratory difficulties (bronchitis and pneumonia). While children living in smoky households do not get asthma as a direct result, they do show an increased tendency toward coughing, increased mucus production, and wheezing. Adults who have respiratory illnesses will certainly have their illnesses both acutely and chronically aggravated by exposure to tobacco smoke. The bottom line is that smoking, smokers, and smoke-filled environments must be avoided whenever possible.

Other airborne irritants that are potentially harmful are cooking odors, aerosol sprays, perfumes and colognes, powders, chemical fumes, auto exhaust, paint odors, other fumes, and any pungent odors. The asthmatic who works in a paint factory is placing himself in a hazardous environment. Nitrogen dioxide, from gas or wood-burning stoves (see page 59, The Kitchen), may cause problems. Formaldehyde, found in particle board, plywood, paper products, floor coverings, and cosmetics, occurs more frequently in mobile homes than in conventional homes, and may also be problematic. In fact, formaldehyde has been identified as a possible component in occupationally induced asthma (see page 53). Become informed about your environment; identify possible aero-allergens; step back and look around you. Carefully consider what's around you!

WEATHER AND POLLUTION

The influence of weather and pollution factors in producing asthma symptoms is unclear. There is considerable controversy surrounding these factors, and for good reason. There are excellent scientific studies supporting opposing views, and many patients report contradictory findings. For example, some people swear that a change in weather causes their asthma symptoms. And they may be correct. There are others who are not at all affected by weather changes. There are considerable individual differences to be found when studying the relative effects of such environmental factors on asthmatics. It appears, then, that the patient himself must be very aware of the possible weather, climate, and pollutant factors that can create a problem for him and must carefully monitor his body's reactions to them. Let's review several factors that one should watch out for.

ADVERSE WEATHER CONDITIONS

Weather has many components including temperature, wind velocity, barometric pressure, and humidity. Some people view weather conditions as a problem because they affect aeroallergens which, in turn, affect asthmatics. For example, high humidity breeds mold. But there are others who view weather conditions as potent culprits in their own right. It doesn't really matter why a certain weather condition affects you; what is important is that you know that it does. As a general viewpoint, it appears that any significant variation away from a comfortable mean may be bad for the asthmatic. Again, here are some general trends

1. In general, cold air is more frequently associated with asthma symptoms than warm air. A rush of cold air may cause bronchospasm in anyone—in the asthmatic, this may be exaggerated.
2. In general, high humidity readings are associated with asthma symptoms.

3. Although the medical literature is full of inconsistent findings, it appears that extreme changes (up or down) in barometric pressure are associated with increased asthma symptoms.
4. It is an ill wind that blows no good to anyone. How true here! A strong wind will blow smog and air pollution away. Unfortunately, it will blow pollen to the allergy sufferer.
5. Rainy conditions tend to help primarily because they wash away aero-allergens, irritants, and pollutants, but warm and humid climates usually work against the asthmatic because such weather conditions facilitate pollen and mold growth.

IONIZATION OF THE ATMOSPHERE

Some weather conditions result in a change in the ionization (loading of positive and negative ions in the molecules of the air) of the atmosphere. Thunderstorms, for example, add electrical charges to the air. The effects of ionization on asthma are unclear. There are some patients who claim they are benefited by negative ion generators in conjunction with air purifying devices.

POTENT POLLUTANTS—OUTDOOR AND INDOOR

Air pollution is bad for asthmatics (as it is for everyone). The air is said to be polluted when the air becomes laden with matter (usually man-made) resulting in increased breathing difficulties. Whether the pollution is industrial smog (usually resulting from fuel combustion and found in such industrial areas as New York, New Jersey, Chicago, and London) or photochemical smog (usually resulting from automobile fumes and sunny environments like Los Angeles and Denver), respiratory problems are aggravated. Certain weather conditions (low wind and temperature inversions) increase the asthmatic's sensitivity to smog. The asthmatic who lives in a highly polluted environment (or downwind of one) is usually looking for and finding trouble.

Although outdoor pollution has received much attention as an annoying irritant for the normal population and has been cited as an aggravating problem or maybe even a trigger for a person with respiratory trouble, indoor pollution, which sometimes goes unnoticed, can be at least as much (or even more) of a nuisance. The average person spends much less time outdoors than he does indoors, so it makes sense for us to investigate potential indoor pollutants and what may be done to decrease their harmful effects.

Indoor pollutants include tobacco smoke, nitrogen oxide (a result of gas stove combustion), woodsmoke (produced by wood-burning stoves), and formaldehyde, a substance used in many building materials and home furnishings. We might be exposed to these pollutants in our homes, our offices, our cars, and maybe even during an airplane trip. The degree to which the indoor pollution affects us will depend upon the indoor concentration of the pollutant, the source of the pollutant, the air exchange rate with the outdoors, as well as the outdoor levels of pollution.

The environment is full of potential troublemakers. Whether they are aero-allergens, irritants, pollutants, or adverse weather conditions, you must be alert and ready to take action against these asthmatic triggers. The action is avoidance: this preventative measure can be extremely helpful. If asthma has made you feel out-of-control, take your revenge. You can gain some control by studying your environment and manipulating it to minimize the quantity of aero-allergens and irritants and their ill effects.

ENVIRONMENTAL CONTROL

When Is It Appropriate to Attempt Environmental Control?

Avoidance of the offending allergen is clearly necessary

1. for the asthmatic who cleans out a moldy basement and becomes symptomatic
2. for the asthmatic who visits his friend who has a cat and develops a tightening of his chest

3. for the asthmatic who wheezes when he goes on a picnic because he is surrounded by external allergens (grass, trees, weeds, pollens, and mold spores)
4. for the asthmatic who just bought a feather pillow and begins to wheeze every night he sleeps
5. for the asthmatic who wheezes at night and is allergic to mites in the bedding

For some asthmatics, the answer is not obvious because the offending allergens or irritants remain obscure. The perennially symptomatic asthmatic who suffers a good deal of the time should be especially interested in pinpointing the allergens that bother him and in experimenting with environmental control. As I mentioned in Chapter 2, the allergist who suspects allergic asthma usually does some preliminary testing to try to uncover the culprits. The patient might react to one or many allergens. At any rate, the results of the testing help pinpoint the triggers. This helps to facilitate environmental control, focusing on the appropriate factors.

Most asthmatics have symptoms which are less extreme. The approach to be taken, then, is to control one's environment as much as possible without going overboard. Total environmental control can be a monumental task, often expensive, inconvenient, and restricting. It requires involvement, both emotional and physical. While it has been clearly documented that environmental control helps, there is no guarantee that you will get back in improved health proportionately what you have invested in time, sacrifice, and money. I recommend attempting to control the environmental variable with moderation as a guiding principle.

What are the alternatives for the patient who doesn't want to bother with environmental control? The asthmatic can take medications to reduce his symptoms. Medication can ease the effects of the allergens or irritants, but as we will see in Chapter 6, drugs can present problems of their own. Many medications have side effects, some more dangerous than others, so they need careful monitoring. In general, we would all like to take a minimum of medication. If the allergen is obvious, avoidance is the best route.

The other alternative might be allergy shots, which will be discussed in Chapter 5. The purpose of shots is to desensitize you to the allergic triggers. Again, it seems obvious that if it is easy to avoid the known allergen, this approach is preferable to weekly visits to the allergist for immunotherapy (allergy shots). When children are involved, it is better to try to control the environment than to cope with the possible trauma and nuisance of allergy shots or the need for medication.

In general, then, environmental control should be attempted when

1. the aero-allergens or irritants have made themselves known through real life experiences
2. allergy testing clearly indicates an aero-allergen that leads to asthma symptoms
3. alternative treatments (medication and/or allergy shots) are less preferable

While environmental control may seem appropriate, there are other factors that must also be considered.

HOW FAR SHOULD YOU GO?

This is not always such an easy question to answer. Patients have their own personalities, with varying degrees of severity of symptoms and their own level of tolerance. It makes sense that if a person has a mild problem and requires minimal amounts of medication, he need not expend a great deal of effort to control his environment.

At the other end of the spectrum is the patient who has tried many approaches to control his asthma with only minimal success. In the moderate to severe asthmatics, stricter environmental control is in order, even if their allergy tests are not all positive.

The answer, then, to "How far should you go?" depends on many factors. Severity of symptoms is very important. Personality factors are also very important. Even the mild asthmatic, who takes a minimum amount of medication intermittently may not be willing to tolerate any wheezing or medication. This individual may be very motivated and willing to go to great lengths to clean up his "space." One of my patients cleans his air conditioner with a Q-tip! Other patients prefer to take any number of pills and suffer any amount of wheezing rather than take the steps necessary to control their environment. Personality factors, tolerance levels, and severity of symptoms interact in any number of combinations.

Other considerations are the expense and inconvenience inherent in implementing environmental control measures. Changing one's heating system, buying and setting up humidifiers, dehumidifiers, and air conditioners can be expensive and inconvenient. You must avoid events where you know you'll be in smoke-filled rooms. You may have to give up Thursday night bingo or other social get-togethers. Telling your child that he cannot go to the circus or zoo may be devastating for him/her. Environmental control measures may come with a price tag, and their cost must be weighed carefully.

If, for example, your child has a mild, brief wheezing spell after an extended exposure to animals that can easily be prevented by the use of a small dose of harmless medication before exposure, then taking the medication is better than taking away such important family activities as going to the zoo. A commonsense logical approach to environmental control is the best policy.

WHERE SHOULD YOU START?

With moderation as our guiding principle, where does one begin? You begin by controlling the environment in which the asthmatic spends most of his time. Usually, this is the bedroom. When this is done, then move to the other commonly used rooms. For the child, it may be the playroom or basement; for the "chief cook and bottlewasher," it may be the kitchen. For the traveling salesman, it may even be the car. Attention should also be paid to the heating and cooling systems that serve the entire house. Finally, some recommendations can be made concerning landscaping and the control of outdoor variables.

If extensive allergy testing has been done, you will want to start your cleanup by focusing on those allergens to which the patient has the most significant reaction. Do not ignore the others. There is a great deal of overlap among aero-allergens. And allergic sensitivities tend to change. One year, mold may be the most significant problem and the next year it may be dust. As long as you are cleaning up your "space," do a thorough job.

Do not forget the airborne irritants such as smoke, paint, strong perfumes, cooking odors, and insecticides. Keep your exposure to these substances at a minimum.

After you have decided on your plan of attack, it is best if the asthma sufferer is absent during and shortly after the cleanup. Whenever the asthmatic is involved in any type of cleanup, a protective mask can be helpful.

The Bedroom

Whenever you approach the chore of cleaning a room, strip it as if you were moving. Vacuum thoroughly and damp mop the walls, including the closets. Remember, we are taking a moderate stance. Some extremists would tell you to do away with all carpeting. If you don't want to do this, then you are obliged to vacuum thoroughly and very frequently. Short pile carpeting is easier to clean and is, therefore, preferable to longer, shaggy styles. Common sense would tell you that if you are sensitive to wool, and your carpeting is wool, it must go! Underpadding must be foam, not felt (animal hairs). If you have no carpeting in the bedroom (or if you have decided to take out the carpeting), the floor needs to be damp mopped frequently.

Everything should be washable: curtains, walls (either paper or painted), window shades, blankets, and bedspreads. There should be as few dust collectors as possible: no stored items under the bed; shades on windows are preferable to venetian blinds (venetians, if used, should be washed in the bathtub regularly); no open bookshelves or knickknacks; no dried flowers; and few if any stuffed animals or toys—which should always be easy to clean. Opt for vinyl, plastic, or other synthetic materials for furniture and car seat covers. Avoid feather (down), kapok, horsehair, or foam stuffings and opt for Dacron/polyester. Foam can sometimes breed mold.

Bedding dust, which contains mites, can be a real problem. Encasing the box springs, mattress, and pillows in nonporous plastic or rubberized cloth is very important. Even the zippers should be sealed with adhesive tape. These coverings should be checked regularly, and they should be vacuumed with every linen change one to two times a week. Plastic casings for mattresses and pillowcases are available. Check with your doctor, surgical supply, or large department stores.

The air in the bedroom should be as clean as possible. During the winter, the amount of heated air should be minimized. During allergy season, keep the windows closed and the air conditioner running.

If you are moving into a new home, do not place the bedroom of the asthmatic above the garage, if possible, or on the side of the house that is most exposed to the wind (because it will be colder and need more heat and will contain more airborne allergens and irritants). Keep the vegetation near this room to a minimum.

After all of this trouble, don't undo all of your good work by allowing smoke, pets, aerosol sprays, or perfumed toiletries in the room. In the case of these irritants, especially in the bedroom, moderation is not good enough. These irritants are just not allowed, with no exception!

Other Rooms

With the major task of purifying the bedroom now complete, it is not unreasonable to wait awhile before proceeding to other rooms. A few weeks should tell you whether your efforts have been worthwhile. If you haven't changed anything else but the cleanliness of the room, and if you are feeling better, environmental control is working for you. Whether you are content with what you've done or are spurred on to conquer other rooms depends on all of the factors we've spoken of previously. If you're ready to proceed, here are some things to look for in several key rooms.

The Kitchen

In the kitchen, make sure there is a good venting system for the cooking odors. These can spread to other rooms and be a problem all over the house. It's a good idea to keep the exhaust fan on while cooking. Obviously, the kitchen should be kept clean and free of dampness (as on windowsills) that breeds mold. Refrigerator drip trays should be cleaned often.

Nitrogen dioxide, produced by gas stoves, can be a potent irritant. Similarly, wood smoke from wood-burning stoves can cause problems. Make sure to keep these ovens well vented and in good working condition to reduce the risk of potential irritants being released into your environment.

The Bathroom

Bathrooms are common breeding grounds for mold because of the dampness. Bathroom tiles, floors, walls, and shower curtains are good spots for mold growth and should be monitored. Unscented disinfectants that reduce mold and mildew can be helpful.

The Basement, Attic, and Crawl Spaces

Basements, attics, and crawl spaces are usually dark and damp and provide the perfect home for mold. They should be avoided by the asthmatic, and kept as dry and clean as possible. If the basement is a play area, a dehumidifier would be a good investment.

For mild mold contamination, these measures will easily handle the problem. For more extensive problems, either get professional help or write to the U.S. Government Printing Office, Superintendent of Documents, Washington, D.C. 20402, and request the pamphlet "How to Prevent and Remove Mildew."

A house that is clean, free of smoke, animal dander, and any other known allergens or irritants is the most suitable home for the asthmatic. Again, when the house is being cleaned, the asthmatic should not be there; when the house is being painted, the asthmatic should be out-of-town—for a week!

Heating, Cooling, Filtering, and Humidifying Systems

The air that circulates throughout the house can be controlled to minimize reactions to aero-allergens. In general, the greater the air disturbance the more chance there is for allergens to circulate. Therefore, forced air heating is not preferable unless it is highly and effectively filtered. If you have this type of heating system, it is very important to add a filtering system (preferably electronic) so that the air that is forced throughout the house is as clean as possible. Vents should be covered with cheesecloth to further filter the air, and in bedrooms the bed should not be near the vent. Electric and hot water heating, and other radiant heating systems are preferable, although these systems do not permit filtering. The optimum temperature is seventy degrees during the day and sixty-five degrees at night.

Air-conditioning is highly recommended, especially for the pollen-sensitive patient. Central air-conditioning is preferable because it lends itself to additional electronic filtration. If, because of cost factors, you must restrict the use of central air-conditioning, an individual unit in the asthmatic's bedroom is suggested. No matter which system is used, the filters must be checked and cleaned often even if they are not very dirty. The entire purpose may be defeated if mold spores are growing on the filter.

There are many different types of filtering systems available for use in one's home. Some filters, like the ones on air conditioners, mechanically trap particles of a certain size. The filters are usually effective for mold spores and pollens, but dust particles, smoke, and animal dander are too small to be trapped. Electrostatic filters also trap particles, but in this case the particles are electrically charged and then trapped. The advantage of electrostatic air purifiers is that they can be mounted onto the furnace and filter the air that flows through the entire house (either heated or centrally cooled air). The disadvantage (which is increasingly being minimized by recent technology) is the production of ozone which can be troublesome for the asthmatic.

HEPA (High Efficiency Particulate Air) filters are most effective because these are capable of trapping very small particles. The disadvantage is that at the present time you cannot filter an entire home with one unit. Therefore, you have to have a HEPA filter unit in each area to be controlled. The purest air is a few feet directly in front of the HEPA filter.

There are many filters on the market today. Some are small, portable units, designed for use in a particular room, at the office, or even in the car. It is best to keep up with the latest innovations by consulting *Consumer Reports,* local stores, or your doctor. Some companies allow you to rent before you buy. If you do buy any equipment, remember, it is a tax deduction.

The optimum humidity in a home is between 40 and 50 percent. Depending upon where you live and the season, humidification or dehumidification may be necessary. Since well-lubricated mucous membranes are important to breathing, there must be moisture in the air. Dry air is very harmful for asthmatics. However, maintaining proper humidity is not always easy or without risk. You must make sure that you are not creating too moist an environment that could promote the growth of mold or mites. Use a humidifier with a humidistat to insure an effective moisture control. You must also clean the humidifier very frequently. Humidifiers can create a new source of mold that will grow very readily in the moist interior of the humidifier. The manufacturers of most humidifiers sell a substance that can be added to the water of the humidifier to inhibit the growth of mold. When you buy a humidifier, be sure to obtain this substance and use it in your humidifier as directed. If the humidifier is moldy, the massive amount of mold spores will then be dispersed into the air along with the moist air. Whether you are using a humidifier or a dehumidifier, controlling the level of moisture in your home is important and keeping the unit clean is crucial.

Tight Building Syndrome

All of the household irritants and pollutants discussed may become more of a problem if your home or office is "tight," or overly insulated. This results from builders' efforts to make buildings as energy efficient as possible. Preliminary research shows that radon, asbestos, insecticides, fungicides, some building materials, and smoke are the probable culprits in causing the "sick building" syndrome. This is characterized by such symptoms as mucous membrane and eye irritations, cough, tightness in the chest, fatigue, headache, and general malaise in the inhabitants of the tight buildings. If these symptoms affect the nonasthmatic, imagine the effects on the asthmatic!

It is important to note that the list of indoor airborne irritants is long. Much more material on this subject is available, but it will help you very little in your detective work. If you find that you are persistently ill in your home, workplace, or any building you frequent, you should consider that some indoor pollutant may be causing the problem for you. If your asthma increases in one building and your nonasthmatic friends and colleagues have other symptoms of malaise, think in terms of indoor pollutants. Since it would be very difficult for you to track the offending substance(s), the Environmental Protection Agency in your city should be able to help you or tell you which engineering firms specialize in that type of "detective work."

Outside the House

You cannot control the environment outside your home nearly as well as you can control the environment inside. However, on your own property you do have more control over some factors that could pose a potential problem. For example, keep the vegetation to a minimum and far away from the house. If you are allergic to some plants, trees, or grasses, eliminate or minimize them as best you can.

Certainly do not let leaves accumulate. Mold thrives on leaf decay. If mowing your lawn causes you problems, either wear a mask or have someone else do it. When possible, the asthmatic should not be around when the lawn is being mowed.

The Car

Unless you happen to spend a great deal of time in the car, the car is not usually a focus of concern. However, when in the car avoid smoking or passengers who smoke. If you are going for a long ride, the close quarters of a car make it very difficult for the asthmatic to bear any irritants. Ask your friends not to wear cologne or perfume that evening. Don't tailgate, especially a diesel, and keep your windows closed so as to minimize fume inhalation. During cold weather, when driving in traffic, wear warm clothing and use the car heater less to minimize fume inhalation. Keep your windows closed and the air-conditioning on during the allergy season or in areas where there are fumes or allergens (fields or farms). If you can, opt for leather/vinyl seat coverings to make cleaning easier. Vacuum seat and floor mats often. Spray moldy areas and clean your engine annually. In warm humid areas, the car air conditioner may become moldy. If you wheeze every time you turn on the car air conditioner, consider having the system professionally cleaned: it may be moldy!

Environmental Control When You're on the Go

Even if your home and car are pure, you still need to interact with the rest of the world. As far as possible, your work setting should be free of aero-allergens and irritants. Now that you have all the facts, reevaluate your job setting. You may want to make some changes. A portable air filter may help control the area around your desk. If your job forces you to deal with some irritants or aero-allergens that are causing your asthma, a change of jobs may be necessary.

In restaurants, ask for the nonsmoking section, the airiest area, and stay away from fireplaces and the kitchen. Take the nonsmoking section on planes as well.

If you are out of your home, consider where you have been before you return home. If you've been visiting a friend who has a dog, your clothing may be bringing trouble into your home's controlled environment. If you've been spending a victorious day in the fields playing baseball, you may be bringing home more than a trophy. Clothes should be removed promptly and laundered immediately.

If you know that you are going to a place where there is the potential of encountering some aero-allergens or irritants, take whatever precautions you can. You may have to increase your medication. If your host for the weekend has a cat, ask him to remove the cat for the weekend and vacuum his home thoroughly. Don't sleep in the cat's favorite room, and simply have the linens changed.

If you are planning a vacation, plan appropriately. If you are pollen sensitive, don't plan a vacation hiking through farm country in August. A cruise may be better! If you are sensitive to animal dander, a dude ranch is a very poor choice of a vacation haven. Don't stay in a hotel or motel that allows pets. Take along your own pillow, or make sure that the pillow is not a feather one, or use several pillow cases if all else fails. Air-conditioning in the summer is helpful.

No Smoking, Please

By far the most common and obvious offender in the outside world is smoke and one of the most difficult problems for the asthmatic is staying away from smoke. It is becoming more acceptable and commonplace for people to ask smokers to curb their habit. The asthmatic must join the bandwagon. He cannot tolerate smoke. Needless to say, an asthmatic who smokes has stacked the deck against himself and has greatly reduced his chances of being helped. Stay away from places where you can't see the No Smoking signs because of all the smoke! Nonsmokers have rights and for the asthmatic it is a matter of "life and breath."

CONTROLLING THE UNCONTROLLABLE: WEATHER AND POLLUTANTS

As I pointed out in the previous chapter, the influence of weather conditions and certain pollutants in causing asthma symptoms is controversial and unclear. If you have become more aware of the possible negative factors in your particular case (as I hope you have by now), then you will take the appropriate steps. For example, if you have found that high humidity works well for you, use humidifiers. If warm weather works against you, use air-conditioning and stay indoors as much as possible. If you are sure that you can reliably predict a cause-and-effect relationship between weather factors and asthma flare-ups, then it may be justifiable to pick and move to an area with the combination of weather conditions most suitable to you. I would caution you, however, that such a drastic change is often unsuccessful. Whenever possible, undergo a trial period of several months.

The relationship between pollutants and asthma is a bit more direct, as you have already learned. Listen to the radio and monitor the air pollution readings to determine the worst levels you can endure. It is true that when eye irritation occurs, respiratory irritation is also probable. The guidelines proposed by the Weather and Air Pollution Committee of the American Academy of Allergy for use by asthmatics during air pollution alerts are as follows:

1. Avoid unnecessary physical activity.
2. Avoid smoking and smoke-filled rooms.
3. Avoid exposure to dust and other irritants such as hair sprays or other sprays, paint, exhaust fumes, smoke from any fire, or other fumes.
4. Avoid exposure to persons with colds and respiratory infections.
5. Try to stay indoors in a clean environment. Air-conditioning may be helpful, if available, as well as charcoal filters and electrostatic precipitators.
6. If it appears that the air pollution episodes will persist or worsen, it may be desirable to leave the polluted area temporarily until the episode subsides.
7. The physician should consider the formulation of specific instructions to be followed by the patient in case of an air pollution alert. The patient should know what medication to use, when to call the physician, and when to go to the hospital.
8. The physician's special guidelines should be kept on an instruction sheet in a readily accessible place.

YOU CAN'T SEE THE FOREST FOR THE TREES

I've been in contact with hundreds of patients who are very committed to controlling their asthma. They are involved, intelligent people, dedicated to helping themselves. However, despite all their major efforts, they seem to deny or overlook the importance of environmental control procedures. They somehow do not believe the potency of aero-allergens or irritants and feel that "a little bit can't hurt." They are doing themselves a tremendous disservice. One severely asthmatic patient, who religiously takes all of her medications, still has four cats. While she has significantly curtailed her life-style choices, she has not eliminated her pets. She does not feel that they are really an ingredient in her asthma. Chances are she is very wrong.

One physician-friend, whose asthma symptoms had just begun to flare up, invited me to dinner. As soon as I entered, I knew just what the problem was. Instead of smelling the aroma of freshly baked croissants, I detected a moldy odor. He had a fine humidifying system, but had never thought to clean the filter.

The mother of another patient complained that her child's asthma had made her a nervous wreck. She had gone from two to three packs of cigarettes a day. Need I say more?

However direct and simplistic the recommendations in this chapter may seem, their simplicity does not mean they are unimportant. You need to take a giant step back and look at your environment objectively. This may very well lead you to take a giant step forward in controlling your asthma.

4

FOOD ALLERGY AND ASTHMA

"You are what you eat" has been heard time and time again. Our society has become very aware of the relationship between the food we eat and the way our bodies function. These days it seems as if nearly everyone is either a calorie-counter, nutrition-minded, or a vegetarian. Whatever the case, much thought is being given to our daily diet.

Most diet-conscious individuals can get away with a little cheating at a cocktail party or on a special occasion. They can repent during the week for their weekend splurges, but such flexibility does not exist for those whose transgressions result in physical reactions (including asthma). Adverse food reactions, which are complex and sometimes confusing, are the topic of this chapter.

Allergic and Nonallergic Food Reactions

Many factors contribute to the confusion about adverse food reactions. Some reactions are allergic and some are not. If the reaction is allergic, an immunological event must have occurred; that is, IgE antibody has interacted with an antigen (the offending food) and has started the chemical chain reaction that I described in Chapter 3. The resulting symptoms can range from a stuffy nose, watery eyes, and scratchy throat, to extensive swelling of the body, migraine headaches, hives, coughing, itchy skin, and the wheezing and breathing difficulty we know as asthma.

The adverse food reactions that are nonallergic (nonimmunologic) are generally referred to as food intolerances. These reactions occur when a molecule in the food causes the release of harmful mediators. Sometimes these mediators are the same as those that are active in the immunological event that defines allergic food reactions. In the case of intolerances, however, there has been no interaction between IgE antibodies and antigens. The resulting symptoms can be the same as in allergic reactions. Two examples that have made the headlines involve monosodium glutamate (MSG) and metabisulfites. MSG is often used in Chinese food. It releases all of the mediators that create problems for the asthmatic, and people who are susceptible to this substance experience severe headaches, itching, sneezing, coughing, and wheezing after eating Chinese food. Although this looks like a classic food allergy, it is really an intolerance.

Metabisulfite has been found on dried fruits, fresh fruit, vegetables, wine, and even in Bronkosol, a solution used in nebulizers or sprays. Individuals susceptible to metabisulfites can have severe bronchial asthma. Once again, it looks like a severe allergic reaction, but it is an intolerance.

To the person who is reacting, it doesn't much matter whether they have an allergy or an intolerance. The effect is the same. To make your reading easier, I will use the term food allergy to cover all adverse food reactions.

Immediate and Delayed Food Reactions

Some food reactions are immediate and some are delayed. Some reactions can even begin when the food is still being chewed. Other reactions may begin as long as twenty-four hours after the food has been eaten.

The immediate reactions leave little doubt about which food is the culprit. If, for example, you eat a peanut and your tongue suddenly swells, you know to avoid peanuts. But while it is nice of your body to let you know so clearly and so soon what food to avoid, immediate food reactions can be intense, even dangerous.

The most severe form of allergic reaction is called anaphylaxis. It is manifested by generalized swelling, hives, wheezing, and choking. In its most severe form, death can result. Steps to take to avoid anaphylactic food reactions will be discussed later on in this chapter.

If for the first time you think you are having an anaphylactic reaction, immediately call for help. Help means any facility with life-support facilities (emergency rooms, police and fire departments, etc.). After you have had an anaphylactic reaction, work out a treatment program with your doctor in case it happens again. You should be equipped with no less than an EpiPen (a premeasured adrenaline-filled syringe designed for easy self-administration) and antihistamines (see p. 167). Even when you are equipped with life-support medication you should still seek medical attention as soon as possible after you administer your medication.

Delayed food reactions are usually not intense, but they can be chronic, annoying, and debilitating. In these reactions your body is not so clear and prompt in telling you which foods to avoid. In fact, the process of finding the troublemaking food can be very difficult, and you may need all the Sherlock Holmes skills you can muster.

Food Allergies Change over Time

Some allergies tend to stay with the individual throughout his life, while others tend to be outgrown. For example, allergies to milk, wheat, corn, and eggs tend to be outgrown, while allergies to fish, shellfish, peanuts, and nuts tend to persist.

Age influences food allergies. From my experience, 10 percent of children and 5 percent of adults have food allergies contributing to their asthma. Food allergy is more common in adults who have had asthma since childhood than it is in later-onset asthmatics who became symptomatic after age forty.

Children tend to be more allergic to milk, wheat, corn, artificial coloring, and flavorings. Adults tend to be more allergic to artificial coloring (especially tartrazine, yellow dye #5); artificial flavorings; aspirin and other anti-inflammatory compounds, such as Indocin, Motrin, Naprosyn, Butazolidin, and Tolectin; benzoate preservatives; metabisulfite; and yeast products.

The Form That the Food Is In

Not only does a particular allergic reaction depend upon the food, but in some instances the form that the food is in can be a determining factor. Some foods become troublesome only after the digestion process releases a substance to which the individual is allergic: Milk allergy is often an example of this kind of food reaction. Cooking or heating food can also change its role as an allergen. Raw shrimp and peas can induce severe anaphylaxis in some patients whereas many of these same people can ingest cooked peas and cooked shrimp with little or no difficulty. Some individuals tolerate warmed milk better while others cannot.

Despite all of this confusion, the simple fact remains that for a portion of the asthmatic population, eating certain foods brings on their symptoms. To touch all bases in treating asthma, the possibility of adverse food reactions must be considered. Surely you will want to know how to find out if food is contributing to your asthma symptoms and you'll also want to know what you can do about it.

How to Deal with Immediate Food Reactions

If you've had an immediate food reaction you will probably have at least a pretty good idea of the culprit food. To help you confirm your suspicion, a RAST blood test (Chapter 2) can be used. A RAST is preferable to skin tests when trying to pinpoint this kind of food reaction because a skin test can cause the very same reaction as the offending food. RAST is usually more helpful when used to test food reactions in children than in adults.

Some foods are notorious for causing immediate food reactions: peanuts, peas, nuts (a peanut is not a nut, it is a legume); bony fish, such as cod, tuna, and bass; shellfish, such as lobster, shrimp, oysters, crabs, and clams; buckwheat, eggs (frequently when eaten by small children); mustard; and monosodium glutamate.

The treatment for immediate food allergy is simple: avoid the food at all costs. Don't try it again. Don't even eat a little. Forget it!

What is not so simple is the degree of caution and constant awareness that is required. Foods come in a variety of forms. If you had an anaphylactic reaction to peanuts, obviously peanut butter would have to go, along with peanut brittle, many candy bars, and some toppings. But you would also have to watch out for foods fried in peanut oil, or foods in which peanut butter may have been used as a thickening agent, and this will require some detective work. For example, you might want to interview the cook in a Chinese restaurant (where peanut oil is often used).

Very recently, peanut and soy oil have been found not to be allergenic. However, I still advise my highly sensitive patients to try the oil under controlled conditions in my office for the first time, and never to use anything but highly purified commercial oils. The problem is that in certain health food stores some soy oils which are prepared by the cold press method, although of high quality and tasty, still have some soy protein in them and are allergenic. If you are peanut or soy sensitive, you probably can safely use the oil. Do *not* do this without discussing it with your doctor first.

Another complicating factor that makes avoidance more difficult is the fact that foods come in families. Peanuts, for instance, are legumes and therefore other legumes might have to be avoided too (i.e., soybeans, peas, carob, etc.). It is important to become familiar with food families; not only will you know what you can't have, but you'll be unafraid to eat the foods that you can have. For example, an allergy to eggs usually does not mean that you can't have chicken or that you must avoid feathers. A list of food families is provided. If you have had some immediate, intense food reactions, consult the list and avoid the culprit and its family!

In the future dealing with food allergy will be even easier. It may be possible within the next few years to take the drug cromolyn sodium in an oral form or drugs of a similar mechanism such as ketotifen (Zaditen) which will prevent food reactions. In the meantime, there is no treatment other than avoidance. While some doctors feel they can neutralize your reactions to some of these foods by prescribing smaller amounts, I have not found this procedure to work well, and I do not recommend it.

The following chart lists various food families and the most commonly eaten foods within the family. I've limited the list to generally popular families. Every effort to ensure that this list is correct and accurate has been made. However, it is possible that there are variations within this list. Therefore, if you have a severe allergy, use this list as a guideline, but be sure to check with your physician to make sure he agrees with the food families. (Note: If you eat rather exotic foods or have had several anaphylactic food reactions, you may need a more comprehensive list, including all food families, foods, extracts, and flavors. Consult your doctor or librarian.)

Family	***Food***
Algae and Fungi	Agar gum, Carrageen
Apple	Apple, Crab apple, Pear, Quince
Arrowroot	Arrowroot
Banana	Banana, Plantain
Beech	Beechnut, Chestnut
Birch	Filbert, Hazelnut, Wintergreen
Brazil nut	Brazil nut
Buckthorn	Jujube
Buckwheat	Buckwheat, Dock, Rhubarb, Sea grape
Cactus	Prickly pear, Tequila
Caper	Caper
Cashew	Cashew, Mango, Pistachio
Citrus	Citric acid, Citron, Grapefruit, Kumquat, Lemon, Lime, Limequat, Orange, Tangerine, Tangelo, Angostura bitters
Coca	Cocaine
Cola nut	Chocolate, Cocoa, Cola nut, Kutira gum, Sterculia
Ebony	Persimmon, Date, Plum, Kaki
Elm	Hackberry

Fungi	Morel, Mushroom, Cheeses (moldy), Truffle, Yeast
Ginger	Cardamom, Ginger, Turmeric
Gooseberry	Gooseberry, Currant (black, red, and white)
Goosefoot	Beet, Beet sugar, Swiss chard, Spinach
Gourd (melon)	Cantaloupe, Cucumber, Casaba, Cassabanana (Curuba), Honeydew, Melon (Spanish, gherkin, and Persian), Pumpkin, Squash, Vegetable marrow, Watermelon, Zucchini
Grains	Bamboo shoots, Barley (malt, whiskey, ale, some liqueurs), Cane sugar (brown and white sugar, molasses, and rum), Corn (includes bourbon, dextrose, and glucose), Millet, Oats, Rice, Rye, Wheat (includes bran, gluten flour, and durum)
Heath	Blueberry, Black buckleberry, Cranberry, Lingonberry
Honey	Honey
Honeysuckle	Elderberry
Iris	Saffron
Laurel	Avocado, Bay leaf, Cinnamon, Sassafras, Cassia
Legume	Acadia, Beans (kidney, green, lima, wax, pinto, and asparagus), Soy bean (soya flour and oil), Carob, Cassia, Fenugreek, Licorice, Lentil, Peas (black-eyed, chick, green, and split), Peanut (and oil), Tamarind, Alfalfa, St. John's bread, Clovers, Guar, Mesquite
Lily	Asparagus, Chives, Garlic, Leek, Onion, Sarsaparilla, Shallot
Linseed	Flax (flaxseed), Linseed
Litchi	Litchi nut
Macadamia	Macadamia nut
Mallow	Cottonseed, Gumbo, Okra, Marshmallow
Maple	Maple (sugar and syrup)
Mint	Basil, Catnip, Artichoke (Chinese or Japanese), Marjoram, Menthol, Mint, Oregano, Peppermint, Rosemary, Sage, Spearmint, Thyme, Pennyroyal tea
Morning Glory	Sweet potato, Yam
Mulberry	Fig, Mulberry, Hops
Mustard	Broccoli, Brussels sprouts, Cabbage, Collards, Kale, Horseradish, Kohlrabi, Mustard, Mustard Greens, Radish, Rutabaga, Turnip, Watercress, Wintercress, Sauerkraut
Myrtle	Allspice, Bayberry, Clove, Eucalyptus, Guava, Roseapple
Nettle	Oregano, Marijuana, Hashish

Nightshade	Chili, Eggplant, Paprika, Ground cherry, Pepper (green, sweet, bell, and cayenne), Pimento, Tabasco, Tomato, Potato
Nutmeg	Mace, Nutmeg
Olive	Olives and Olive oil
Orchid	Vanilla, Guaiacum gum
Palm	Coconut, Date, Sago
Papaya	Papaya, Passion fruit, Papain
Parsley	Anise, Carrot, Black cumin, Seeds (caraway and celery), Chervil, Coriander, Cumin, Dill, Fennel, Parsley, Parsnip, Sweet cicily
Pepper	Pepper (black and white)
Pine	Pine nut
Pineapple	Pineapple
Plum	Almond, Apricot, Cherry, Peach, Nectarine, Plum, Prune, Wild cherry, Sloe
Pomegranate	Pomegranate
Poppy	Poppyseed and Oil
Rose	Raspberries (black and red), Boysenberry, Dewberry, Loganberry, Strawberry, Rose
Seaweed	Kelp, Dulse
Sesame	Sesame (seed and oil)
Spurge (tapioca)	Tapioca, Castor bean
Sunflower	Artichoke, Chamomile, Chicory, Dandelion, Endive, Escarole, Lettuce, Sunflower seed, Tarragon
Tea	Tea (green and pekoe)
Walnut	Walnuts (black and English), Butternut, Hickory nut, Pecan
Water chestnut	Water chestnut

Anaphylactic Emergencies

If you have ever experienced an anaphylactic reaction, you certainly would not want it to happen again. Since severe anaphylaxis does not afford you the time to get to a doctor or emergency room, you must have an emergency treatment that you can use. I would strongly recommend carrying Adrenalin since it can be administered easily (after training) and is available in a portable kit called EpiPen (ask your doctor). It also might be prudent to discuss with your physician which antihistamine to have available for you to use after Adrenalin at the first sign of trouble. I usually recommend Benadryl or Chlor-Trimeton. Remember that EpiPen just buys you the time to get to a medical treatment facility.

TESTING FOR DELAYED FOOD REACTIONS

It isn't easy to be sure that your asthma symptoms are the result of delayed adverse food reactions. Most of the time we think of allergic reactions as immediately observable. The asthma symptoms that occur when we're not eating are not usually associated with food. But they can be! In fact, the chronic asthmatic who has not found significant and consistent relief by using asthma medications or by controlling the environment may very well find that food is a contributing factor.

Our search would be made easier if testing for food allergies through skin tests or blood tests were reliable. Unfortunately, as I have mentioned previously in Chapter 2, this is not the case at this point in time. Current testing procedures do not always provide us with RELIABLE answers. If you have a hunch as to what food or foods cause you grief, the investigative work might be shortened. If you have no idea, or if you suspect many foods, it would be wise for you to go on a multiple elimination diet to help you find the culprits. First, let's deal with the easier case, when you have a hunch.

TESTING YOUR HUNCH

Do some thinking about your experiences with asthma as it relates to the foods that you've been eating. If you've been symptomatic after thick shakes, think about an adverse food reaction to milk. Sometimes your favorite food turns out to be a major troublemaker. Think about the foods you love and eat often or in great quantity. Sometimes, the "hidden" food allergy comes to the surface during the discussions I have with my patients. Three examples come to mind.

One patient had the feeling that food was causing her asthma symptoms, and she came with a long list of suspects. She had adverse reactions to certain cheese crackers, cottage cheese that was served in a restaurant, some fish, some delicatessen salads, and deviled eggs. One night she dined on chicken paprikash in a Hungarian restaurant. Later that evening she had severe wheezing and shortness of breath. As she recounted these events we hit upon the possibility that paprika, which had been used in everything she had reactions to, either as an ingredient or a garnish, was the culprit!

One case was solved after an off-the-cuff comment made by the patient. She was describing the constancy of her asthma symptoms and commented that the only time she felt well during the last few months was during the Jewish holiday Passover. She followed the traditional customs of this holiday and by doing so, had in fact placed herself on a food elimination diet by avoiding a large number of the yeast products she was used to eating. She had discovered her hidden food allergy accidentally.

Another patient recalled that she always became more symptomatic after an evening out with her sister and brother-in-law because she would laugh too much. The more she laughed, the more she coughed. Later, on the way home, her wheezing would continue to worsen. When we discussed this further, she mentioned that the foursome often went out for Chinese food. As it turned out, it was the monosodium glutamate (MSG) in the food that caused her problem and not her laughter.

So it is important to carefully think about food and asthma. If you have come up with one or two strong suspicions, you will want to check them out by going on what I will call a simple elimination diet. First I'll outline the "simplest" elimination diet, which eliminates only one food. Then I'll outline a "simple" elimination diet, which eliminates two foods.

One interesting phenomenon I have noticed recently is that a small number of my patients who never suspected yeast as a problem (mostly the adult patients) have had great success on the simple yeast-free diet. Even if you haven't suspected yeast as a problem, you might want to try this before going on to anything more complicated.

THE SIMPLEST ELIMINATION DIET (ELIMINATING ONE FOOD)

This is the diet you are going to attempt if there is one food that you have decided to eliminate. If your suspect food is milk, wheat, corn, eggs, yeast, or salicylates, on one of the following pages (pages 80–133) you will find information about what foods to avoid, different names under which your eliminated food might be disguised, and a few sample meals to get you started. If your suspect food is not one of the common food allergens I have included, you can make up your own information page for your suspect food.

You must eliminate all forms of your forbidden food for your particular diet for ten days. I have tried to include as many of the common avoidance foods under each category as possible. This doesn't mean that you can't come up with some of your own entries. Don't stop with my list. Especially in this crucial time of testing, you might find additional things that you can eat or that you must avoid by asking questions, reading, and using your own common sense. For example, I have listed candy as a forbidden food for those on a salicylate-free diet since most candy has artificial coloring and flavoring. It doesn't mean that if you have found a totally natural, salicylate-free brand of candy that you shouldn't go ahead and enjoy yourself. What I am getting at is that my information chart is just a place to begin. You have to play detective on your own. And, of course, avoid all foods that you already know cause allergic reactions.

Once you have started on any one of the elimination diets, don't have even the smallest amount of the culprit food. If your aunt just baked your favorite sour cream coffee cake, and you are on a milk-free diet, freeze it until you have finished checking out your possible milk allergy. A taste might ruin the whole attempt to find out your hidden food allergy.

If after ten days you are feeling much better, then chances are you have struck it rich! Let your doctor know that you have improved. You then have to check your findings by trying the food you eliminated one more time. If after staying away from it for a while, you try it again and you become symptomatic, then you have found your problem. Sometimes, when you have avoided a problem food for a while, you might have a worse reaction than usual when you reintroduce it. Discuss this possibility with your doctor, and be sure to have appropriate medication available in case you need it. If the food you are going to eliminate contains an important nutrient, consult with your doctor for his advice on how to supplement this missing nutrient in your diet.

If after ten days you feel no different or if you are only slightly better, chances are you've guessed wrong. If you're still suspicious, try one more week, but you've probably eliminated the wrong food. Another possibility is that you have chosen only one of many problem foods and eliminating just one of them didn't do the trick. If you still feel certain that food is a problem, then go ahead to the multiple elimination diet. If you would rather avoid such a strict diet, you might try one week of a yeast-free diet (if yeast wasn't the original food you've already eliminated). Some patients have done well on yeast-free diets even when they never even considered yeast as a possible problem. At this point your options are: to give up the food idea (I think it would be a bit soon for that); go on a yeast-free diet for a week; or go directly to a multiple elimination diet.

SIMPLE ELIMINATION DIET (ELIMINATING TWO FOODS)

If you are attempting to eliminate two foods instead of one, you must be a bit more cautious in your plan. At first, you simply eliminate both foods for a week.

If after the week or ten days of being on the two-food simple elimination diet you are feeling significantly better, then you know that either one or maybe both of the foods you have been eliminating are your food allergens. If you tried to add both foods back into your diet simultaneously and you became symptomatic, you would not know which one had caused the problem. So, add back only one of the foods you have been eliminating. If after three days there is no reaction, then that particular food is not producing your allergic reaction. Then reintroduce the second food and see if a reaction occurs. If there is a reaction to the first food you reintroduced, then you know that you are allergic to that food. Stop eating it and wait until you are symptom-free (about three days, but maybe more). Then add the second food and see if you react to it. Remember, if you are reacting to a certain food, stop eating it immediately. Don't wait to see how sick you can get. Let reactions fade over a period of three days before adding anything else.

If there are no significant differences in your symptoms, then either you are not allergic to those foods or perhaps these two foods are only a few of the many that you are allergic to. At this point, you might discount the food connection entirely or go on to a bit more detective work. You have two choices. One, you could go on the multiple elimination diet for a week to ten days. This diet is a rigorous diet which eliminates many foods at once so that you would have a better chance of eliminating the culprit or culprits and discovering your hidden food allergies. The other choice is to try a yeast-free diet, as mentioned previously. So, you may either go on the yeast-free diet (found on pages 125–127) and then if it doesn't work, go on to a multiple elimination diet, or you may go directly to a multiple elimination diet. (It is more common for adults to have problems with yeast. So if you are dealing with a child and the simple elimination diet didn't work, I would go directly to the children's multiple elimination diet.)

Relief from food allergies is not subtle. It is dramatic. The patient improves remarkably. If after I ask, "Did you improve on the diet?" the patient has to think for a while, I know that it was not successful. Usually there is no doubt about the failure or success of the diet (as long as the patient has not cheated). While the process may have taken considerable time, effort, and sacrifice, the results will be very clear and well worthwhile.

We hope your hunches have been correct and you've managed to test and corroborate your hidden food allergy. Now on to the diets that will be used if either the simple elimination diets failed or if you never had any hunches to begin with.

Yeast

There has been much ado about the yeast-free diet. There are some who say it is a surefire cure for everything from warts to melanomas; and others who say that the whole thing is ridiculous because yeast is a normal inhabitant of the body, and except in rare individuals (those with severe forms of leukemia and other cancers), it couldn't possibly harm you. Yet we are faced with the puzzling fact that a small group of patients' symptoms are improved immeasurably when they are on a yeast-free diet. Who is right?

Based on my experience, I think too much can be made of the so-called yeast connection. I really doubt that yeast or candida could ever alter the course of most illnesses. I doubt in most people that it causes lethargy, symptoms of insanity, or most of the other things candida is imputed to do. But I do know that in a small group of patients, with asthma, hives, eczema, and sinus disease, remarkable changes occur when they are on the yeast-free diet.

Now, for the next surprise. I really don't think that patients who are helped by the yeast-free diet are overgrown by candida, or even are allergic to yeast. They certainly are not helped by taking antifungal agents such as nystatin, Mycostatin, or, even worse, ketoconazole. The latter drug can cause liver damage, so not only won't they be helped by this drug but they might instead be harmed.

What I think is happening is that the yeast-free diet eliminates many foods from that individual's normal diet, which in effect significantly limits his menu. In fact, the principle of the multiple elimination diet suggested in this book is very similar. I think that certain individuals are harmed by some foods that they ingest, and when many different foods are eliminated, this simplifies their diet, often eliminating the offending foods. When this happens, they feel better. I'm not sure if this has anything to do with allergy, but there is some harmful factor in some foods that causes a problem in some individuals.

We all know that certain foods make us feel miserable each

time we eat them. For example, after I eat bananas, I find myself getting more and more fatigued. This has nothing to do with allergy, but is probably related to some of the vasoactive substances that are in bananas. Foods are very complex and there are many substances in them that actually act as drugs. For example, certain poisonous mushrooms contain atropine, a substance which, if taken in large quantities, will cause cardiac arrhythmias, high temperature, dilated pupils, and in excessive amounts, could result in death. That, of course, is an extreme example of a food that could harm everyone who takes it. However, the substance in banana that makes me sleepy may not affect most other individuals adversely.

No one understands why some foodstuffs will harm certain individuals. I read an interesting article in the *New England Journal of Medicine* which may help explain some of the reasons. Eons ago our hunter-gatherer ancestors were not exactly faced with a wide variety of food. As a matter of fact, food was scarce, and if one counted all the different kinds of seeds, grains, and meats they could hunt or gather, perhaps they had twenty different kinds of food. Today there are thousands of varieties of food.

However, if I was placed back in time, in an area of the world where banana was a major food, I would not do too well. I never would be able to write this book, as I'd be asleep! Of course I couldn't hunt or gather food and I'd probably die. I certainly would not have an important place in society. My genes would not be passed on to future generations. The people in that self-enclosed area who could eat all of the foods without adverse effects would survive while those who couldn't tolerate the foodstuff in that area would die out. Thus, everyone surviving could eat all of the foods and would continue to have offspring who could eat all of the foods.

This was the way the world was for many centuries, and it is only recently that people have been able to emigrate all over the world, and foodstuff can be flown in from anywhere in the globe at any time. However, genetic changes take millennia to produce profound changes in our race; therefore, we may be prepared to eat only certain foods, but we are now faced with many foods which we may not be genetically prepared to cope with.

My ancestors were Lithuanian and Austrian. They didn't have bananas. They also didn't have tuna fish, but I have no problem with tuna fish. We can tolerate most of the foods to which we are exposed, but there are some foods with which we have difficulty. Some people have much more difficulty than others. Thus, when you go on a multiple elimination diet or a yeast-free diet, you may remove certain of the foods from your diet that bother you. If this is the case, you will feel well on the diet. However, most of the foods you eliminated are probably not bothersome to you, and you may find as you add foods back into your diet that some of those foods contain certain forms of yeast.

MULTIPLE ELIMINATION DIET (YOU HAVEN'T GOT A CLUE)

This diet is for the patient who has suspected food as a trigger for his or her asthma symptoms, but doesn't know where to begin. Maybe you tried a simple elimination diet in which you eliminated one or two foods, maybe you tried a yeast-free diet and you found no relief. At any rate, this diet is for the patient who is tired of guessing and is willing to bite the bullet and put food allergies to the final test.

HOW A MULTIPLE ELIMINATION DIET WORKS

The idea of a multiple elimination diet is to eliminate the usual food allergens (plus of course any other food which you might suspect) for ten days to see if your symptoms do noticeably decrease (I say noticeably because if in fact you do have food allergies, eliminating the offending allergens will make a significant difference, rather than a slight difference).

If after ten days of the multiple elimination diet, there is no difference in the severity of your symptoms, either you did not eliminate the right foods or food is just not a problem. You might very well give up the idea of food-related asthma symptoms or you might try an even stricter diet. Most patients will not attempt the stricter diet.

On the other hand, if after ten days on the multiple elimination diet, you do feel significantly better, then you know that some food or foods might be a problem for you. You will then try to find out which ones they are. After enjoying your better breathing for the ten days while you were on the multiple elimination diet, you will now want to add back foods methodically one at a time, to pinpoint which foods are causing you grief. In other words, if after you add back a food you are still well, you add another and another and another, until you hit the ''jackpot'' by finding the one or two foods causing major symptoms.

Now that you understand the basic idea behind the multiple elimination diet, you must know how to go on it. I will tell you what you may eat, and I will provide you with a suggested day-to-day menu to help you along the way. Since sometimes the hardest part of a special diet is having the allowed foods on hand, I will also provide you with a shopping list for one week's worth of food. Of course, this will not be the only possible list, but it might help some of you who are very busy and don't have the time or perhaps the inclination to do it yourself.

Once I have explained how to go on an elimination diet, I will explain the process of adding back the suspected foods.

Since children and adults do not totally coincide on the list of usual food allergens, and adults and children usually do not share similar likes in foods, I will recommend a multiple elimination diet for children and a slightly different one for adults.

THE MULTIPLE ELIMINATION DIET (CHILDREN'S VERSION)

The foods children most often react to are milk, wheat, chocolate, eggs, corn, and salicylates. Salicylates can be found naturally in some foods and can also be man-made chemicals. It is the man-made chemicals that you should avoid. These include such items as aspirin, aspirin compounds, artificial flavoring, and artificial coloring. Since salicylate-sensitive people usually react to yellow dye #5 (tartrazine) and the benzoates, I would avoid these also. I would further suggest avoiding culprits such as monosodium glutamate (MSG), metabisulfites (preservative used in dried fruits, on salad bars, and in red wines), too many spices (I would stick to salt, pepper, and garlic powder), and condiments loaded with additives. In other words, in addition to eliminating the basic foods I have mentioned, I would keep the rest of the diet as plain as possible.

Allowed Foods for Children's Multiple Elimination Diet

BEVERAGES
Spring water (glass bottles are preferable to plastic)
Seltzer (no artificial color)
Iced tea (made from all natural black tea)
Pure bottled or freshly squeezed juices
Soybean Milk (corn-free, check label)

FRUITS AND VEGETABLES
Fresh untreated not overripe fruits and vegetables (make sure these have not been sprayed with chemicals and wash all fruits and vegetables well).
Canned fruits and vegetables (no corn syrup, no additives and packed in its own juices, no sugar added).

GRAINS
Barley
Oat
Rice
Rice cakes (without wheat)
Rye

MEAT AND FISH
Fish (fresh or fresh-frozen)
Chicken
Turkey (fresh, no nitrites or preservatives or MSG)
Veal
Beef
Pork
Lamb

DESSERTS, SNACKS, AND SWEETS
Potato chips (in soybean or safflower oil)
Banana chips (no metabisulfites)
Coconuts (fresh)
Nuts (no preservatives or corn syrup)
Dried fruits (not treated with metabisulfites)
Cookies (milk-free, wheat-free, egg-free, and corn-free, color- and preservative-free)

FATS
Soy margarine
Kosher margarine (labeled pareve without artificial coloring)
Oil (soybean, safflower, and sunflower)
Egg-free mayonnaise

MISCELLANEOUS
Baking powder (cereal-free, sold in health food stores)
Potato flour
Potato meal
Vinegar (pure white or red—check that it doesn't contain metabisulfites)
Tapioca
Salt
Pepper
Soups (homemade)
Natural gelatin
Natural jelly
Baking soda (for brushing teeth, no toothpaste)

Shopping List for Children's Multiple Elimination Diet

Sometimes the hardest part of a diet is having the allowed foods available. What follows is a suggested shopping list for enough food for one child who will be following the multiple elimination diet for one week. Of course, depending upon your child's appetite, the amounts may vary.

BEVERAGES
1 gallon freshly squeezed or bottled fruit juice (orange, tomato, grapefruit, pineapple, cranberry, etc.)
1 gallon pure bottled water
1 quart natural club soda (seltzer)
Decaffeinated tea (not artificially colored or flavored)
2 quart bottles natural soda (Natural 90 soda is good)

FRUITS AND VEGETABLES
3 bananas
3 grapefruits
1 head lettuce
3 or 4 tomatoes
1 package soup greens (contains celery, carrots, parsnips)
1 bunch fresh dill
1 package carrots
5 lb bag white potatoes
2 sweet potatoes
1–2 green peppers
2 lb fresh vegetables (zucchini, string beans, broccoli, etc.)
2 apples
a few stalks of celery
2 or 3 lemons
2–3 oranges
melons (if in season)

Any fruit or vegetable the child likes best may be substituted for any of those on the above list.

MEAT OR FISH
2 whole chickens (quartered) plus extra backs (1 package)
2 chicken cutlets (breasts or thighs)
1 chicken breast
Lamb chops, veal chops, or pork chops
Natural turkey breast (no nitrites or preservatives)
Natural luncheon roast beef
1 lb chopped meat
½ lb flounder or sole

CANNED FOODS
2 cans tuna fish packed in water
2 cans fruit (packed in its own juice—no corn syrup or added sugar)
Baked beans (Health Valley, found in health food stores)
1 large can whole tomatoes (suggested brand: Health Valley)

GRAINS, CRACKERS, AND COOKIES
1 box cream of rice
2 packages rice cakes (no wheat)
1 package mini rice cakes
2 boxes cookies with no wheat, milk, corn, or eggs (suggested brand: Harvest Farm)
Quaker Oats oatmeal

2 boxes oat mix (available in health food stores)
1 box rice flour mix
Soy flour (available in health food stores)
1 box white or brown rice

FATS
Egg-free mayonnaise (Hain mayonnaise or homemade*—follow recipe)
Soy margarine (suggested brand: Willow Run)
Olive oil
Soybean, safflower, or sunflower oil

SNACKS AND MISCELLANEOUS
Cookies (Harvest Farm makes milk-free, wheat-free, corn-free, and egg-free natural cookies)
1 large bag potato chips
1 or 2 bags banana chips (no preservatives)
1 box raisins (check that these don't have metabisulfites)
1 bag natural peanuts
Natural instant soup (suggested brand: Miso-Cup; Edward & Sons)
Canned fruit (in its own juice—not corn syrup)
Salt, pepper, garlic powder
Natural applesauce (unsweetened or sweetened with sugar, but not corn syrup)
Natural gelatin (no colors)
Natural ices or sorbet
1 small jar natural peanut butter
1 jar natural jelly
Honey
White distilled vinegar
Baking soda

This list should cost about $80. This is initially expensive, but once you know which foods your child prefers, you can eliminate the ones he/she doesn't like. After the first week, you will also have a better idea of the accurate quantities you need. If you keep receipts of what you spend, you should be able to deduct special foods that are not part of your usual shopping from your taxes (check with your doctor and your accountant!)

Children's Seven-Day Suggested Menu Plan

What follows is a seven-day suggested menu. Every item which either requires an explanation of some sort or a recipe will have an asterisk next to it. Recipes appear at the end of the chapter.

DAY #1

Breakfast

Any juice (freshly squeezed or pure bottled)
Cream of rice (soy margarine and sugar)
Rice cake with natural jelly

Snack

Banana

Lunch

Tuna Fish Surprise*
Potato chips
Carrot sticks
Mini rice cakes

Snack

Cookies and juice

Dinner

Half a grapefruit
Salad with oil and vinegar dressing
Roast chicken (seasoned with salt, pepper, and garlic powder)
White rice
String beans

Bedtime Snack

Baked Apple*

DAY #2

Breakfast

Fruit juice (freshly squeezed or pure bottled)
Oatmeal (soy margarine and sugar)
Rice cake with natural jelly

Snack

Quartered orange (melon, if in season)

Lunch

Natural peanut butter and jelly sandwich (on oat bread made from mix or rice cakes)
Canned fruit (in its own juice, no corn syrup allowed)
Seltzer

Snack

Natural ices (summer) or natural instant soup (winter)

Dinner

Chicken Soup* (save the chicken for tomorrow's chicken salad)
Hamburger
Mashed potatoes (mashed with soy margarine*, salt, and pepper)
Cooked carrots (use fresh carrots)

Bedtime Snack

''Chocolate'' (really carob) cookies
Juice or tea

DAY #3

Breakfast

Banana Pancakes*
Fresh fruit salad

Snack

Tomato juice with a lemon slice (make it look pretty)

Lunch

Chicken Salad Surprise* (use chicken from yesterday's soup)
Potato chips
Carrot sticks

Snack

Natural gelatin

Dinner

Potato Soup*
Chicken Marengo*
Rice
Cooked zucchini

Snack

Cookies and juice

DAY #4

Breakfast

Fruit juice
Rice muffins (follow recipe on rice flour mix) and jelly
Applesauce

Snack

Nuts and raisin mix (use natural peanuts and raisins)

Lunch

Rolled up turkey or roast beef
Potato salad with egg-free mayonnaise or potato chips
Baked beans (Health Valley brand)

Snack

Canned fruit in its own juice

Dinner

Melon or half a grapefruit
Meatballs and Rice*
Cooked carrots

Snack

Cookies and juice

DAY #5

Breakfast

Fruit salad
Cream of rice
Mini rice cakes

Snack

Banana chips and juice

Lunch

Tuna fish salad with egg-free mayonnaise on oat bread
Natural ices (summer) or leftover chicken soup (winter)

Snack

Celery filled with *natural* peanut butter

Dinner

Salad with oil and vinegar
Lamb chops, veal chops, or pork chops
Baked potato
String beans

Snack

Cookies and juice

DAY #6

Breakfast

Fresh fruit juice
Oatmeal (with soy margarine* and sugar)
Applesauce

Snack

G.O.R.P. (Good Ole' Raisins and Peanuts) or tomato juice with lemon

Lunch

Turkey sandwich on oat bread or rice cake (use egg-free mayonnaise)
Natural gelatin with drained canned peaches

Snack

Potato chips

Dinner

Half a grapefruit
Hamburger
Sweet potato
Broccoli

Bedtime Snack

Cookies and juice

DAY #7

Breakfast

Quartered oranges
Applesauce pancakes (top oat mix pancakes with applesauce)
Natural decaffeinated iced tea

Snack

Banana chips

Lunch

Natural peanut butter and jelly on oat bread or rice cakes
Fruit juice

Snack

Fruit salad

Dinner

Tomato juice with lemon slice
Baked or broiled flounder or sole
Candied Sweet Potatoes*
Zucchini

Snack

Cookies and juice

ADULT ELIMINATION DIET

In addition to some of the allergens which are common to many children, adults are often allergic to yeast products. Therefore, for the adult going on a multiple elimination diet, I have excluded yeast and foods containing yeast, as well as those foods eliminated from the children's diet. The following list contains the foods that the adult is allowed to eat.

Allowed Foods

BEVERAGES

Spring water (bottled)
Seltzer (no artificial coloring)
Coffee (not instant or cleared with eggs)
Freshly squeezed or pure bottled juice
Soybean milk (corn-free, check label)

FRUITS AND VEGETABLES

Fresh untreated fruits (no preservatives; wash well)
Fresh untreated vegetables (EXCEPT mushrooms; no preservatives)
Fruits and vegetables (canned, no corn syrup sweetening)

GRAINS

Barley
Oat
Rice
Rice cakes (without wheat)
Rye

MEAT AND FISH

Fresh fish
Chicken
Turkey (fresh, no nitrites, preservatives, or MSG)
Veal
Beef
Pork
Lamb

DESSERTS, SNACKS, AND SWEETS
Potato chips (soybean, safflower or sunflower oil)
Coconuts (fresh)
Nuts (no preservatives or corn syrup)
Natural gelatin
Cookies (special brands without milk, eggs, corn, wheat, or color)

FATS
Soy margarine
Kosher margarine (labeled pareve without artificial coloring)
Oil (soybean, safflower, and sunflower)
Homemade mayonnaise (without egg and vinegar—see recipe)

MISCELLANEOUS
Baking powder (cereal-free, sold in health food stores)
Potato flour
Potato meal
Honey
Natural jelly
Sugar
Salt
Pepper
Homemade soups
Tapioca
Baking soda and salt (for brushing teeth, no toothpaste)

Shopping List for Adult's Multiple Elimination Diet

The following is a suggested shopping list which should provide you with enough food for the first week of the multiple elimination diet (if you are following the recommended daily menu plan which follows). Needless to say, you can make up your own menus and your own list if you have the time. If you have trouble finding any of the items in the grocery store, try a health food store.

BEVERAGES
1 gallon freshly squeezed or bottled fruit juice
1 gallon pure bottled water
1–2 quarts natural club soda or regular soda (Natural 90 is a good brand)
Coffee (if it is decaffeinated, make sure that the decaffeinating process does not involve chemicals)

FRUITS AND VEGETABLES (not overripe)
2 grapefruits
3 bananas
3 apples
3 oranges
2 lemons
1 melon (if in season)
1 pint strawberries (if in season)
2 sweet potatoes
1 5 lb bag potatoes
1 head lettuce
4 tomatoes
½ lb string beans
½ lb zucchini
1 bag carrots
1 stalk celery
1 package soup greens
1 bunch fresh dill

CEREALS, GRAINS, AND BREADS
Oatmeal (no flavors or additives)
Cream of rice (no flavors or additives)
Barley
Rice cakes (2 packages—check that these do not contain any corn or wheat)
Oat mix—you can make oat bread, oat muffins, or pancakes (if you like these, you can buy 2 packages, if you don't like these, buy extra rice cakes)
1 box white or brown rice
Soy flour

CANNED FOODS
1 can tuna fish in water
1 can sweet potatoes (not in corn syrup)
1 large can whole tomatoes

MEATS AND FISH
1 lb chopped meat
½ lb filet of sole
½ lb filet of flounder
½ lb turkey breast
½ lb sliced roast beef
2 lamb chops or veal chops
2–3 chicken cutlets
2 whole chickens quartered plus one package extra backs

FATS
Soy margarine (Willow Run is good)
Oil (sunflower, safflower, soybean)

SNACKS AND MISCELLANEOUS
1 box cookies (Harvest Farm or Barbara's—READ LABELS)
Natural ices or natural sorbet
1 box raisins (no metabisulfites)
1 package peanuts (no additives)
Potato chips (soybean or safflower oil)
Banana chips
Instant soup (Miso-Cup; Edward & Sons)
Natural applesauce (unsweetened)
Honey
1 jar natural jelly
Egg substitutes

The following is a seven-day, day-by-day menu for an adult to follow. An asterisk appears next to the courses for which I offer a recipe (that may be found at the end of the chapter). Beverages may be chosen from the allowed list of beverages above.

DAY #1

Breakfast
Half a grapefruit
Cream of rice (add soy margarine, salt, and sugar)
Rice cake with jelly

Snack
Tomato juice

Lunch
Tuna Fish Surprise*
2 rice cakes
Beverage

Snack
Banana

Dinner
Salad with oil and lemon
Roast chicken (season with salt, pepper, and garlic powder)
Baked potato with margarine
Carrots
Beverage

Snack
Cookies and juice

DAY #2

Breakfast
Orange juice (bottled or freshly squeezed)
Oatmeal (soy margarine, salt, and sugar)
Rice cakes

Snack
Baked Apple*

Lunch
Melon
Turkey breast on rice cakes
Potato chips
Carrot and celery sticks

Snack
Instant soup or a piece of fruit

Dinner
Potato Soup*
Broiled filet of sole
Rice
String beans
Beverage

Snack
Fresh fruit salad

DAY #3

Breakfast
Quartered orange
Oat muffins with jelly

Snack
Tomato juice with lemon

Lunch
Roast beef, lettuce, and tomato sandwich on rice cakes
Natural soda

Snack
Fresh fruit cup

Dinner
Chicken Soup*
Chicken Marengo on Rice* (save some sauce for Day #5 Lunch)
Beverage

Snack
Cookies and juice

DAY #4

Breakfast
Cranberry juice
Cream of rice (soy margarine, salt, and sugar)
Rice cakes with jelly

Snack
Orange

Lunch
Tomato juice
Chicken salad sandwich (use last night's chicken from soup on rice cakes and homemade mayonnaise*)
Carrot and celery sticks
Potato chips

Snack

G.O.R.P.* (Good Ole' Raisins and Peanuts)

Dinner

Half a grapefruit
Hamburger
Candied Sweet Potatoes a la Shirl*
Steamed zucchini
Beverage

Snack

Frozen honey-nut banana*

DAY #5

Breakfast

Apple slices
Oatmeal (soy margarine*, salt, and sugar)
Rice cakes

Snack

Banana chips or celery with peanut butter

Lunch

Fresh fruit salad
Rice with Chicken Marengo Sauce (left over from Day #3)

Snack

Cookies and juice

Dinner

Half a grapefruit
Broiled filet of sole
Baked white potato with margarine
Peas
Beverage

Snack

Sorbet or natural ices

DAY #6

Breakfast
Grapefruit juice
Oat muffins with jelly

Snack
G.O.R.P. (Good Ole' Raisins and Peanuts)

Lunch
Instant soup (natural)
Tuna Surprise*
Celery and carrot sticks
Baked Apple*

Snack
Potato chips

Dinner
Salad with oil and lemon
Veal or lamb chops
Baked potato
Steamed carrots
Beverage

Snack
Cookies and juice

DAY #7

Breakfast
Pineapple juice
Banana Pancakes with Honey*

Snack
Any fresh fruit

Lunch
Tomato juice
Turkey, lettuce, and tomato sandwich (on rice cakes or oat bread)

Snack

Celery sticks with peanut butter

Dinner

Salad with oil and lemon
Meatballs and Rice*
Zucchini
Beverage

HOW TO ADD BACK FOODS ON A MULTIPLE ELIMINATION DIET

Once you have survived this first week or ten days, you have made it through the worst part. You now must evaluate your symptoms. As I have already mentioned, if an improvement has occurred, it should not be a slight one. If you have improved considerably, then you are ready to start adding back foods. But if you are still a bit symptomatic, you may want to stay on the elimination diet for another few days or even for another week. There are individual differences as to how long the ill effects of allergens last.

Before you begin the adding back process, you should contact your physician to let him know. You will want to be clear on what he would want you to do about medications and contacting him if you react to a food that you add back. Sometimes when one has not had a food allergen for a while, the reaction that occurs is a bit more severe than when the food was being eaten continuously.

Since milk is an important source of nutrition and because it is found in so many foods, you might want to start by adding back milk and milk products in their PURE form. Many milk products have artificial coloring and even preservatives. (The FDA does not require a listing of all ingredients on dairy products, and so you should be cautious that you have not added milk with coloring or preservatives). I would add foods such as whole milk, natural, uncolored, and unprocessed cheese, and pure butter. (I have found that Land O Lakes butter is one of the purest and, if you'll notice, the palest, indicating no coloring is used.) Heavy cream or sour cream might have other ingredients that would cause a problem, and so if you did react, you would not know what caused the reaction. The idea is to conduct as controlled an experiment as possible. Welcome to the world of scientific experimentation! Eat large enough quantities of the food so that you can test the true effects. If you don't have a reaction to milk within three or four days, then assume that it is a safe food and continue having it. You will then be ready to add back the next food. If you did react to milk, check it off as a probable allergen and stop eating it. Totally eliminate milk and milk products from your diet. You cannot proceed to the next food until your symptoms are under control. Don't rush this process because you might confuse the results of the reaction to the next food you will be adding.

To repeat, either you had no reaction to milk or you have waited a sufficient amount of time for the reaction to subside. Either way, you are now ready to continue the adding back process. Probably, wheat should be added back next.

In adding wheat, make sure that it is in the pure form, such as cream of wheat or wheat flour. If you are dealing with a child who is allowed yeast, you could add bread if the child did not react to milk and the bread has milk, or you can add bread if the child was allergic to milk, but the bread has no milk in it. Read the labels on the bread and make sure that there are no other forbidden ingredients. If you are an adult, adding back wheat must be kept separate from adding back yeast. Be sure that you make the distinction. Once again, if your symptoms stay the same, then wheat is not a problem food for you. If you did react, stop eating wheat, check it off as a probable allergen, and wait until you are feeling as well as you were prior to eating wheat before you add back the next food.

Continue adding back each food you originally eliminated, making sure that you never proceed until you are as good as you were before you began the adding back process. Depending on how many foods you reacted to and how long your individual reaction period is, this process could take several weeks.

You might be thinking "I'll never be able to do this" or "I'll never get my eight-year-old to do this.'' You'd be surprised at how easy it will become to avoid some foods if all of a sudden you are breathing better than you ever had before. If you are dealing with a child, explain everything to him ahead of time. Make it a game. Tell him that even though there are many things that he will not be able to eat for a while, he is going to be eating some new things that he never ate before. Let him help you with some of the preparation, and if he is old enough to read, give him some recipe books to look through. If you tell someone else in front of him, ''Poor Johnny has to go on this disgusting diet which I don't even think will make a difference,'' you can't expect a whole lot of enthusiasm from the child. If, on the other hand, you say, ''This is going to be an exciting and somewhat weird week. Johnny is going to eat lots of new foods. We're going to take to the kitchen, try new recipes, and hopefully he will feel a lot better,'' you can expect that your optimism will rub off. Your attitude and encouragement can often make the whole difference. Don't try to change your child's entire diet and think that you can keep it a secret. Even a one- or two-year-old will know that something is different.

For the adults, try to avoid having a dinner party at this time. It's hard to serve vichyssoise, chicken kiev, and mousse au chocolat to guests while you're eating cream of rice and oat bread. If you can't avoid these situations, just keep your sense of humor and know that you are doing something that may be very important for you. Make sure you continue to keep your doctor informed and call him if you have any questions or certainly if you have any serious reactions.

NATURAL MEDICATIONS

Many over-the-counter drugs and most prescription drugs have artificial colors and flavors. Besides the patients who know that they are allergic to artificial ingredients, I feel that all asthmatics should try to avoid the colored and flavored medications whenever possible. Before taking over-the-counter medications, make sure you check the ingredients, just as you do when buying any food product. Make sure that all of your doctors are aware that you would like natural medication. Ask the physician to prescribe a medication that is not colored or flavored. Your pharmacist can help you select brands. Even when you're at the dentist's office, ask the hygienist to use some other cleansing agent besides toothpaste, which is filled with artificial ingredients. Don't be embarrassed to speak up!

Alcohol

Many people think they are allergic to alcohol. It is true that everyone will have an adverse effect to alcohol if they drink enough of it, but there are many people who will have difficulty even with small amounts of alcohol. Alcoholic beverages are extremely complex mixtures of chemical substances. For example, red wine contains many irritating constituents. In addition, histamine exists naturally in some red wine. A preservative used in red wine, especially younger wines and Beaujolais Nouveau, is metabisulfite. Metabisulfites can have a devastating effect on some asthmatics.

Ethyl alcohol is a powerful drug. It is a very strong vasodilator (causes blood flow to increase) and can nonspecifically cause asthma and sinus problems. People with a tendency toward sinus disease and/or asthma very often have attacks after drinking. These attacks may not be the result of an allergy to alcohol but to this same biochemical effect.

Skin testing will not elucidate who will have trouble with alcohol. If we drink, it should all be in moderation, but certainly asthmatics and allergic people in general should be very careful when they drink. If you find that alcohol triggers an asthmatic attack, don't drink. Nobody can give you a shot or neutralize your body to alcohol. Some asthmatics can drink hard liquor and not wine, rarely vice versa. It may pay to experiment in order to find the appropriate substance that you can drink. Remember if you drink, don't drive, and be sure to find out whether or not it is safe to combine alcohol in your body with your medications.

Vitamins

I'm a very strong believer in the scientific method. I will on some occasions give you opinions in this book based on my experience, and when I do so I will tell you that I am giving you my opinion. Almost everything in this book is based on scientific fact, fact carefully developed by allergy scientists over many years using very carefully controlled studies. Why have I chosen this point in the book to give a lecture on the scientific method? Because the scientific method was used to establish the dose and the need for certain key coenzymes, very vital to the body, known as vitamins. There is a myth that has developed around vitamins, that in large doses they are miracle drugs against everything. I disagree with this. Since many of my patients may be on a diet or have health problems, I recommend that they have a good balanced diet, or as balanced a diet as possible, and take normal doses of multivitamins, not mega doses of vitamins. As this book goes to press there is no good study that demonstrates that using vitamins in anything that exceeds the recommended doses is good for asthma. In summary, save your money. Have a good balanced diet and, if need be, supplement that diet with prescribed normal doses of vitamins.

ASTHMATICS BEWARE

It should certainly be clear at this point that each asthmatic is unique and that for each food-sensitive asthmatic there is a unique list of problem foods which he must avoid. However, there are a few substances which have received media attention lately since they have become notorious troublemakers for many asthma sufferers. Some of these substances have caused very severe reactions and sometimes deaths. These substances are (1) monosodium glutamate, MSG, often used in Chinese and kosher cooking and as a seasoning and preservative in many prepared foods; (2) aspartame, the artificial sweetener known as Nutrasweet, found in a multitude of diet beverages and diet foods; (3) aspirin and aspirin-containing medications (Anacin, Fiorinal). Some medications, which are aspirin related, are commonly prescribed for problems with arthritis or gastrointestinal disorders. Among these are Advil, Motrin, Alka-Seltzer, Indocin, Naprosyn, Butazolidin, Tolectin, etc. These are called nonsteroidal anti-inflammatory drugs, or NSAID; (4) metabisulfite. Metabisulfites and other sulfiting agents can often be found in the following foods:

Avocado dip and guacamole
Beer
Cider
Cod (dried)
Cooking sherry
Fruit (cut-up fresh or dried)
Fruit juices, purees, and fillings
Gelatin
Potatoes (cut-up fresh, frozen, dried, or canned)
Salad dressing (dry mix)
Salad bar salads
Sauces and gravies
Sauerkraut and cole slaw
Shellfish (fresh, frozen, canned, or dried clams)
Soups
Vegetables (cut-up fresh, frozen, canned, or dried)
Wine vinegar
Wine, wine coolers

It's not always known if the reactions to these substances are food intolerances or food allergies, but there are often devastating effects. It would be best, whenever possible, for the asthma sufferer to avoid these culprits. If it is important to you to have any of these, it would be wise to consult with your physician and arrange for some way to test your sensitivity (this could either be a challenge test done in the office or perhaps a bit of experimenting on your own *under your physician's supervision,* by eating the foods in small quantities and taking note of any possible ill effects). In general, it would be best to avoid these whenever possible, especially when you are on special elimination diets and you are trying not to confuse your results.

Eliminating Foods: A Guide to Survival

While we may have reached the initial goal of finding the hidden allergy, we now have the ultimate goal of living without the food or foods so that symptoms will continue to be reduced or eliminated. Your initial ecstasy at pinpointing the culprit might be short-lived when you realize what you may have to do without for the rest of your life. While your doctor may be patting you on the back, you may be lamenting a life without chocolate chip cookies. Much of your work lies ahead. Let me offer some survival guides.

It is not easy to deprive yourself, nor is it easy to cope with asthma. You must make a total commitment to stay on the food avoidance or elimination diet. The stakes are very high and success is completely under your control. Assuming that you are totally committed, here are some suggestions.

1. Expect frustration at the beginning of your diet. Feelings of deprivation, hostility, anger, and probably hunger can be expected too. If you are the parent of a child who must do without many of his favorite foods, you might expect some hard times in the beginning. If you are dealing with a child, it would be a good idea to explain that the diet is designed to help him feel better; this may lessen his feelings of hostility. Don't be wishy-washy with the child and promise him that he can eat the food that he's allergic to once in a while. You are not sure of this. The idea is to be firm but understanding and loving. Combining these two is not always an easy job.
2. Treat yourself well! When you know what you cannot have, stock up on what you can have. Spend a little extra if you have to. Since the diet forces you to deprive yourself, it is a good idea to pamper yourself in other ways. If you have done without chocolate bars only because they contain artificial flavors, how about a box of all natural expensive chocolates once in a while?

3. Educate yourself! Learn everything you can about the food you are avoiding. Did you know that yeast is found in many vitamins and that mustard is in mayonnaise? Learn the brands that you can have. Learn the names your food can be called; for instance, tartrazine is yellow dye #5; vanillin, which sounds like vanilla, is an artificial flavor, not a natural extract. Learn to read labels carefully and skeptically. Small amounts of one ingredient are not always required to be listed. Watch out for collective terms such as spices and natural flavors. You cannot be sure which spice or which flavor you are eating. When you order 7 Up that has no artificial ingredients, you can and may often easily be served similar drinks which do. General terms can be a problem. Don't be misled into thinking that all healthy foods are natural foods. If artificial coloring is a problem for you, and if your physician is writing a prescription for you, remind him that you must have uncolored medication. These are not always easy to find. I have some patients who have to empty the contents of some capsules into clear capsules. Your pharmacist can be helpful too. Vitamins and prescription medications are often artificially colored.
4. Be aggressive! Wherever you are, you have the right to ask about the food that you are eating or buying. When you go to a restaurant, ask the waitress about the ingredients before you order. If she doesn't know, ask for the manager or chef. You will find that most people are very eager to help. If no one knows the ingredients or if you do not have faith in the answers you have gotten, do not eat. The consequences are too great. If you are invited to a dinner party at someone's home, call ahead of time, explain your problem, and inquire about the menu. In a supermarket, ask about their meat, fish, and produce. Some meats may be colored and some fruits may be sprayed with metabisulfite or other preservatives. If you are not sure about the ingredients in a product, and if you're worried that you might react to it, call the company

and make some inquiries. If you are invited to a wedding, call the caterer ahead of time and find out what will be served. If you find yourself in any of these situations, remember to remain diplomatic. Don't say, "Your product almost killed me. What is in it?" For sure you will not get the whole story. Rather say, "My family always enjoys your product, but I have some allergies and I need some information." For the caterers at a wedding, call at a time when they are not likely to be busy. Know when you are licked. Sometimes you might not be able to get all of the information you would like. Try again at another time.

5. Be prepared! If you know you are not going to be able to eat as much as everyone else, be prepared by either eating something beforehand, or by bringing along something you can nibble on. If you cannot have prepared salad dressings, bring a little of your own. If this will be inappropriate, prepare yourself psychologically to be hungry.
6. Stick to your guns. Don't be pressured into cheating!
7. Don't let down your guard! One case study illustrates this point very well. One patient who is allergic to MSG frequented a local delicatessen and always ordered their brisket, which the manager said contained no MSG. One evening after her usual meal, she became very symptomatic. When she called the restaurant, the manager was embarrassed and apologetic and explained that their new cook had changed the recipe to include MSG. The patient should not have let her guard down.

   Constant caution is needed for another reason. Not only can recipes change, but your body's sensitivities can also change. It is possible to develop new food allergies or intolerances and if you suspect this, you must check it out. If you become more symptomatic, even though you have stayed on the same diet for a while, perhaps a week-long elimination diet might set you straight again.
8. Spread the word! Particularly in the case of children, everyone must be made aware of the child's food restrictions. This includes teachers, coaches, aunts, uncles, grand-

parents, and friends and their parents. Be very specific. Give brand names that are allowed whenever possible, saying, ''My child is on a natural diet,'' is not enough. Many brands proudly advertise that one of the ingredients is natural, whereas the other ingredients might be artificial. Give exact brand names and make it easier for everyone. Make sure special arrangements are made for your child at school parties and at birthday parties.

9. Consider a rotation diet. Some patients, who might not be able to tolerate certain foods in large amounts eaten frequently, do well when the food is eaten every fourth day (at most). What is happening is that there isn't enough of a food buildup to cause an allergic reaction. On a rotation diet, the patient does not feel totally deprived. He can have his favorite foods as long as he does not ''pig out'' day after day. This diet does not work for everyone and certainly not for someone who reacts to a certain food no matter how infrequently he eats it. Ask your doctor about a rotating plan. If you are food-sensitive, it is not a good idea to overeat any one food. Play safe!
10. Pick a vacation spot that gives you some flexibility. If you have many food allergies, think twice before going on a vacation to a country where they speak another language. Either change your plans or learn how to say ''Hold the tomato'' in Italian.
11. Remember that extra expenses for special health-related diets as prescribed by a doctor can be a tax deduction. Save your receipts from the health food store.
12. Always bring enough medications, just in case there is a slipup.

This text, when used in conjunction with the food elimination diet, offers you a wealth of information. You and your doctor can formulate a plan tailored to suit your needs. Dietary management of food allergies can be quite demanding, but it's vital for your health.

The diet plans are set up for you to be able to ''do it yourself.''

However, only your doctor knows your state of health and state of nutrition. Review all of your treatment and diet plans with him.

Milk-Free Diet

OTHER NAMES FOR MILK
whey
milk and nonfat milk solids
casein
caseinate

DO NOT EAT THE FOLLOWING FOODS:

BEVERAGES
milk
cream
shakes
malteds
any beverage made with milk or milk products

FRUITS AND VEGETABLES
Vegetables prepared in cream or butter

CEREALS AND BREADS
Cereal (cold with milk or cooked with milk)
Many breads, crackers, and baked goods

MEAT, EGGS, FISH, AND CHEESE
All cheese
Some luncheon meats
Eggs (prepared with milk or butter)

DESSERTS, SNACKS, AND SWEETS
Many cookies
Most chocolates
Ice cream
Sherbert
Custards
Puddings

FATS
Butter

MISCELLANEOUS
Creamed soups
Sauces (made with milk, cream, or butter)

SAMPLE MENUS

SAMPLE #1

Breakfast
Juice
Oatmeal with margarine
Graham crackers

Snack
Apple

Lunch
Tuna fish salad sandwich on bagel
Potato chips
Carrot sticks
Iced tea

Snack
V-8 and milk-free cookies (read the label)

Dinner
Salad with oil and vinegar dressing
Hamburger or steak
Baked potato with margarine
Carrots with margarine or honey

Snack
Natural ices or sorbet
Juice

SAMPLE #2

Breakfast

Half a grapefruit
Two eggs any style in margarine
2 rice cakes with jelly

Snack

Banana

Lunch

Tomato juice
Turkey sandwich on pita bread
Soda or iced tea

Snack

Popcorn

Dinner

Salad with oil and vinegar dressing
Roast chicken
Spaghetti with cheeseless tomato sauce
String beans with margarine
Coffee, tea, or soda

Snack

Milk-free angel food cake
Coffee, tea, or juice

Wheat-Free Diet

OTHER NAMES FOR WHEAT
Flour (wheat and gluten)
Semolina
Durum
Bran
Farina

DO NOT EAT THE FOLLOWING FOODS:

BEVERAGES
Postum
Malt
Beer

FRUITS AND VEGETABLES
Any fruits or vegetables prepared with breading or in a sauce with flour as a thickener

CEREALS AND BREADS
Many cereals
Most breads
Many crackers
Most baked goods

MEAT, EGGS, FISH, AND CHEESE
Meat loaf (with bread crumbs)
Breaded cutlets
Luncheon meats
Some hamburgers
Some meatballs

DESSERTS, SNACKS, AND SWEETS
Most cakes and cookies
Donuts
Some chocolates
Some cheesecakes

FATS
No restrictions

MISCELLANEOUS
Many soups
Many sauces

SAMPLE MENUS

SAMPLE #1

Breakfast

Juice
Oatmeal with butter
Rice cakes with jelly

Snack

Orange

Lunch

Tuna Fish Surprise*
Potato chips
Coffee, tea, or juice

Snack

Wheat-free cookies (health food stores will have these)
Juice

Dinner

Half a grapefruit
Roast chicken
Baked potato with butter or margarine
Zucchini

Snack

Ice cream

SAMPLE #2

Breakfast

Juice
2 eggs in butter or margarine
2 rice cakes with jelly

Snack

Banana

Lunch

Large fresh fruit salad
Coffee, tea, or juice

Snack

Wheat-free cookies and juice

Dinner

Potato Soup*
Broiled flounder
Rice
String beans with almonds
Beverage

Snack

Cheese Cake*
Coffee or tea

Corn-Free Diet

OTHER NAMES FOR CORN
Syrup (usually means corn syrup)
Sorbitol (usually made from corn)
Dextrose
Glucose
Whiskey
Bourbon
Baking powder (usually made with cornstarch)

DO NOT EAT THE FOLLOWING FOODS:

BEVERAGES
Many carbonated beverages
Some soybean milk
Sweetened fruit juices
Instant tea or coffee
Beer
Gin

Instant formulas
Any beverage in waxed cartons

FRUITS AND VEGETABLES
Corn
Canned and frozen fruit with sweeteners
Vegetables in waxed containers
Succotash
Hominy
Candied fruits

CEREALS AND BREADS
Most presweetened cereals and commercial breads
Graham crackers
Hominy grits
Corn flakes
Pancake mixes
Anything baked on a surface sprinkled with corn (pizza dough)

MEAT, EGGS, FISH, AND CHEESE
Luncheon meats
Hot dogs
Some fish (canned and packed in corn oil)

DESSERTS, SNACKS, AND SWEETS
Ices
Many ice creams
Gelatin desserts
Many candies
Brown sugar
Cake mixes
Anything with baking powder (many cakes)

FATS
Corn oil and foods fried in corn oil

MISCELLANEOUS
Jams
Jellies
Dressings with corn oil
Some peanut butters
Some aspirins

Capsules
Some vitamins
Monosodium glutamate (MSG)
Adhesives (don't lick envelopes or stamps)

SAMPLE MENUS

SAMPLE #1

Breakfast

Bottled or freshly squeezed fruit juice
Cream of rice
Toast with butter or margarine

Snack

Banana

Lunch

Half a grapefruit
Tuna fish salad sandwich on bread (make sure it has no corn)
Brewed coffee, tea, or juice

Snack

Tomato juice
Cookies without corn or baking powder (read the label)

Dinner

Salad with oil and vinegar dressing (don't use corn oil)
Chicken cutlets fried in soybean oil or olive oil
Linguini with tomato sauce (sauce must not have corn sweeteners)
String beans
Beverage

Snack

Ice cream without corn sweeteners (many of the better brands do not contain sweeteners)

SAMPLE #2

Breakfast
Melon (if in season) or an orange
2 eggs (any style)
Bagel with butter or margarine

Snack
Cup of tomato juice (pure and bottled)

Lunch
Cottage cheese and lots of fresh fruit
Carr's TableWater Crackers

Snack
Cookies (without corn)
Coffee, tea, or juice

Dinner
Salad with oil and vinegar dressing (don't use corn oil)
Roast beef seasoned with salt and pepper
Baked potato with margarine or butter
Carrots
Beverage

Snack
Baked apple

Egg-Free Diet

OTHER NAMES FOR EGG
Albumin (processed or dried)
Meringue

DO NOT EAT THE FOLLOWING FOODS:

BEVERAGES
Eggnogs
Egg creams
Malteds

Root beer
Some coffee (cleared with eggs)

FRUITS AND VEGETABLES
Souffles
Quiche
Fritters

CEREALS AND BREADS
Breads (made with egg or brushed with egg white)
Egg noodles
Pancakes
Waffles
French toast
Breaded foods (first dipped in egg)
Some pasta

MEAT, EGGS, FISH, OR CHEESE
Eggs (fresh or powdered)
Meat loaf
Meatballs
Any meat mixtures
Croquettes
Sausage
Cutlets

DESSERTS, SNACKS, AND SWEETS
Meringues
Cream pies
Custards
Icings
Many baked goods
Some candies
Pretzels
French ice cream

FATS
No restrictions

MISCELLANEOUS
Mayonnaise (unless it is egg-free)
Sauces (tartar and hollandaise)
Some soups

SAMPLE MENUS

SAMPLE #1

Breakfast

Half a grapefruit
Cereal and milk
Toast (bread without egg) and jelly

Snack

Banana

Lunch

Tuna salad sandwich on bread (tuna must be made with egg-free mayonnaise which can be bought in most health food stores)
Carrot sticks
Juice or soda

Snack

Popcorn

Dinner

Salad with oil and vinegar dressing
Roast chicken
Sweet potato
Zucchini

Snack

Ice cream (check label for egg)

SAMPLE #2

Breakfast

Orange juice
Oatmeal with margarine or butter
Toast and jelly

Snack

Tomato juice

Lunch

Half a grapefruit
Turkey breast sandwich
Potato chips
Coffee, tea, or soda

Snack

Baked apple

Dinner

Potato Soup*
Broiled flounder (with lemon and butter)
Rice
String beans
Coffee, tea, or soda

Snack

Apple pie (check that crust hasn't been brushed with egg)

Salicylate-Free Diet

OTHER NAMES FOR SALICYLATES

Aspirin
Tartrazine
Yellow Dye #5
Artificial color
Artificial flavor
Flavor enhancers
Antioxidants

DO NOT EAT THE FOLLOWING FOODS:

BEVERAGES

Most soft drinks (7-Up is okay)
Tea mixes
Wine
Diet drinks
Beer

Birch beer
Gin
Distilled beverages (except vodka)

FRUITS AND VEGETABLES
Some frozen fruit and vegetables which contain coloring (the ingredients do not have to list coloring)
Frozen french fries
Fast food french fries
Fruit toppings (artificially colored)

CEREALS AND BREADS
Cake mixes
Colored cereals
Cereals with preservatives (BHA and BHT)
Most whole wheat breads
Breads with additives

MEATS, EGGS, FISH, AND CHEESE
Luncheon meats (with nitrites)
Hot dogs
Meat prepared with tenderizers
Cheese (processed and colored)
Some frozen fish

DESSERTS, SNACKS, AND SWEETS
Jell-O
Some cakes and cookies (with artificial ingredients)
Gum

SAMPLE MENUS

SAMPLE #1

Breakfast
Half a grapefruit
Oatmeal
Toast (check bread) with natural jelly

Snack

Celery with natural peanut butter

Lunch

Tossed salad with oil and vinegar dressing (you can easily make your own—if you use bottled, check the label)
Turkey sandwich (use naturally prepared turkey on natural bread)
Coffee, or tea, or natural juice

Snack

Popcorn

Dinner

Chicken Soup*
Roast beef
Baked potato
String beans
Natural 90 soda

Snack

Breyers ice cream

SAMPLE #2

Breakfast

Pineapple juice
Pancakes (made from Hungry Jack Pancake Mix)
Natural pancake syrup

Snack

Tomato juice and natural crackers

Lunch

Half a grapefruit
Hamburger
Plain potato chips (not barbecued or flavored)
Carrot sticks

Snack
Orange

Dinner
Tossed salad with natural dressing
Broiled flounder
Rice (no additives)
Cooked carrots
Natural 90 soda

Snack
Pepperidge Farm cookies

Yeast-Free Diet

OTHER NAMES FOR YEAST
Leavening

DO NOT EAT THE FOLLOWING FOODS:

BEVERAGES
Malt drinks
Milk fortified with vitamins
Ginger ale
Root beer
Black tea
Wine
Whiskey
Vodka
Rum
Buttermilk
Frozen and canned juices

FRUITS AND VEGETABLES
Dried fruits (prunes, raisins, etc.)
Mushrooms
Chili peppers
Tomato sauce

CEREALS AND BREADS
Breads
Many cereals (those with malt or fortified with thiamine, niacin, and riboflavin)

Most crackers
Pasta
Farina

MEATS, EGGS, FISH, AND CHEESE
Cheeses
Sausage

DESSERTS, SNACKS, AND SWEETS
Cookies
Cakes
Pretzels
Candy with malt

FATS
Mayonnaise
Sour cream

MISCELLANEOUS
Soy sauce
Sauerkraut
Vinegar
Dressings
Catsup
Pickles
Horseradish
Many vitamins and medications

SAMPLE MENUS

SAMPLE #1

Breakfast
Half a grapefruit
Cream of rice with butter
Rice cakes with jelly

Snack
Apple

Lunch

Turkey and roast beef slices
Rice cakes
Carrot sticks
Coffee or club soda

Snack

Popcorn

Dinner

Lettuce and tomato salad (oil and lemon dressing)
Roast chicken
Baked white potato
String beans
Coffee or soda

Snack

Natural ice cream

SAMPLE #2

Breakfast

Freshly squeezed orange juice
2 eggs, (any style)
Rice cakes with jelly

Snack

Banana

Lunch

Tomato juice
Hamburger
French fries
Carrot sticks

Snack

Corn or potato chips

Dinner
Potato Soup*
Broiled flounder or sole
Rice
Zucchini
Coffee or soda

Snack
Sherbert

Recipes

BAKED APPLE WITH RAISINS (1 serving)

Ingredients
1 large baking apple
1 tablespoon light brown sugar (check for colors and preservatives)
2 teaspoons soy margarine
⅛ teaspoon cinnamon
⅛ teaspoon nutmeg
1 teaspoon raisins
¼ cup water

Procedure

1. Preheat oven to 375 degrees.
2. Wash and core apple and place in a small baking dish.
3. Combine remaining ingredients (except water) and fill apple with mixture.
4. Pour water around the apple.
5. Bake for 50 minutes or until tender, basting with syrup in dish occasionally.

BANANA PANCAKES

Follow the recipe for pancakes on the box of the oat mix. Mash up ⅓ to ½ of a fairly ripe banana and mix into the pancake batter. Cook pancakes as indicated on the box.

CANDIED SWEET POTATOES Á LA SHIRL

Ingredients

1 large can of yams (not sweetened)
honey
2 tablespoons margarine

Procedure

1. Melt margarine and pour over yams which have been placed in a baking dish.
2. Dilute honey with a little water and pour over yams.
3. Bake at 350 degrees for about 1 hour.
4. Baste every once in a while.

CHEESECAKE

Ingredients

5 eggs
1 pint sour cream
1 pound cream cheese
1½ cups sugar
1 teaspoon vanilla
4 tablespoons cornstarch

Procedure

1. Mix all ingredients in a food processor.
2. Pour into cheesecake pan.
3. Bake at 375 degrees for 1 hour.
4. Leave oven door open for 1 hour after baking is completed.

CHICKEN MARENGO (2–3 servings)

Ingredients

3 chicken breasts, skinned and boned
¼ stick margarine
½ green pepper
½ small onion, julienned
1 small fresh tomato
¼ cup olives (adults should omit these)
12 ounces whole canned tomatoes
¼ cup olive oil (adults use an allowed oil)
garlic powder (no preservatives)
salt and pepper

Procedure

1. Cut chicken breasts into filets and flatten (or buy precut filets at your grocery).
2. Sauté lightly in margarine until light brown on each side.
3. Pour off excess margarine.
4. Add pepper, onion, olives, and fresh tomato to chicken.
5. Meanwhile in blender, mix canned tomato, olive oil, garlic, salt, and pepper, and puree. Pour over chicken.
6. Simmer until vegetables and chicken are tender.

CHICKEN SOUP (This will give you about 8–10 servings. The broth comes in handy in many recipes and the chicken can be used in chicken salad).

Ingredients

1 whole chicken, cut in quarters, and a few extra backs
soup greens (a few carrots, a few stalks of celery, one onion peeled, and one parsnip)
fresh dill (⅓ bunch, soaked in water before using)
3 quarts of water
1 tablespoon salt

Procedure

1. Fill a 6–8 quart pot with water and boil.
2. Add all ingredients to boiled water and bring to a second boil.
3. Cover and simmer for about 2 hours (until chicken is tender).
4. Strain soup and pour into jars; refrigerate overnight.
5. Skim most of the fat off the top and heat to serve.

FROZEN HONEY-NUT BANANA

Roll a peeled banana in honey and then in finely chopped walnuts. Freeze overnight. Defrost slightly before eating.

MAYONNAISE

Ingredients

1 cup salad oil
egg substitute equivalent to 2 eggs
2 tablespoons lemon juice
1 teaspoon sugar
½ teaspoon salt

Procedure

1. Pour ¼ cup of the oil into processor or blender and add the egg (substitute), lemon juice, sugar, and salt.
2. Process or blend (at high speed) for about 10 seconds.
3. While machine is running, carefully add remaining oil.
4. Process or blend until thick and smooth.

MEATBALLS (2 servings)

Ingredients

½ pound chopped meat
¼ cup soy flour
equivalent to 1 egg of egg substitute
garlic powder
salt
pepper
Homemade Tomato Sauce* (See recipe below)

Procedure

1. Mix soy flour, egg substitute, and spices in a mixing bowl.
2. Add chopped meat and combine well.
3. Meanwhile, heat tomato sauce in a 4–6 quart saucepan.
4. Form meatballs and gently place in sauce.
5. Bring to a boil for a few minutes and then simmer for 1 hour over low to medium flame.
6. Serve with rice.

POTATO SOUP

Ingredients

4 cups raw cubed potatoes
2 cups coarsely sliced celery
1 cup coarsely chopped fresh onions
2 cups water
½ stick margarine
1 teaspoon salt
pepper
fresh parsley

Procedure

1. Place potatoes, celery, and onions in a large kettle and add salt and water.
2. Cover and cook over medium heat until vegetables are tender, about 15–25 minutes.
3. When vegetables are tender, put undrained vegetable mixture through a food processor or blender.
4. Return to pot and add margarine, salt, and pepper.
5. Garnish with parsley and serve hot.

TOMATO SAUCE

Ingredients

2 medium onions
1 large green pepper
1 clove garlic
¼ cup oil
2–3 pounds tomatoes
1 teaspoon salt
1 teaspoon pepper

Procedure

1. Peel and coarsely chop the onions.
2. Coarsely chop the green pepper.
3. Chop the garlic finely.
4. Heat the oil in a large pan; add the garlic and vegetables and sauté them until limp and tender (10 minutes).
5. Peel the tomatoes (by dipping them briefly in boiling water to loosen skins) and chop them.
6. Add the tomatoes to the pan with the salt and pepper.
7. Simmer uncovered about 2 hours or until thick.

TUNA FISH SURPRISE (This can be made with chicken salad) Take a large tomato and cut off the top quarter. Scoop out the inside. Make tuna fish salad with tuna and either homemade or an allowed mayonnaise and fill the tomato with the salad. Garnish with parsley to make it look pretty.

5

IMMUNOTHERAPY

Immunotherapy, also known as hyposensitization, is another approach that's available to help you control your asthma. Immunotherapy involves a series of allergy shots whereby the patient is injected with small amounts of extracts of the offending allergens to lessen his sensitivity during future exposures. Less sensitivity means fewer allergic reactions, fewer symptoms, and less trouble.

Immunotherapy has been used since 1903. At first, it was thought that the extracts were antitoxins. Later, it was believed that when the extract was injected, it induced the production of a blocking antibody that formed a complex with the allergen, preventing the allergic chain reaction from developing. This theory was only part of the truth. In addition to blocking antibodies, it is believed that the extracts facilitate the production of suppressor T cells. These cells suppress the production of antibodies (IgE), thus stacking the cards against the allergic chain of events. Whatever the underlying mechanism, immunotherapy is very useful in many cases.

Allergy Testing

Your candidacy for allergy shots will depend upon several factors including the outcome of a complete case history, physical examination, the severity of your symptoms, the area in which you live, and the course of your asthma. If your history reveals obvious allergens that can be eliminated or significantly reduced by environmental control measures, I recommend attempting this control approach first. If your symptoms are severe or worsening, and if no obvious allergens are revealed, allergy testing is in order. Based on my understanding of all of the facts about my patient, I will decide whether a full allergy workup or just a limited number of tests are required. Once this decision is made, I decide which type of allergy test to administer.

Skin Tests

One way of testing for allergies is the use of skin testing, in which the patient's skin reactivity to various allergens is measured. There are two types of skin tests, epicutaneous (on top of the skin) and intradermal (under the skin). Epicutaneous skin tests can either consist of a scratch test or a puncture test. In the scratch test, a series of scratches are made on the surface of the skin and the extracts of suspected allergens are rubbed into the scratches. In the puncture skin test, a drop of allergen is placed on the skin and then the skin is punctured slightly with a needle. The doctor looks at the resulting scratch or puncture to determine the presence of a reaction that comes in the form of itchy, red, and swollen skin. Usually, any swelling more than one fifth of an inch in diameter is considered to be a positive reaction. This type of testing is very specific. If you react positively, chances are you are allergic to that substance. Epicutaneous tests are specific, but often fail to detect some allergies.

Intradermal skin testing is administered by injecting small amounts of the allergy extract under the top layer of skin. The skin reaction the doctor is looking for is the same as in the epicutaneous tests. While these intradermal tests are not as specific as the epicutaneous tests, they are more sensitive. They will not miss any allergies, but they may report some false positive reactions. Many doctors will use a combination of these two types of skin tests to get a more reliable allergy profile.

RAST

In the last twenty years a new approach to allergy testing has developed that allows doctors to test sensitivities outside of the patient's body (in vitro testing). The most popular type of in vitro testing is called the RAST, or Radioallergosorbent Test. This blood test measures the amount of specific IgE in your blood against the substance for which we are testing. For the most part, the amount of IgE antibody for a particular substance determines the individual's sensitivity. If I am testing for ragweed, the RAST can tell me the exact amount of antiragweed IgE in your blood. Because the amount of IgE for each substance in your blood is so small, it could not be measured until the advent of the RAST technique, which in effect magnifies the substance so that it can be measured. The further benefit of the RAST is that it not only tells whether a patient is allergic, but also tells how sensitive the patient is. The RAST can take the place of approximately sixty skin tests.

The RAST is not perfect, however, since there are times when it gives an indefinite answer. At these times, a skin test may have to be done as well. Even when the RAST does not clearly demonstrate that an allergy is present, it still supplies information about the level of sensitivity with very little discomfort to the patient. I use this information to prepare the most appropriate dosage at which to begin allergy testing. When the skin testing is used alone, I have to begin with low dosages and work up slowly. The RAST shortcuts this process.

My Standard Procedure

Once a careful history has been obtained, a physical examination done, and the determination made that allergy testing is needed, I do a RAST. If the RAST results are positive, that is as far as I need to go. If the RAST is negative or equivocal but I still suspect that the person has an allergy, then I do skin testing. But I only do the skin tests on the few substances about which I have some remaining questions. I also have the advantage of having information from the RAST about the most appropriate levels to use in testing. I rarely need more than six skin tests after doing the RAST (as opposed to the more than sixty when skin testing is done alone). Based on all of my findings, I list those substances to which the patient is allergic.

Are You a Good Candidate for Immunotherapy?

With the list of allergens in hand, I must decide if immunotherapy is appropriate for the patient. If any of the culprits can realistically be removed from the patient's environment, I urge this course of action. If you can clean up the environment, get rid of offending foods, or use simple medications to bring your symptoms under control, this may be the way to go. If you can't, then you may well have to consider immunotherapy.

If your symptoms are mild and do not last long (less than one month) you may still be able to avoid allergy shots. For example, if you are pollen-sensitive, and you know that September is going to be a miserable month, you may choose to take simple medications, confine yourself to indoor activities, or spend a month cruising on the high seas instead of getting allergy shots year-round.

Many of you will not be so lucky. Your allergic asthma symptoms may be of longer duration than a month. Simple medications may not control your symptoms or you may be faced with side effects from the medication. At any rate, if you suffer for a good part of the year, and if your symptoms are not easily tamed by environmental control, diet, or drug therapy, then you are a good candidate for immunotherapy.

There are a few other factors that would increase your chances of being helped by allergy shots. Immunotherapy is much more successful with some allergens than with others. It is effective in reducing allergic reactions to pollen, dust, mites, mold, and animals. Food immunotherapy is not effective. Immunotherapy is most successful in children age five or older and remains highly effective until late middle age when its effectiveness begins to diminish.

Administration Alternatives

Allergy shots can be administered under one of two plans. A ''seasonal'' approach would be indicated for those patients whose symptoms occur only during a very specific season. Some doctors treat these patients with immunotherapy three or four months prior to the individual's ''bad'' season. This pattern must go on year after year. I prefer the other approach, a ''perennial'' program. In this plan, patients receive allergy shots all year round. The goal is to establish a maintenance level for a period of time and then to phase out the allergy shots completely. My rule of thumb is that if a patient can be kept virtually symptom-free for two to three years while receiving allergy shots only once in three to four weeks, he no longer needs allergy shots. The average treatment time is four to seven years and can be longer for more severe asthmatics.

The Serum

The ''serum'' used in allergy shots is a highly purified aqueous solution of an extraction of the offending allergens. Thus, grass extract is actually an extraction of grass pollen and cat extract is an extraction of cat dander. The doctor uses your test results and his knowledge of common allergens to prescribe the appropriate mixture for you.

The ''serum'' must be refrigerated but never frozen. I prefer that extracts not be out of the refrigerator for more than twenty-four hours. However, they can be out for up to ninety-six hours without any real problem. After that it is not dangerous, but they do lose some of their potency. The bottle should also be labeled with an expiration date.

Who Gives You the Injections?

Injections are usually administered in the allergist's office by a nurse. On very rare occasions a patient could have a severe reaction (wheezing, swelling, or even shock) and emergency treatment may be needed. Therefore, the doctor must always be present. For various reasons you may opt to have your injections in a medical office other than your allergist's. Make sure your allergist sends complete instructions regarding your serum dosage and schedule to your doctor. In this situation, you may be responsible for your own serum vials. Make sure to keep the serum refrigerated between trips unless your own physician will keep the serum in his refrigerator. In rare situations certain patients (on long-term maintenance therapy with no previous history of reactions to their shots) may receive allergy injections from a nurse or a family member. Of course injectible Adrenalin and antihistamines must be available. This method is not suitable for most patients, but if you think it applies to you, discuss it with your physician.

The Schedule

The usual schedule for allergy shots is once a week. This continues until a maintenance level is reached, usually between six months and a year. The dose is usually in increments of 0.05–0.10 milliliters each week.

Sometimes this schedule is disrupted, perhaps either because of a reaction or a missed appointment. If you miss an injection, and the period of time between this injection and the preceding one is less than two weeks, your dosage can still be increased according to schedule. However, if the period of time between the preceding injection and this one is more than two weeks, but less than four weeks, the preceding injection should be repeated.

If you exceed four weeks, your dosage must be reduced according to a general rule of thumb of 10 percent every week beyond four weeks that the dose was not given. If you miss more than three months, you probably will have to start again, although you can be increased more quickly than the first time.

After a year of immunotherapy, it is important for me and the patient to evaluate progress. If there has been no improvement, I will usually stop immunotherapy. If things are going well, the program should be continued with an effort to cut back the frequency of injections to every two to four weeks over the next year or two. I normally maintain a patient on allergy injections for a minimum of two to three years after he has been relatively symptom-free while receiving injections on a monthly basis.

No one has any absolute figures on when to discontinue immunotherapy or how often symptoms recur after immunotherapy has been discontinued. However, if you have been symptom-free for two years while on a monthly maintenance when allergy injections are discontinued, there is a greater than 50 percent chance that you will remain symptom-free within the first few years after discontinuing shots. I feel that it is very important to try to discontinue shots in order to see if a patient can do without them; therefore, constant reevaluations are important.

Reactions

The most annoying aspect of weekly allergy shots is the standard policy of having the patient wait *thirty minutes* after receiving the shot. This waiting time is very important, however. If there is going to be a severe adverse reaction, it usually occurs within thirty minutes and it will need immediate medical attention. If this happens, you'll be very glad that you waited.

This reaction can almost always be reversed providing you are in the doctor's office. In addition, it is very important for your local reaction to be evaluated. The next dose is guided by your reactivity to your previous shot. The most common reaction is a local one, characterized by an itchy, raised, circular reddened area around the injection site, known as a wheal. If the wheal is large enough (quarter size or larger), the dose may have to be repeated or even reduced for the next injection.

The most serious reactions are not local but systemic. These reactions can include sneezing, chest tightening, asthma, hives, swelling, difficulty in swallowing, nausea, stomach pains, fainting, or even collapse. (On rare occasions death has occurred.) These reactions may require Adrenalin, antihistamines, or a tourniquet to slow down the absorption of the offending substance. Fortunately, these reactions are very rare.

Sometimes systemic reactions occur twelve to twenty-four hours after the injection. This should be reported to your doctor, who may prescribe antihistamines or other medications, depending on the severity of the reaction.

What You Can Expect from Immunotherapy

Immunotherapy is an inexact science, at best. It is a rare person who will have a one-hundred-percent cure with allergy injections. On the other hand, if skin testing or a RAST is done carefully, leading to the preparation of the correct serum to immunize you against the appropriate set of allergens, and if you are in the age range where good response is more common, there is an excellent chance that more than 50 percent of you will achieve almost complete control of the symptoms that immunotherapy was designed to control.

One great misunderstanding about allergy injections comes from the belief that immunotherapy will cure the asthma. It does not. It may cure your reaction to ragweed or to cats or to dust. Depending upon how important this is in your constellation of symptoms, immunotherapy may considerably relieve your symptoms. If a person is allergic only to cats, but refuses to get rid of his cats, and I treat him and he is lucky enough to get almost a one-hundred-percent response from the shots, then I will in effect have almost "cured" his asthma. But this is unusual.

Asthma, as you know by now, is a very multifactorial disease. Immunotherapy can be very important to people with asthma, although it can be a tedious process. To the extent that their asthma symptoms are of an allergic nature, allergy shots can reduce the amount, frequency, and severity of symptoms. Once this happens, it becomes easier to control the other aspects of asthma. The individual may require less medication for example, but still have some symptoms. In the future, a few injections a year may be sufficient to control the patient's symptoms. For now, we must be satisfied with this imperfect but often very helpful adjunct tool in the treatment of allergic asthma.

6

PHARMACOLOGICAL MANAGEMENT OF ASTHMA

SEARCHING FOR THE MAGIC POTION

Countless thousands of asthma sufferers constantly search for a magic potion to cure their disease. They cannot be cured by swallowing one pill, but the medications available today are becoming increasingly effective and will make a tremendous difference for the asthmatic. Since the preparation of the original *Asthma Handbook,* there have been numerous beneficial changes. I was amazed at how much of the drug information in the Future chapter five years ago could be transferred to this chapter on drugs. Thus we should be optimistic about new and helpful drugs that will soon become available. You should always be in close contact with your physician, not only to monitor your present drug regimen, but also to make sure you are aware of all innovations in drug therapy.

Drug therapy, removing substances to which one is allergic, avoiding substances to which one reacts, and being hyposensitized to substances that one cannot avoid will lead to almost complete control of symptoms in most asthma sufferers.

Asthma medications can be very complicated. There are scores of medications, many of them very similar, available for the treatment of asthma.

If you are unfamiliar with the differences among these medications, you will have a situation similar to walking into a classy French restaurant and ordering from the menu without having a knowledge of French. Bluffing your way through the menu may result in choosing six different courses of potatoes. Uneducated selections of asthma medications may have a much more disastrous outcome.

The purpose of this chapter is to discuss the facts concerning the selection and use of asthma medications. It is not meant for you to use to medicate yourself. That could be a sure road to disaster. It is meant for you to use in conjunction with your physician's instructions. An educated patient and a knowledgeable physician are the best team. You will find that when you know the facts of your illness, you will be able to work with your physician in a more effective manner.

Underlying Principles

Whether asthma is looked at from the standpoint of anatomy, physiology, or metabolism, it is a very complicated disease. As much as we currently understand about asthma and as much as we continue to learn every year through active and ongoing research programs, we truly do not understand all of the basic mechanisms underlying its causes. The disease is caused in large part by an inadequate supply of a chemical known as CAMP (cyclic adenosine 3'5'-monophosphate) within the various cells of the body. CAMP is found in the cells of almost every major organ system in the body. In the muscle cells of the lung, CAMP is important since its presence serves to prevent the bronchoconstriction that results in asthma. In the circulating mast cells of the blood, its absence serves to increase the tendency of the mast cells to release histamine and other harmful substances that cause allergic reactions. CAMP is broken down by an enzyme (phosphodiesterase) into the chemical AMP (adenosine monophosphate), while its production can be stimulated with the help of another enzyme, adenyl cyclase, from the predecessor chemical ATP (adenosine triphosphate). In general, drugs that inhibit the action of phosphodiesterase tend to increase the level of CAMP within the cells, and thereby help to decrease the incidence and severity of asthma attacks and of allergy reactions in general. Theophylline medications are helpful in preventing and treating asthmatic attacks perhaps in part because of their ability to inhibit the action of the enzyme phosphodiesterase, thus decreasing the breakdown of CAMP into AMP. Although we do know that theophylline medications are extremely helpful in the treatment of asthma and that they inhibit the enzyme phosphodiesterase, we cannot be certain that the above-mentioned process is the way in which it works.

Whereas the breakdown of CAMP into AMP (which is not good for the asthmatic) can be stimulated by the enzyme phosphodiesterase, the production of CAMP from ATP (which is good for the asthmatic) can be stimulated by the enzyme adenyl cyclase. The action of this enzyme can be stimulated by a class of drugs known as sympathomimetic drugs that are in essence modifications of Adrenalin and function in ways similar to that molecule. The primary advantage of the sympathomimetic drugs that are used in place of Adrenalin is that they are effective when taken orally, whereas Adrenalin must be injected. However, Adrenalin is extremely effective in treating acute asthmatic attacks precisely because it is so effective in helping to stimulate the production of CAMP within those cells involved in the asthmatic attack.

Even in the presence of inadequate amounts of CAMP, the allergy reaction cannot occur unless adequate amounts of calcium are able to flow through the cell membranes. A class of drugs containing cromolyn sodium inhibit enzymes that allow the flow of calcium across the mast cell membranes and this inhibits the release of mediators, for instance, histamine. These drugs are therefore useful in treating asthma.

One of the reasons why asthmatics have less CAMP than necessary may be because adenyl cyclase (the enzyme that stimulates the production of CAMP from ATP) does not function well and is blocked. Because of this blockade, the sympathomimetic drugs cannot stimulate the action of adenyl cyclase and help to transform ATP into CAMP. Corticosteroids break through this blockade and allow adenyl cyclase to be effective in producing

CAMP in a more normal fashion from the precursor molecule, ATP. Corticosteroid medications have an important and complex role in the treatment of asthma.

To summarize then, there are four major ways in which the CAMP molecule can be made to exist in increased levels in the various cells controlling the allergic or asthmatic reaction within the body, thereby generating four strategies to follow in managing asthma with medication. We will examine the theophylline drugs, the sympathomimetic drugs or Adrenalin-like drugs, cromolyn sodium and the corticosteroid medications in sequence. In discussing each class of drugs, I will describe the major characteristics of the class, the general guidelines for the administration of these drugs and also dosages, side effects, and relative precautions. At the end of the chapter you will find a chart which summarizes in a readable way information on each medication available at your pharmacy.

Theophylline

I will begin with the theophylline drugs because they are the mainstay of therapy programs in this country. The drugs in this class include theophylline, Slo-Bid, Theo-Dur, Theo-24, Uniphyl, Theolair, Slo-Phyllin, Bronkodyl, Theophyl, Elixophyllin, Somophyllin, Choledyl, aminophylline, and many others. Aminophylline and Choledyl are not pure theophylline and are usually used only in special circumstances.

SHORT-, INTERMEDIATE-, LONG-, AND TWENTY-FOUR-HOUR ACTING THEOPHYLLINE

Theophylline medications are available in four different forms: short-acting, intermediate-acting, long-acting, and twenty-four-hour. Short-acting drugs have their maximum effect after about two hours and generally are out of the body after about four hours. These drugs are taken every four to six hours. Intermediate-acting theophylline drugs peak after about four hours and are generally out of the body after eight hours. These drugs are taken every eight hours, more or less. Long-acting theophylline drugs may not reach their peak action for two or three days and the contents of an individual pill may not be out of your body for sixteen hours or longer. These long-acting theophylline preparations work somewhat differently from the short or intermediate theophylline because they have a cumulative effect and must be taken on a regular basis every twelve hours to be effective. There are now medications which can be taken once a day, every twenty-four hours. They may not reach their peak action for four days. During a twenty-four-hour period they will peak eight to twelve hours after the pill was taken, reaching a low level twenty-four hours after the pill was taken.

Brand names of the short-acting drugs include Aminophyllin, Bronkodyl, Quibron, Slo-Phyllin, Elixophyllin, and Somophyllin-T. The intermediate-acting drugs include Theophylline-S.R., Slo-Phyllin-S.R., Theolair-S.R., Theophyl-S.R., Quibron-S.R., and Elixophyllin-S.R. When you see S.R. (or T.R.) after the drug name, it means sustained release (or time released) which implies that you have an intermediate-acting drug.

Long-acting preparations include Theo-Dur, Constant-T, and Slo-Bid. The long-acting preparations work by building up a sustained blood level of theophylline after two to three days and then maintaining a more or less constant level as long as the drug continues to be taken regularly. The brand names of the twenty-four-hour theophylline are Uniphyl and Theo-24.

WHICH ONE SHOULD YOU USE?

For the mild asthmatic who is symptomatic only on an intermittent basis, or who is in the midst of an acute attack, I usually recommend short- or intermediate-acting drugs.

For the asthmatic with moderate or severe symptoms of a more chronic nature, I usually prescribe the long-acting (every twelve hours) drugs. My best experience has been with Theo-Dur and Slo-Bid. I have found Slo-Bid especially useful. The most important features of Slo-Bid include the following: (1) There is less gastric irritation. Patients who could not take other forms of theophylline have no difficulty with Slo-Bid. (2) The granules can be taken out of the capsule and given to children and adults who cannot swallow pills. Even when the granules are taken out of the capsule, the long-acting characteristic of the pill is maintained. This is also true of Theo-Dur Sprinkles, but the Theo-Dur product has a very erratic absorption for patients under the age of six.

These long-acting theophylline drugs are usually useless if taken during an acute attack or if taken only once a day (if you take these drugs only once a day, you will never build up a therapeutic level in the bloodstream).

Next, let me explain the twenty-four-hour acting theophylline. For those patients in whom this medication lasts the full twenty-four hours, the drugs are helpful, convenient, and appropriate. However, my experience with my more severe patients tells me that these medications do not last beyond twenty to twenty-three hours. Those few hours can be very critical, especially if they occur early in the morning. Some of my patients were getting severe attacks at that time, whereas when they were on Slo-Bid or Theo-Dur (long-acting), they were not. It is best to use these medications with older patients because their metabolism is slow. Since children have rapid metabolisms, they are not good candidates for twenty-four-hour acting theophylline medications. When appropriately prescribed and used, these drugs are effective in approximately 65 percent of patients.

DOSAGE

In children on a short-acting drug, I usually use about 1.8 milligrams per pound of body weight every four to six hours four times a day as a starting dose. I prefer that the starting dosage not exceed 100 milligrams per dose (400 milligrams a day, total) in a child or adult.

If this achieves a positive result, I would have the patient take the medication during an acute attack and then continue for up to one to two weeks after his symptoms have improved. Many people tend to go off their medication as soon as the acute symptoms end. You must realize that once you have an asthma attack, whether it is related to an infection or not, your lungs are in a "twitchy" state. Even though the patient feels well, it is often best to stay on medication up to a week after the attack is over.

In a slightly more chronic patient, I might use an intermediate-acting theophylline. For a child, I would give roughly 2.4 milligrams per pound of body weight as a starting dose usually every eight hours not to exceed 125 milligrams per dose (375 milligrams per day). For an adult, the starting dosage is 125 milligrams per dose. Basically, the only time I use shorter- and intermediate-acting medication is to treat intermittent acute attacks. These drug preparations are very beneficial for people who wheeze occasionally. These starting doses (short- and intermediate-acting) can be increased if not effective. Discuss the schedule with your physician. Once medication is required on a fairly regular basis or on a chronic basis, then the long-acting drugs are the ones I recommend.

With long-acting theophylline in a child, the initial dosage is 16 milligrams per kilogram or 7 milligrams per pound of body weight per day. In an adult I would normally start with 200 milligrams of Theo-Dur every twelve hours. If there is no problem (headache, tremulousness, anxiety, nervousness, stomachache, or jitteriness) after three days, and if the symptoms are not alleviated, I would go to 300 milligrams every twelve hours; and once again after three days if there are no adverse reactions and no significant relief, I might increase the dosage to 400 milligrams every twelve hours. At this point I usually recommend that a blood level be taken.

Some patients find that they become symptomatic before they are due for the next dose of the long-acting drug (ten hours after the last dose). In these cases I sometimes divide the total daily dose into three doses every eight hours instead of twice a day, every twelve hours. This often achieves satisfactory results. Children under the age of twelve are very fast metabolizers, and tend to do much better on every eight-hour dosing.

If my patient has heart disease, liver disease, or is over fifty years of age, I might recommend not exceeding 200–300 milligrams every twelve hours without a blood level.

Two relatively new medications, Theo-24 and Uniphyl, are convenient because they can be taken just once a day, in the morning. Uniphyl comes in 200- and 400-milligram tablets. Theo-24 comes in 100-, 200-, and 300-milligram capsules.

Doses that exceed 900 milligrams a day absolutely must be taken on an empty stomach. If food is taken within one hour (especially a fatty meal), the absorption of theophylline is enhanced and toxic levels can ensue.

Theo-24 and Uniphyl are formulated differently. Instructions vary for each of these pills; even different strength pills of the same type have different instructions. I will tell you how I use these drugs, but be aware that your doctor may use them differently and achieve the same results. As I've mentioned previously, I find twenty-four-hour theophylline preparations not helpful in most cases. When I utilize them in a patient who has used a twelve-hour theophylline preparation and whose total daily dose does not exceed 900 milligrams, I merely add up the total dose. If my patient uses Theo-Dur 400 milligrams every twelve hours, the total would be 800 milligrams for the day which can be given in the morning. If the total exceeds 900 milligrams, I start with 900 milligrams and build up (after 900 milligrams the relationship of the two drugs changes). Then depending on the blood level I increase the dose by 100-milligram increments, measuring the blood level *at least four days* after each increment. This drug requires two blood levels taken four days after there is no variation in the dose of the medication. The first level is measured at twelve hours and the other at twenty-three hours. I then raise the amount of medication until the patient is comfortable or asymptomatic. Unfortunately the twelve-hour level is often too high and the twenty-three-hour too low. However, when the drug works it is a convenience and is the drug of choice for that patient.

If I had a patient who was not on any previous theophylline drug and I wished to begin treatment with Uniphyl, I would start with a twelve-hour preparation and titrate the patient to his appropriate level of theophylline, and then switch over to Uniphyl as described in the preceding paragraph. These drugs are normally given in the morning. Some patients get into trouble several hours before the twenty-four hours are over, placing them in jeopardy in the early morning hours when they are most likely to be asleep, or just upon awakening when they would naturally want to function well. In order to avoid this "dipping" problem, Uniphyl may be given immediately after dinner (if the dose doesn't exceed 900 milligrams). However, there is some debate about when the drug should be taken. Please check with your doctor. This method offers an important and potentially promising use of Uniphyl.

THEOPHYLLINE LEVEL IN THE BLOOD

The level of theophylline in the bloodstream (blood or serum theophylline level) can be measured. This measurement provides very important information, and it can guide the physician in the proper use of theophylline in his patient. In general, we attempt to avoid theophylline levels in excess of 20 micrograms/milliliters since these can be toxic. Some people experience beneficial effects from theophylline with blood levels as low as 5 micrograms/milliliters but most people seem to require dosages of theophylline that result in blood levels in excess of 10 micrograms/milliliters. Therefore, the "therapeutic range" of blood theophylline for most patients is considered to be between 10 and 20 micrograms/milliliters. That simply provides a level that extremely few people will find too high to be tolerated, but which most patients will find high enough to provide adequate relief.

A blood theophylline level is a very precise measurement that I depend upon to advise me as to how much of the drug to administer to any particular patient. It is very important to know the exact relationship between the time the dose of medication is taken and the time the blood is drawn to measure the level of the drug. When measuring blood theophylline in a patient taking a short-acting medication, the blood is generally drawn two hours after the previous dose. When taking an intermediate-acting theophylline drug, the blood is generally drawn four hours after the last dose.

In measuring blood theophylline levels in patients taking long-acting Theophylline medications, the situation is more complicated. The patient should have taken the medication every twelve hours for three consecutive days without missing a dose. The blood is then drawn between three and eight hours after the previous dose. In Theo-24 (ultra-long-acting, once-a-day drug), the blood is drawn twelve hours after taking the medication. In the case of Uniphyl, the blood may be drawn eight to twelve hours after taking the medication. If the precise timing is not followed or if dosages have been missed, the blood level may be inaccurately interpreted, since the assumption behind the interpretation of the measurements will be invalid. For example, if a patient misses a dose and a low blood level is recorded, one may mistakenly conclude that the medication dosage should be increased, resulting in toxic levels. In preparing to obtain blood theophylline level measurements, it is essential to follow the instructions of your physician.

Once the appropriate level of theophylline is achieved, the dosage should be stabilized and the blood level should be checked every six months to one year or when the patient is experiencing adverse side effects or increased asthma symptoms. Your metabolism and, therefore, your level of theophylline may be influenced by a number of factors that are important to understand.

Factors Affecting Theophylline Metabolism and Bloodstream Levels

YOUR METABOLISM

Under certain conditions, theophylline metabolism is altered and theophylline medications are metabolized differently, either more slowly or more quickly. You may, therefore, need more or less of the drug. Children tend to metabolize the drug faster than adults;

therefore, they require more drug per pound of body weight. If you smoke, you metabolize the drug more quickly. Your doctor should be aware of your smoking habit when prescribing this drug. By the way, if you are asthmatic and need theophylline, you certainly should not be smoking anyway! Theophylline is not distributed into the body fat. Therefore, the dose is calculated for "ideal weight," not real weight. Excessively overweight people do not require much more theophylline than their leaner counterparts. If you are obese, it is not a bad idea to lose some weight: this would make breathing easier.

Theophylline drugs are metabolized more slowly (thereby requiring less of the drug per pound of body weight) in individuals with congestive heart failure or with liver disease. A once-a-day dosage of long-acting theophylline may be sufficient. If you contract a viral infection or fever, you tend to metabolize more slowly, thereby increasing your theophylline level. If you should get such an infection while on theophylline, inform your doctor. Flu vaccines may also increase theophylline levels by decreasing theophylline metabolism. Some theophylline drugs, Uniphyl, and Theo-24, metabolize more slowly and have a reduced excretion after a very fatty meal; thus the serum theophylline level can rise, sometimes to dangerous levels.

Some drugs alter the elimination of theophylline. Therefore, if you are taking a new medication and if you are also taking theophylline, notify your doctor. For example, erythromycin decreases the metabolism of theophylline and you might need less theophylline while taking erythromycin. Cimetidine (Tagamet) commonly increases theophylline levels; ranitidine (Zantac) very rarely does. It is unclear at this time whether steroids slow down the metabolism of theophylline, thereby increasing the theophylline level. Therefore, when you are on both theophylline and steroids, you will need to work closely with your physician to monitor your theophylline level and your symptoms.

Not only do some medications affect the metabolism of theophylline, but theophylline affects the metabolism of some other medications. For example, theophylline, when taken with Inderal (propranolol), interferes with its effect. Patients who are on lithium should be aware that theophylline will increase their secretion of lithium. It is always important to check with your doctor about whether your medications interact and influence each other. If the metabolism of theophylline is altered, you may begin to have some side effects. You must communicate their presence to your physician.

SIDE EFFECTS

The side effects of theophylline are headache, stomachache, shakiness, nervousness, and a rapid heart rate. One patient said that her five-year-old would see her taking her pill and say, "Oh-oh, Mommy's taking her crabby pill again."

Some of my patients report that the irritability or jitteriness they experience is reduced when the drug is ingested after food. It has also been shown that caffeine acts in a similar fashion to theophylline. In fact, caffeine may be transformed into theophylline in the body. Therefore, drinking coffee or tea while taking theophylline is not a good idea as it could increase the theophylline level in your bloodstream. However, if you suddenly become symptomatic and you're caught without your medication, try drinking two cups of coffee.

Theophylline is an excellent drug and is highly effective and tolerated well, most of the time. Its side effects are minimal and manageable. It is a potentially toxic drug and must be administered and monitored carefully, under the supervision of your physician. If, however, you have any adverse side effects, report them to your doctor. Do not continue taking your prescribed dosage if this occurs. It may be possible to reduce the dosage for a few days and then try again, but your doctor must decide this. Used appropriately, it is a wonder drug.

Sympathomimetic Drugs

For many people, theophylline is sufficient. However, another class of drugs has for years played a very active role in asthma care. This class consists of the sympathomimetic drugs, which have an Adrenalin-like effect and work with the sympathetic nervous system. The sympathetic nervous system is part of the autonomic nervous system, where the defect of asthma lies. As you remember, the autonomic nervous system helps keep your lungs open and allows you to breathe easier. The most important drug in this class is Adrenalin (epinephrine).

Earlier in this chapter you learned that Adrenalin stimulates the enzyme adenyl cyclase to increase the production of CAMP from ATP. The more CAMP, the better. So it makes sense that Adrenalin and Adrenalin-like drugs are important.

EPI

The most important sympathomimetic drug is epinephrine, also known as Adrenalin. Adrenalin does not have a place in everyday treatment of asthma; rather, its most frequent application is in the emergency room. It is extremely effective during an acute attack. In the emergency room, Adrenalin or epinephrine is known to its friends as epi. If you've ever had emergency treatment of asthma and you were given a shot in a small syringe that made you feel jumpy, nervous, and possibly headachy, but allowed you to breathe better without wheezing, that was epi. It worked! I will discuss epi and its use in the section on acute attacks.

Sympathomimetic medications come in various forms: inhalant sprays, tablets, syrups, and liquids which can be nebulized into a fine mist. Depending upon the age of the patient and the severity of the symptoms, your physician will make his choice as to which form or forms would be the most appropriate for you. In the following sections I will discuss what is currently available in the sympathomimetic medications and the form that each of these drugs comes in.

ALBUTEROL

This drug has the brand name of Proventil, or Ventolin. The names Proventil and Ventolin are very optimistic sounding names, suggesting that they promote ventilation. They are excellent drugs.

These drugs have slightly more beta-2 action, which means that they are helpful for the lungs and less harmful for the heart. However, they still have a slight adverse effect on the heart, and therefore, are not usually used by patients with cardiac problems. Your physician may decide that the spray form is safe for heart patients.

I usually recommend taking the spray form as the first line of attack. In general, the inhaled form of albuterol gives more benefits with less side effects.

SPRAY

In mild asthmatics I would recommend that the spray be used on an as-needed basis (two sprays at most every four hours). For the mild asthmatic who needs more, or for the moderate or severe asthmatic, I would recommend that he take two sprays four times a day on a regular basis. The action of the spray can often lasts as long as four to six hours. A total of twelve sprays within twenty-four hours is usually considered to be a safe upper limit.

One of the dangers of the spray form of this drug is the temptation to overuse it. Even though very few people would ever consider taking more than a prescribed dose of a pill form of a drug, they might not take sprays seriously enough. Especially since there is often immediate relief, it is tempting to take an extra puff. However, just as there is a specified dosage of drugs in pill form, there is a specified dosage of drugs in spray form. If you begin to overdose on the spray, there is often a rebound effect in which, rather than causing bronchodilation, you get bronchospasm. This is called "locked lung syndrome." Needless to say this is not a good state of affairs. Albuterol (Proventil and Ventolin) has much less of a tendency to cause this syndrome than do the older sprays.

The best way to use sprays is to first exhale, slowly and deeply, and then place your lips around the spray. Breathe in, slowly and deeply, and spray at the beginning of this inhalation. Inhale the spray slowly and deeply into your lungs and hold it for ten seconds. It is very important to take your time and breathe the medication in deeply. Do not swallow it! It was not designed to work that way. If you are told to spray twice, wait one minute before you spray a second time. Do not spray twice and then breathe in. Each spray must be taken individually and correctly.

Make sure you keep your spray container clean; wash the mouthpiece often. Make sure you always have a clean spray container available. The spray containers come with covers; use them. At night, be careful about overusing it. Place it just out of reach so that you cannot reach for it when you are half asleep. Sprays are very safe if they are used correctly. When used incorrectly or abused, they can be dangerous.

SPACERS

The effectiveness of sprays has recently been enhanced by the use of a spacer, a small tube which you attach to the mouthpiece of the inhaler to increase the distance from the mouth to the spray. This increased distance allows the aerosol to break up into smaller particles that seem to penetrate more deeply into the respiratory passages of the lungs. The spacer also may reduce the incidence of fungal overgrowth and hoarseness (side effects of inhaled medications).

In addition to increasing effectiveness, the spacers have been a great help to young children and the elderly who have trouble coordinating the spray medication and their breathing. This lack of coordination often leads to incorrect use of the spray. The spacer suspends the aerosol for a while, giving the child a chance to inhale a few times and receive an effective dose of the medication. Common spacers currently used are the Monaghan Aerochamber and Inspirease. Discuss the appropriateness of your using a spacer with your physician.

NEBULIZED LIQUID

Albuterol also comes in a liquid form that can be nebulized. This means the liquid is put into a machine that turns the liquid into a fine mist so it can be breathed in easily. This device has been very helpful for the very young child, the elderly, or anyone who is too ill to manage the spray device. The use of the nebulizer has kept many children out of the emergency room. DeVilbiss is a popular brand of nebulizing machine. If you get a prescription from your physician, it is often possible to receive reimbursement for this purchase from your insurance company. The purchase of this equipment is also tax deductible.

Albuterol liquid, which comes in individual little bottles, is poured into the nebulizer. The unit bottle contains 2.5 milligrams of albuterol in a saline solution. This is the correct dose for adults and children over twelve years old. There is no hard and fast rule for the doses used with younger children. For children three to six years of age, I usually use one quarter of the dose, and for children six to twelve years of age, one half the dose. Although research data on children is limited, I do find this preparation to be the most effective of all the nebulizer solutions. As the mist comes out, breathe in slowly and deeply as best you can. Do not breathe in and out faster than you normally would. It should take you about ten to fifteen minutes to inhale all of the medication. You should stop if you feel that your heart is racing or if you experience a tingling sensation in your fingers. Your doctor should give you an adequate explanation of the use of the nebulizer. If you do not get excellent results from the nebulizer, contact your physician.

TABLET

The tablet dosage is 2 to 4 milligrams taken three to four times a day. If this dose does not work, and if the patient is not having any adverse effects, the dose may be cautiously increased to 8 milligrams four times a day, as tolerated. A long-acting tablet is called Albuterol Repetabs.

Albuterol Repetabs are available in a 4-milligram dosage. When a patient is taking the short-acting preparation, I merely add up his twenty-four-hour total dose and divide by two. Thus, if my patient is taking Albuterol tabs four times a day, the total would be 16 milligrams. I would give 8 milligrams (two 4-milligram tablets) every twelve hours. The starting dose for adults and children over twelve is 4 to 8 milligrams every twelve hours. The maximum dosage is 32 milligrams per day. The side effects can be jitteriness, tremulousness, and an increased heart rate.

SYRUP

Proventil syrup is available to be used for ages two and older. Your doctor will decide what he wants to do for children younger than two years old. The usual starting dose for adults and children over fourteen years old is one teaspoon (2 milligrams) to two teaspoons, three to four times a day. If the patient is still symptomatic and there are no side effects (such as nervousness, racing heart, jitteriness, muscle tremor), the dose may be increased cautiously up to 4 teaspoons four times a day. Children six to fourteen years of age start with one teaspoon, three to four times a day and slowly increase up to three teaspoons four times a day. For children two to six years of age, start with 0.1 milligram/kilogram of body weight, three times a day, not to exceed one teaspoon three times a day. Once again, following the same rules, the dose may be increased to 0.2 milligram/kilogram three times a day, not to exceed two teaspoons three times a day.

METAPROTERENOL (ALUPENT OR METAPREL)

Among the widely used sympathomimetic drugs used today is metaproterenol. The two brand names are Alupent and Metaprel. These medications are available in spray form, liquid for nebulizer (only Alupent), tablets, or syrup.

SPRAY

The spray form of metaproterenol can be taken on an as-needed basis for the mild asthmatic, one or two sprays every four hours as needed with a maximum dose of twelve inhalations in a twelve-hour period. If this as-needed basis is not controlling the mild asthmatic, or for the moderate or severe asthmatic, the spray is often prescribed regularly, two to three inhalations every three to four hours (not to exceed the maximum of twelve inhalations per twelve-hour period).

All of the precautions and helpful hints in using a spray form of a medication are the same as those under the spray section for albuterol on pages 156–157. Spacers, such as discussed in the albuterol section, also apply to the metaproterenol sprays.

NEBULIZED LIQUID

Metaproterenol liquid can be easily nebulized into a fine mist inhaled by very young or very old patients who have trouble with the coordination of the hand-held metered dose spray. The machine used is the same as is described in the nebulized liquid section under Albuterol.

Metaproterenol liquid for nebulizing comes in a premixed solution contained in an ampule. For children younger than three, I recommend half an ampule. For children older than three, or for adults, I recommend a full ampule. If you don't have the premixed Alupent, then use 0.2 milliliter for children under the age of three and 0.3 milliliter for children over the age of three and adults. Dilute with saline to make approximately 2.5 cubic centimeters of total solution. Important: see page 275 for discussion of the use of the sympathomimetic sprays in children.

TABLETS AND SYRUPS

Neither Alupent nor Metaprel are generally advised for children under six years of age. While it is not believed that these drugs are dangerous for children under six, they have not been adequately studied, and the Food and Drug Administration (FDA) cannot make a ruling on the safety of these medications. If, however, your youngster is ill enough to require it, your physician may opt to prescribe its use. This is something you and he must consider carefully.

In children from ages six to nine, or who weigh under 60 pounds, the usual dose is one teaspoon (10 milligrams) three or four times a day. In children over nine years of age, or who weigh over 60 pounds, 20 milligrams three or four times a day (one 20-milligram tablet, or two teaspoons, four times a day) is advisable. The usual adult dose is 20 milligrams three or four times a day.

The oral form of this drug is usually not recommended for anyone who has hypertension, coronary artery disease, congestive heart failure, arrhythmia, hyperthyroidism, or diabetes. These are all relative contraindications. Since your physician knows your case, he will make the final decision on the use of this medication for you.

In its oral form (tablet or syrup), metaproterenol does have some side effects. Extreme shakiness of the skeletal muscles and increased cardiac activity are its major adverse symptoms. The effect on the skeletal muscles usually wears off after a week or two. Certainly a person with cardiac disease would take the drug in its oral form only in very unusual, carefully considered, cases.

TERBUTALINE SULFATE (BRETHINE OR BRICANYL)

Terbutaline Sulfate, also known as Brethine or Bricanyl, is a beta-2 sympathomimetic drug that is available in oral form and in an inhaler. Both are very similar to either Metaprel or Proventil. Some patients seem to do better with one of these medications than the others. Terbutaline is felt to be the safest spray for pregnant women.

The same kinds of stipulations apply as with the other drugs. Terbutaline is not officially recommended for children below the age of twelve. It is not generally used by people who have cardiovascular disease, hypertension, congestive heart failure, arrhythmia, or diabetes. This drug may also cause the familiar side effects of shakiness, headaches, and muscle cramps. Most of the time the side effects diminish after taking the drug for a few days.

The dose is normally 2.5 to 5.0 milligrams every six to eight hours three times a day. When there are side effects, the dose can be reduced to 1.25 milligrams three times a day, and in some people this reduced dose can still be very helpful. The dosage

(2.5 milligrams three times a day) is the recommended dose for children from the age of twelve to fifteen. No one should take more than 15 milligrams a day.

Honorable Mention

There are two drugs that you might have heard of or read about in older books. They were used a great deal at one time, but now have been replaced by more effective and less problematic medications. Despite their problems and relative inefficiency, they were the best we had at the time and they deserve honorable mention.

Ephedrine was a very important drug eighteen years ago when I first started my practice. While it opened up the airways in the lungs (bronchodilation), it often had unpleasant side effects. It made some people nervous and caused occasional severe headaches, and did not help enough to make coping with the side effects worthwhile. Today ephedrine is rarely used in the treatment of asthma.

Isoproterenol is the drug used in the Mistometer, Medihaler-Iso, and in a host of other sprays. These drugs were very helpful livesavers for many, many years. They were quite beneficial in terminating an acute attack. They were sometimes prescribed in a linguet (a tablet placed under the tongue, usually at a dosage of 10 to 15 milligrams), rather than swallowed. Despite its years of useful service, isoproterenol's heyday is over. It had more cardiac effects and fewer beneficial pulmonary effects in comparison with today's newer medications. As with ephedrine, these are retired with honor.

Summary

In summary, the oral sympathomimetic drugs work well to complement theophylline medications; except in children one to two years of age where they may be used as primary medications, or also in conjunction with theophylline. The inhaled sympathomimetic agents can work as a primary medication in mild asthma at all ages or in conjunction with theophylline when theophylline alone is inadequate.

Theophylline-Sympathomimetic Combination Drugs

There are several medications that contain both theophylline and a sympathomimetic agent in a fixed and predetermined combination. Examples include Primatene "P" Formula, Tedral, Bronkotabs, and Marax. If some of those names sound familiar, it is because they are over-the-counter preparations, some of which are advertised to the general public. While it is true that the combination of theophylline and a sympathomimetic drug is useful in treating asthma, I generally do not recommend any of these medications. I find that patients often do not take the over-the-counter medication seriously enough, and therefore, their use may not be monitored by a physician. These medications can be abused with devastatingly adverse consequences. (The combination of these two drugs in a fixed proportion is not helpful.) Asthma drugs should be combined in the proportions appropriate to each patient. It is difficult, if not impossible, in a fixed drug combination to obtain the appropriate combination for a majority of patients. Second, the sympathomimetic drug used is ephedrine which, as I have already indicated, is no longer generally used in the treatment of asthma. Third, added to the combination of theophylline and ephedrine is either phenobarbital or an antihistamine, hydroxyzine hydrochloride, with a sedating side effect. Phenobarbital is not used in the treatment of asthma, and sedation is something we try to avoid.

Cromolyn Sodium (Intal)

Cromolyn sodium (Intal) was discovered approximately twenty-three years ago and was believed to protect against an allergic reaction. When it was introduced in the United States about seventeen years ago it was hoped that the long-sought-after elusive cure for asthma was finally here. Initially, Intal was used to treat any type of asthma, chronic bronchitis, and emphysema in the country. It didn't work on most patients, and was a great disappointment, falling quickly into disuse.

Fortunately, it did not stay there long. As we began to understand how it really worked, we started to use it on the appropriate patients. It works wonderfully on patients with mild allergic asthma, and in younger patients (five years to thirty-five) with exercise-induced asthma. However, it was cumbersome to use.

The Intal capsule was placed into the inhaler and punctured by sliding a cylinder on the top of the inhaler down and then back. The mouthpiece of the inhaler was then placed in the patient's mouth, loosely held by the lips between the teeth (do not bite down on it). The patient leaned his head back and took a rapid, deep inhalation, directing the powder over the tongue. After removing the device, the patient held that position for approximately ten seconds, then exhaled. After a second inhalation, the patient then checked the capsule to make sure that all of the powder had been used (three to five inhalations might have been necessary). Since the powder has a lactose base (which may cause cavities), the patient had to rinse his mouth after using Intal. As you can see, you practically had to suck the powder into your lungs.

Nevertheless, if you had mild asthma or exercise-induced asthma, and you didn't choke while taking the medication, it was almost like a cure and had virtually no side effects. The old Intal capsule couldn't be used during the acute attack because it was irritating; and small children, in whom it should work best, didn't have the coordination to use it.

Then four things happened, three already discussed in the first *Asthma Handbook*. The fourth, *hot off the press,* is brand new and has changed our concept of asthma, and will be introduced here. The changes are as follows:

First, several years ago, Intal became available in a liquid form that can be administered by using the nebulizing machine, which converts the liquid medicine to a fine mist that can be inhaled easily (without requiring much coordination on the part of the patient). The dosage is one ampule (20 mg cromolyn sodium in 2 milliliters purified water) four times a day for adults and children, age two and over.

Second, Intal became available as a spray. The dose is two sprays four times a day. No longer is the cumbersome spinhaler necessary for most people. This is the most dramatic change because the drug is so easy to use now. A small minority of patients are bothered by the spray.

Third, and in conjunction with the second improvement, for both little children and anyone else who could not coordinate the use of a spray (metered dose inhaler), there is the spacer discussed on page 157 that enables almost anyone from age two to ninety to use the medication.

So now anyone who should use the drug can use it. This brings us to the fourth and most important change. The mechanism of the drug is much clearer. At first it was thought it worked by stabilizing the mast cells and by preventing calcium from entering the cell. Calcium is an important ingredient in the breakdown of the CAMP and in the release of histamine from the mast cell. Intal appears to ''paralyze'' the mast cell, preventing the release of histamines and other harmful substances.

Although the preceding mechanism is important, it is now known that cromolyn blocks both the inflammatory response and the late phase reaction. These are two new concepts, so let me explain them. Everyone knows what inflammation looks like. When you get an infection the area around it gets swollen, red, hot, and tender. That's exactly what happens in the lung in an allergic reaction. After the allergic reaction occurs, the blood vessels bring lots of blood into the area. The blood carries white cells to protect the body. But they cause a great deal of damage as they try to protect the body. We've already explained that the body's response to an allergic reaction is a mistake. So there are all of these white cells attacking the lung tissue to protect it, which would be fine if they were protecting it against pneumonia bacteria; but if it's just dog dander, then the white cells are really killing their own allies (the lung tissue) for nothing. Dog dander is, after all, harmless. Once the inflammatory response occurs it is not easily reversible.

The other concept is the late phase reaction. We used to think if you breathed in some dust to which you were allergic, you would have an attack for a few hours and then get better. Not true! When you have an allergic reaction to dust, you get sick immediately. But the reaction doesn't go away immediately; the inflammatory response then occurs and can continue for days. This is the late phase response.

The late phase response is the severest aspect of asthma; it causes the most serious prolonged attacks, which are not responsive to sympathomimetics, anticholinergics, or theophylline medication. And that's why we are talking about the late phase response in this section. There are only three modalities that prevent the late phase response: (1) allergy injections, (2) corticosteroids, and (3) *Intal*.

So we see Intal is a very versatile and useful drug. (Although Intal sometimes takes one or two months to obtain a therapeutic level, it's often worth the wait). I use Intal when sympathomimetic drugs are not sufficient to control asthma. I often use it before theophylline and often in conjunction with theophylline. It is useful at any age, but the younger the better. It can be nebulized for babies as young as one year of age. It is a useful drug to prevent exercise-induced and allergic asthma. In fact, if you arrange to take your Intal dose about half an hour prior to exercise, you will probably be able to engage in physical exertion with fewer symptoms. And finally, I very often use it now in treating severe asthmatics, with the hope that it will blunt that inflammatory response.

Antihistamines

There is a myth that antihistamines cause asthma. Many doctors are reluctant to give antihistamines to asthmatic patients, for fear that it will dry up the secretions. However, antihistamines are sometimes very useful in asthma. If you have a cold or concurrent allergies, such as nasal congestion, itching, or hives, there is no reason why you cannot take an antihistamine, as long as it is only taken in normal doses and it makes you feel better.

This has been well borne out. As a matter of fact, in certain forms of bronchitis, antihistamines are used as a form of treatment. Also, antihistamines can be helpful as a primary drug among a small group of asthmatics. Therefore, if you are having difficulty with some of the other asthma drugs, and if they are not working, then perhaps your physician can try antihistamines. We are not going into great detail about antihistamines in this book because they are not usually important in the treatment of asthma and are discussed in books on allergies.

Iodides

Another class of drugs is the iodides. It is not known how they work, but they can be very effective. Potassium iodide (SSKI) is a liquid usually recommended in a dosage of five to ten drops three times a day for adults. Side effects include the suppression of thyroid activity, skin rashes, an irritated stomach, and swollen salivary glands. If one develops an underactive thyroid, the drug is usually stopped and often not resumed.

Corticosteroids

I am presenting the next class of drugs, the cortisone drugs, also called steroids, last because they are used when all else seems to fail. These drugs are always used in conjunction with other medications.

It is important for you to remember that help for the asthmatic lies in the proper functioning of the adenyl cyclase enzyme cycle; in asthma, this cycle does not function well. Under certain conditions (for instance, when you have an infection) or at certain times, possibly during an acute attack, adenyl cyclase appears to be completely inactive, as if its action is blocked. The corticosteroids have the unique ability to break through this blockade and get the adenyl cyclase system working again to stimulate the production of CAMP.

There are many types of cortisone that are not always interchangeable. The types that I prefer to use are Prednisone and Medrol. These are short-acting, have few side effects, and lend themselves to use on an alternate-day basis, which is important and will be elaborated upon later. Decadron, Celestone, and Aristocort are longer-acting drugs and have limitations. Cortisone also comes in a spray form as beclomethasone (Vanceril and Beclovent), as triamcinolone Acetonide (Azmacort), and as flunisolide (AeroBid). These sprays have a great deal to offer the asthmatic. They will be discussed later.

SHORT-TERM USE

The majority of asthmatics can be treated very well on a combination of the medications I have previously described. However, there are specific times when symptoms seem out of control for reasons that are not always obvious. At these times I recommend a short "burst" of cortisone. For example, if you develop a bad infection or have an acute attack, your doctor may use a high dose of cortisone (for instance, forty to sixty milligrams of Prednisone a day for three or four days). Then he will either tell you to stop the drug abruptly, or taper down over a few more days. If you find yourself in this position a few times each year, it is all right. There are always side effects from cortisone, but when used in short bursts, the side effects are minimized. Using cortisone on a short-term basis is effective in relieving the acute symptoms, allowing you to function, and even preventing hospitalization.

LONG-TERM USE

Some asthmatics are plagued by symptoms that are chronic enough and severe enough to require cortisone drugs on a very regular basis. If you need to take cortisone on a long-term basis, there are several things you should know.

First, the way to keep your body functioning as normally as possible is to take cortisone every other day, preferably every other morning, to minimize the side effects. Cortisone drugs suppress the normal secretion of the adrenal hormones. This is something you want to minimize. If you take cortisone every day you are, in effect, telling your body that it does not have to do its normal job of producing its own cortisone.

Now there is no choice between taking the long-acting or the short-acting (Medrol and Prednisone) forms of cortisone. The longer-acting drugs (Decadron, Celestone, and Aristocort) inhibit your body's normal hormone secretion for too long a time. The only way to go is to take the short-acting drugs on an alternate-day basis.

The second thing to know about taking steroids, is that the adverse side effects are minimized if the entire dose is taken early in the morning. The morning is the best time to supplement the body's cortisone production. Introducing cortisone at any other time gives the body a false signal that confuses and suppresses the cycle.

The starting dosage of a cortisone drug to be used over a long period of time varies, depending upon the severity of your symptoms. With the understanding that cortisone is always used with other medications, our goal is to keep you comfortable and functioning well. Forty milligrams of Prednisone every other day is a reasonable dosage. This may sound like a lot, but it really isn't because forty milligrams every other day may cause fewer side effects than ten to twenty milligrams of Prednisone every day. Once again, your symptoms will be the best guide. If, for example, you are quite symptomatic on the day you are not taking cortisone, or even on the night before your next dose, the every-other-day dosage may need to be raised (or in some cases, extended to a short burst of everyday doses). You must tell your doctor how you are doing.

Once you are comfortable and functioning well, my strategy is gradually to reduce your dosage to the least amount of cortisone that keeps your asthma under control. You will have to rely on your doctor's judgment for prescribing the appropriate amount of cortisone. Doses too small to control symptoms are not helpful, and doses in excess will produce unnecessary side effects.

SIDE EFFECTS OF CORTISONE

If it weren't for the side effects of corticosteroids, this might be "the" magic potion. But there are serious, long-range side effects that make this drug the last one to try and the first one to eliminate.

Corticosteroids, then, are not to be used lightly, but when they are necessary, use them. An alternate-day dosage helps reduce or eliminate side effects when the drugs are used on a long-term basis. When you need the drugs only occassionally in the bursts I have described, it usually does not have many side effects. There may be some sudden weight gain, hunger, swelling from fluid buildup, and loss of potassium. A potassium supplement may be taken, especially if your doctor prescribed a diuretic to reduce the swelling that may also cause a loss in potassium.

Long-term use of corticosteroids in children (even when the proper precautions are taken) causes reduction in growth. In children and adults, cortisone tends to produce cataracts, ulcers, nutritional deficiencies that lead to loss of bone substance, muscle weakness, striated and thin skin, the masking of infection, and abdominal problems. In addition to the alternate-day dose, there are steps to be taken to minimize each of these side effects.

Eyes: If you are on cortisone on a fairly regular basis, you should have your eyes checked at least once a year for glaucoma and cataracts.

Ulcers: Taking cortisone with food and the use of antacids (when there is stomach discomfort) help reduce the chances of getting an ulcer.

Nutritional Deficiencies: Patients on cortisone should often supplement their diet with calcium and vitamin D. Be sure you discuss with your doctor all of the supplements you are taking, as excess vitamin D and calcium are also dangerous.

Another adverse side effect of the long-term use of cortisone is known as osteoporosis, a loss of calcium in the bone matrix that makes the bone weak and vulnerable to collapse. This can be rather severe especially in older people. Patients on cortisone for a long period of time who develop severe back pain around their spine could have spinal collapse, something to be taken seriously. There are new calcium fluoride medications available for patients with severe osteoporosis. Consult your physician.

If the loss of potassium becomes significant, you may feel weak, tired, lethargic, and experience muscle cramping. If this is not controlled, you can also develop a cardiac arrhythmia that could be serious indeed. Therefore, your doctor may want you to have your potassium levels monitored by a blood test. Depending on your blood potassium level, your physician will advise you either to take a potassium supplement or increase your intake of potassium-containing food.

There are several varieties of potassium supplements, such as K-Lyte/Cl and Klorvess. They are to be taken by dissolving them in four ounces of cold water and swallowing them. Klorvess has no coloring and may be used by those who are allergic to food coloring. Potassium can be irritating to the stomach and should always be taken after meals. For those of you who cannot tolerate the potassium supplements, Slow-K (a coated tablet that bypasses the stomach and goes on into the small intestine where it is absorbed) is recommended. It, too, has side effects, and therefore, I do not recommend it unless my patient can absolutely not tolerate potassium in any other way.

Some foods that contain potassium are dates, figs, peaches, dried apricots, tomato juice, blackstrap molasses, peanuts, raisins, flounder, bananas, baked potatoes, sunflower seeds, oranges, orange juice, and cranberry juice.

Cortisone tends to mask signs of infection and suppress fever. Patients often tell me that they feel as if they had a fever of 102 degrees, but they don't register this on the thermometer. There is also a tendency for cortisone to mask abdominal problems. If you have the least suspicion that you have an infection or if you are vomiting or having diarrhea or stomach pain of any type, notify your doctor.

AN AGREEABLE ALTERNATIVE

Fortunately, another way of taking cortisone is now available. There are four sprays that are inhaled—Vanceril, Beclovent, Azmacort, and AeroBid. Vanceril and Beclovent contain beclomethasone clathrate, nonabsorbable cortisone in a crystalline form that you breathe into your lungs. The cortisone crystals are not absorbed into your body until they exceed a certain dose. Azmacort contains triamcinolone acetonide, a slightly different compound which may work for those who cannot tolerate Vanceril or Beclovent. Azmacort comes with its own spacer device. You can therefore have the benefits of a fairly high dosage of steroids without the side effects of the oral medication. Beclovent and Vanceril have been used for about ten years, and there seem to be no severe side effects. We will have to wait and see if there are any side effects farther down the road.

The typical dose for these sprays is two sprays four times a day. You can go up to four sprays, four times a day with minimal absorption, and therefore, minimal to no systemic side effects. However, two sprays four times a day is the top dose that probably does not produce side effects in a child less than twelve years old.

AeroBid is a flunisolide spray. It is supposedly more potent than the other sprays and is used twice a day. Start with two sprays twice a day and go to four sprays twice a day, if needed. Children six to fifteen years of age should not exceed two sprays twice a day. I do not find that AeroBid is any better than the other three sprays, and AeroBid's terrible taste is a severe drawback. All of the sprays can be used twice a day in patients with mild asthma.

These drugs are meant to be used on a daily basis for the

chronic patient. They are useless during an acute attack because they cannot get to the absorbing surface of the lung because of the mucus produced. Other, more potent steroid sprays may be available in the future. The increased potencies of these drugs will significantly reduce the number of times a severe asthmatic will have to spray each day. It is also hoped that these drugs will enable the patient to reduce or eliminate the dosage of oral steroid medications.

It is tempting when you feel great on Vanceril (Beclovent or Azmacort) to stop taking the oral cortisone. Although this is an eventual goal, it must not be done suddenly; *this has been fatal in some patients. You must taper your dose of oral cortisone very, very slowly.* This allows your adrenal cycle to adjust. While you are reducing your dosage of oral cortisone according to your doctor's orders, you may experience some melancholia and some general achiness. Be prepared. Oral cortisone may give you a false "high" feeling and coming off of it may give you a real "low" for a while.

CORTISONE IN SPECIAL SITUATIONS

As I have mentioned, steroids suppress the adrenal gland. Cortisone taken orally every day is most suppressive; every-other-day oral dosages are less suppressive; and cortisone sprays are the least suppressive. This suppression may last anywhere from three to eighteen months after cortisone is discontinued. Therefore, your adrenal system is not going to work for you efficiently, especially when it is needed in some special situations.

During surgery, emergency medical care, or even some dental work, you depend upon the adrenal glands to work quickly to produce protective hormones. Suppressed adrenal glands will not do this and they must be supplemented. You must inform whoever is in charge of your medical or dental care that you are taking or have taken cortisone, your dose, and how long you have been taking it. If your adrenal gland is not functioning, you must get additional steroids or death can result.

If you have taken more than about 10 milligrams of Prednisone per day (Medrol—8 milligrams, Decadron—1.5 milligrams,

Celestone—1.2 milligrams, and Aristocort—10 milligrams) for more than a week, or for ten nonconsecutive days in any month, or use any of the steroid sprays on a regular basis, then you are considered steroid dependent. The degree of dependency and therefore the need for supplementary cortisone has to be determined by your physician. Most patients who use steroid sprays are not steroid dependent unless they have used systemic steroids in the last eighteen months. However, steroid dependency in these individuals is related to dose and medical status. Once again check with your own physician. Therefore, if you are cortisone dependent, you must carry a card in your wallet. Write your present dose, the length of your treatment, and your doctor's name and telephone number. You should add any significant allergies, especially drug allergies.

The reason for this is that you have the ability to tell your doctor or dentist about your need for cortisone prior to surgery or dental treatment. You will not be able to do this if you are injured or unconscious in a car accident. Ask your doctor about a Medic-Alert bracelet. This identifies you, your medications and special needs, and your doctor. The Medic-Alert bracelet can be obtained by writing to Medic-Alert, P.O. Box 1009, Turlock, California 95381-1009.

I may have made steroids sound like horrible and dangerous drugs. They are quite effective, but their effectiveness costs! Prednisone is a small, white pill, usually much less expensive than other asthma drugs. It may be ironic that such a little, innocent-looking pill can be so helpful and yet so harmful at the same time. Use it when it is needed and appropriate, but strive to reduce the dose of steroids to the lowest possible level (preferably zero) so long as you are comfortable and functioning well.

NEW DRUGS

Atrovent (ipratropium bromide) has been found to be useful in some mild and moderate asthmatics, and not as helpful with severe patients. It comes in a spray form and is used as a maintenance therapy for bronchial asthma and never for the acute attack. I do not use it alone because albuterol (Proventil and Ventolin), theophylline, or cromolyn sodium (Intal) are so much better. I use it in combination with other drugs.

TAO (troleandomycin) is an antibiotic, but not a very good one. Thirty years ago it was noticed by scientists at the National Jewish Hospital that very severe asthmatics who were also on Medrol (a steroid), when treated for infection with TAO, became miraculously better. They soon discovered that the improvement had nothing to do with the antibiotic effect of TAO, but rather with its ability to enhance the effects of Medrol without the side effects. Unfortunately, TAO is toxic to the liver, which created a stumbling block to its use. Scientists at the National Asthma Center discovered that smaller doses of TAO are effective and not toxic. Therefore, for severe asthmatics who cannot come off daily doses of steroids, TAO may be an answer.

Methotrexate is a drug used in treating cancer, arthritis, and other illnesses. It has recently been found to be useful in allowing the dose of Prednisone to be lowered in certain asthmatics. This drug needs further study before it becomes widely used, but it is promising.

Gold is a drug used in treating rheumatoid arthritis. An oral form of this drug was recently invented and also appears promising in allowing steroids to be tapered in certain asthmatics. It, too, needs further study.

Sample of Drug Treatment Regimens

In my effort to carefully explain each drug separately, we run the risk of losing sight of my overall plan of attack for individual situations. What follows is a sampling of several drug treatment regimens which I recommend. These are applicable to the ''average'' asthmatic, i.e., one between the ages of ten and sixty, who is healthy, not pregnant, and not lactating. I am also assuming that the proper laboratory and allergy workup has been done.

The first type of patient is well most of the time but has some intermittent attacks. I usually start this patient on albuterol spray and tell him to use it whenever he gets an attack. I only suggest this to a patient who gets a few spasms a week and is always completely relieved by the spray. This type of patient often has mild exercise-induced asthma and is instructed to use the spray prophylactically. This is the mildest form of asthma.

A similar type of patient to the one above has few attacks that are easily handled by albuterol spray, unless he gets an upper respiratory infection. At that time his whole world falls apart and he can be sick for weeks. This type of patient requires the early use of theophylline, antibiotics, steroid sprays, and even short, high doses of steroids. He needs to be on theophylline and sympathomimetic sprays and probably steroid sprays for at least several weeks after the upper respiratory infection because his lungs are unstable after this type of attack. This is very important because if the medicine is stopped prematurely, he will have more attacks. The patient is instructed to continue to take the sprays and theophylline for at least two to four weeks after the attack. It varies from patient to patient. Incidentally the resultant lung instability may be present in many different types of patients and one must be constantly alert to it.

The next gradation of patient is one who has mild wheezing all of the time. The first thing I try is the albuterol spray on a regular basis. If this prevents the problem and returns the pulmonary functions to normal, then this is the only treatment I use. If there is an infectious element whenever a URI (upper respiratory infection) occurs, I treat in the same manner as in the case of a patient with infection-induced asthma.

The next step is the same patient who is not completely controlled on albuterol spray alone and needs something extra, although his uncontrolled attacks are not severe. In this case I have three choices. Most likely I would start him on a long-acting theophylline, such as Slo-Bid or Theo-Dur, while continuing the albuterol spray. I would increase the dose of theophylline (as described on page 150), until either the patient got toxic symptoms because his serum theophylline level became too high, or the problem was under control. In this scenario we will assume the problem is under control.

The next option would be to add Intal spray. If the symptoms were not too severe, I would add two sprays of Intal four times a day to be used after two sprays of albuterol. Since it can take several weeks for Intal to work, I might have to use theophylline in the meantime. However, if the patient improved, I would withdraw the theophylline. If the patient continued to have no difficulty, I would keep him on the albuterol-Intal combination. If he got worse when the theophylline was withdrawn, I would know that it was the theophylline that was helpful and withdraw the Intal. In rare cases the patient will get worse again, and then I know it was a combination of the Intal and theophylline that was effective, and I would maintain the patient on albuterol, Intal, and theophylline. However, in this example, we will assume the Intal worked with the albuterol and that is what our patient will be maintained on.

The next option would be to add Atrovent spray. I rarely do this, but in some cases the combination works and I would maintain the patient on the combination of the two sprays (albuterol and Atrovent).

From the above three examples you can see that in the group of patients that I call mild to moderate, most of the treatment is a combination of two to three medications, all of which have minor side effects. If one combination doesn't work, I try another and sometimes come up with a combination of all three. I favor the Intal-albuterol combination or Intal alone, if I can get away with it, because Intal has the least side effects of all the other medications used for asthma. Incidentally, we have now covered the needs of approximately two-thirds of all the asthmatic patients.

Now we get to the group that I call moderate asthma. In this group the above measures are not fully effective. Here I continue to use whatever combination of medication appears to work, and I add a steroid spray to the patient's regimen. I start with two sprays four times a day and will go as high as five sprays four times a day to control the symptoms. If this works, I will reduce the steroid spray to the lowest level that keeps the patient comfortable. This type of patient very often has breakthrough attacks that may require the use of systemic steroids on an intermittent basis. I have discussed the principles of how I use steroids in this fashion, but here it is again. I advise the patient to take 1–2 milligrams/kilogram per day (not to exceed 60 milligrams per day) or 40 to 60 milligrams per day for two to three days; and then I have the patient reduce the dose by 10 milligrams a day trying to discontinue the steroids in one week. I have the patient continue his other medications and certainly continue it after the steroids are withdrawn. In most patients, a few courses of steroids a year are all they need. However, there are patients who are on oral cortisone drugs more than they are off them. This small group of patients constitutes the severe class.

In the severe patient the above measures do not work and we must add oral steroids to the other medications. I normally start with a burst of steroids and then find the level that controls my patient. I then double the dose on one day and continue the controlling dose on the next day. I will use hypothetical dosages here for the sake of clarity. Let's suppose I controlled my patient's asthma completely at 15 milligrams per day. If I attempted to go lower than that, the patient would have symptoms. Once he is stable I would give him 30 milligrams the first day and 15 milligrams the second day; 30 the third and 15 the fourth, 30, 10, 30, 10, 30, 5, 30, 5, 30, 2.5, 30, 2.5 and then 30 milligrams of Prednisone every other day. Once the alternate dose is established, I will then try to find the lowest possible dose that will control his symptoms. If I can keep the patient on 10 milligrams or less of everyday Prednisone, I do not bother with alternate-day dosing. The patient is instructed to take the medication upon awakening preferably before 8:00 A.M., every other morning. On the occasions he has an attack, he can take an extra dose or go on everyday dosage for a few days and then quickly come back to alternate-day dosage.

We've now taken care of 95 percent of the asthmatic population. The last 5 percent need everyday Prednisone, and if I can't keep the dose below 20 milligrams a day I try low dose TAO or possibly send them to an asthma center for further evaluation.

Summary

I have spent a great deal of time informing you about the management of asthma with medication. You must be knowledgeable so that you and your doctor can work together. Do not use the information in this chapter to self-medicate! Use it to be an effective member of the team.

An effective drug program is part of an overall program to identify the triggers of your asthma and to reduce or eliminate their ill effects whenever possible. Your doctor, with your help, designs this program and you must understand it and monitor it, evaluating successes and failures. Don't alter the drug program without your doctor's knowledge and approval. Do not play with over-the-counter drugs. Ask about the long- and short-term side effects of each drug and get specific recommendations on how to administer them. Learn what to expect from each drug. Go home, follow the plan, and monitor your body's reactions. Keep a written record.

If you are being treated by another physician for a nonasthma problem, tell him what drugs you are taking and ask if any drugs he is prescribing may either be incompatible with your condition or may interact adversely with your medications. Do not assume that he will remember what medications you are on, or even that you are asthmatic. If you are unsure or uneasy about his recommended medications, consult your asthma doctor. At all costs, know yourself and be aware! The magic potion is available and it works well. It is complex and may produce side effects, but when used properly, it is very effective.

The Most Commonly Used Medications in the Treatment of Asthma

COMMERCIAL (GENERIC NAME)	DESCRIPTION	ACTION	INDICATIONS	ADVERSE REACTIONS	DOSAGE AND ADMINISTRATION	PRECAUTIONS, WARNINGS
Aero-Bid	*Metered Dose Inhaler:* 250 mg of flunisolide each activation	Corticosteroid	Patients who require corti-costeroids to con-trol bronchospasm	Bitter taste See Azmacort	*Adults:* 2–4 sprays twice a day *Children (6–15):* 2 sprays twice daily	See Azmacort
Alupent (metaproterenol sulfate)	*Tablets:* 10 or 20 mg *Metered Dose Inhaler:* 0.65 mg per actuation *Syrup:* 10 mg/ 5 ml *Inhalant Solution for nebulization:* 5% or 0.6%	Bronchodilator	Relief of Reversible Bronchospasm	Nervousness, tachycardia (fast heart rate) tremor, nausea, hypertension (high blood pressure)	*Tablets:* *Adults:* 20 mg 3–4 times a day *Children 6–9 years:* 10 mg 3–4 times a day *Children over 9 years:* Adult dose *Syrup:* See tablets *Metered Dose Inhaler:* *Adults and Children 12 years and older:* 2–3 inhalations every 3–4 hours (maximum 12/day)	Contraindicated in arrhythmias, (irreg-ular heartbeat); caution in hyper-tension, coronary artery disease, hy-perthyroidism, or diabetes

					Inhalant Solution 5%: Adults and Children 12 years and older: via compressed air nebulizer. 0.2 ml to 0.3 ml diluted in 2.5 ml of saline solution or other diluent 3–4 times a day *Inhalant Solution 0.6%* Each 2.5 ml vial is equivalent to 0.3 ml 5% solution in 2.5 cc diluent	
Aminophyllin (aminophylline) (not recommended by me)	Each tablet contains 100 mg or 200 mg aminophylline dihydrate which contains 85% theophylline anhydrous by weight (short-acting)	Bronchodilator	Relief of Reversible Bronchospasm	GI distress, irritability, seizures, arrhythmias	See Slo-Phyllin	See Slo-Phyllin

COMMERCIAL (GENERIC NAME)	DESCRIPTION	ACTION	INDICATIONS	ADVERSE REACTIONS	DOSAGE AND ADMINISTRATION	PRECAUTIONS, WARNINGS
Atrovent (ipratropium bromide)	18 mg of ipratropium bromide per inhalation	Anticholinagic	Bronchodilator for maintenance treatment (never for the acute attack. More useful in chronic obstructive pulmonary disease than in asthma	Palpitations, nervousness, dizziness, headache, rash, nausea, vomiting, tremor, blurred vision, dry mouth, cough	2 inhalations 4 times a day for adults; not indicated for children. Maximum 12 inhalations per day	Should be used with caution in narrow-angle glaucoma, prostatic hypertrophy, or bladder-neck obstruction. Also, caution not to spray in eye which causes temporary blurring of vision
Azmacort (triamcinolone acetonide)	Each inhalation delivers 100 mg triamcinolone acetonide	Corticosteroid	Patients who require corticosteroids to control bronchospasm Patients who require a spacer	Sore throat, adrenal suppression, candida, rarely increased wheezing, cough, facial edema	*Adults:* 2 inhalations 2–4 times a day. Maximum 16 inhalations per day *Children 6–12 years:* 1–2 inhalations 3–4 times a day	Caution in transferring steroid dependent asthmatics due to risk of adrenal insufficiency. Monitor patients for HPA suppression, dry mouth, oral thrush, hoarseness

Beclovent (beclomethasone diproprionate)	Each inhalation delivers 42 mg beclomethasone diproprionate	Corticosteroid	Patients who require corticosteroids to control bronchospasm	See Azmacort	*Adults:* 2 inhalations 3–4 times a day Maximum 20 inhalations per day *Children 6–12 years:* 1–2 inhalations 3–4 times a day. Maximum 10 inhalations per day	See Azmacourt
Brethaire (terbutaline sulfate)	Each inhalation delivers 0.2 mg of terbutaline	See Proventil	First choice for inhaled bronchodilator during pregnancy See Proventil	See Proventil	2 inhalations repeated every 4–6 hours	See Proventil
Brethine (terbutaline sulfate)	*Tablets:* 5 or 2.5 mg terbutaline sulfate *Injections:* 2 ml ampules 1 mg/ml	Bronchodilator	Reversible Bronchospasm	Nervousness, fast heart rate, tremor, nausea, high blood pressure	*Tablets:* *Adults:* 2.5–5 mg 3 times a day *Children 12–15 years:* 2.5 mg T. I. D. *Injection:* 0.25 mg injected subcutaneously into lateral deltoid area. Second dose may be administered in 15–30 minutes. Maximum dose is 0.5 mg within a four-hour period	Contraindicated in irregular heartbeats, caution in high blood pressure, coronary artery disease, hyperthyroidism, or diabetes

COMMERCIAL (GENERIC NAME)	DESCRIPTION	ACTION	INDICATIONS	ADVERSE REACTIONS	DOSAGE AND ADMINISTRATION	PRECAUTIONS, WARNINGS
Bricanyl (terbutaline sulfate)	See Brethine	Bronchodilator	Reversible Bronchospasm	See Brethine	See Brethine	See Brethine
Choledyl (oxtriphylline)	Each tablet contains 200 mg or 100 mg oxtriphylline. Each tsp. of the elixir contains 100 mg in ethanol 20% (Short-acting) *Pediatric Syrup:* 50 mg/5 ml (Short-acting)	Bronchodilator	Bronchitis, bronchial asthma, asthmatic bronchitis, pulmonary emphysema, or similar chronic obstructive lung disease. Produces slightly less gastric distress than other xanthines. Rarely used today	Gastric distress, palpitations, CNS stimulation (agitation)	See Slo-Phyllin	See Slo-Phyllin
	S.A. Tablets: 400 or 600 mg oxtriphylline (Long-acting) (100 mg oxtriphylline is equivalent to 64 mg anhydrous theophylline)				See Slo-Bid	See Slo-Bid

Constant-T	Scored sustained release tablets contain 200 mg or 300 mg anhydrous theophylline (Long-acting)	Bronchodilator	Reversible Bronchospasm	GI distress, palpitations, CNS stimulation (agitation)	See Slo-Bid	See Slo-Bid
Elixophyllin	*Elixir:* contains 80 mg anhydrous theophylline in 20% ethanol per 15 ml tablespoon	Bronchodilator	Reversible Bronchospasm	GI distress, irritability, seizures, arrhythmias	See Slo-Phyllin	See Slo-Phyllin
	Capsules: contain 100 mg or 200 mg anhydrous theophylline (Short-acting)					
	S.R. Capsules: contain 125 mg or 250 mg anhydrous theophylline (Intermediate)				See Slo-Phyllin SR	See Slo-Phyllin SR
	GG Liquid: 15 ml contains 100 mg anhydrous theophylline and 100 mg guaifenesin (Short-acting)				See Slo-Phyllin	See Slo-Phyllin

COMMERCIAL (GENERIC NAME)	DESCRIPTION	ACTION	INDICATIONS	ADVERSE REACTIONS	DOSAGE AND ADMINISTRATION	PRECAUTIONS, WARNINGS
Intal-capsules (by Fison) (Cromolyn sodium)	Each capsule contains 20 mg cromolyn sodium	Inhibits the degranulation of sensitized mast cells. Inhibits the release of histamine and other mediators	Cough, wheeze, throat irritation, bad taste, nausea, allergic rashes (side effects are rare)	Adjunctive therapy in the management of patients with bronchial asthma and to prevent exercise-induced asthma (side effects are rare)	For inhalation only: *Adults and children 5 years and older:* 1 capsule 4 times daily at regular intervals with its inhaler. One capsule inhaled approximately 15 minutes before exercise	Hypersensitivity to cromolyn. Has no role in the treatment of an acute attack of asthma. Use with caution in patients with impaired renal or hepatic functions
Intal nebulized liquid (by Fison5) (cromolyn sodium)	Each ampule contains 20 mg cromolyn sodium in 2 ml purified water for inhalation	See Intal capsules	See Intal capsules	See Intal capsules	1 ampule nebulized 4 times a day	See Intal capsules
Intal spray (by Fison5) (cromolyn sodium)	Each metered spray delivers 800 mcg of cromolyn sodium	See Intal capsules	See Intal capsules	See Intal capsules	2 sprays 4 times a day or 2 sprays 15 minutes prior to exercise	See Intal capsules

Marax (Not recommended by me)	*Tablet:* Contains Atarax (hydroxyzine HC1) 10 mg; ephedrine sulfate 25 mg.; theophylline 130 mg. *Syrup:* Each 5 cc. contains Atarax 2.5 mg.; ephedrine sulfate 6.25 mg. theophylline 32.5 mg.	Bronchodilator	Acute attack of bronchial asthma and in the prophylactic therapy of the disease	Drowsiness, excitation, tremulousness, insomnia, nervousness, palpitation, rapid heart rate, tachycardia, vertigo, dryness of nose and throat, headache, sweating precordial pain (chest pain), cardiac arrhythmias	*Oral: Tablet:* *Adults:* 1 tablet 2 to 4 times daily *Children over 5 years:* ½ adult dose *Syrup: Children over 5:* 1 tsp 3 to 4 times daily *Children 2–5 years:* ½ to 1 tsp 3 to 4 times daily *Children under 2:* Not recommended	Use with caution in patients with enlarged prostrate. Caution patients against driving or operating machinery if drowsiness occurs. Contraindicated in patients with hypertension, cardiac disease, hyperthyroidism, diabetes. Contraindicated in pregnancy
Metaprel (metaproterenol sulfate)	*Tablets:* contain 10 or 20 mg (scored) *Syrup:* 5 ml. contains 10 mg *Metered Dose Inhaler:* Delivers 0.65 mg per inhalation	Bronchodilator	Reversible Bronchospasm	Tachycardia (rapid heart rate), tremor, agitation	*Syrup and Tablets:* *Adults:* 20 mg 3 or 4 times daily *Children over 9 years:* 20 mg 3 or 4 times daily *Metered Dose Inhaler:* 2–3 inhalations every 3–4 hours (maximum 12 per day)	See Alupent

COMMERCIAL (GENERIC NAME)	DESCRIPTION	ACTION	INDICATIONS	ADVERSE REACTIONS	DOSAGE AND ADMINISTRATION	PRECAUTIONS, WARNINGS
					Inhalant Solution: Hand Bulb Nebulizer: 10 inhalations 3–4 times a day *Compressed Air Nebulizer:* 0.3 ml diluted in 2.5 cc normal saline 3–4 times a day	
Primatene (Not recommended by me: over-the-counter. Use only if recommended by a phvsician.)	*Mist:* Delivers 0.2 mg epinephrine per inhalation *Mist Suspension:* Delivers 0.3 mg epinephrine bitartrate (equivalent to 0.16 mg epinephrine base) per inhalation	Bronchodilator	Bronchial Asthma	Bronchial irritation, insomnia, agitation, GI distress (for oral tablets)	*Mist and Mist Suspension:* 1–2 inhalations every 4 hours. Only use this product with a physician's advice	Use with caution in patients with hyperthyroidism, hypertension, (high blood pressure), acute coronary disease (heart disease), and cardiac asthma

	Tablets (P Formula): theophylline 130 mg, ephedrine HCL 24 mg, phenobarbitol 8 mg *Tablets (M Formula):* Pyrilamine maleate 16.6 mg is substituted for phenobarbitol				*Tablets:* *Adults:* 1 every 4 hours *Children-(6–12):* One-half above	Use with caution in presence of cardiovascular disease, severe hypertension, hyperthyroidism, prostrate hypertrophy (enlarged prostrate), glaucoma (Also has antihistamine)
Proventil (by Schering) (albuterol)	*Inhaler:* Each spray delivers 90 mcg albuterol	Bronchodilator	Relief of reversible bronchospasm, prevention of exercise-induced asthma	Nervousness, tachycardia (rapid heart rate), tremor, nausea, hypertension (high blood pressure)	*Inhaler:* *Adults and children over 12 years:* 2 inhalations every 4–6 hours	Contraindicated in arrhythmias (irregular heartbeats), caution in hypertension (high blood pressure), coronary artery disease, hyperthyroidism or diabetes

COMMERCIAL (GENERIC NAME)	DESCRIPTION	ACTION	INDICATIONS	ADVERSE REACTIONS	DOSAGE AND ADMINISTRATION	PRECAUTIONS, WARNINGS
	Tablets: (short-acting) contains 2 mg or 4 mg albuterol as the sulfate salt			*Tablets:* (short-acting) *Adults and children over 12 years:* 2–4 mg 3 to 4 times a day (maximum 32 mg a day)		
	Tablets-Repetabs (long-acting): 4 mg tablets			*Tablets-Repetabs* (long-acting): *Adults and children over 12 years:* 1–2 tablets every 12 hours maximum 3–4 tablets a day		
	Syrup: 2 mg in 1 teaspoon			*Syrup: Adults and children over 14 years:* 1–2 tsp 3–4 times a day (maximum 4 tsp 4 times a day) *Children 6–14 years:* 1 tsp 3–4 times a day		

	Children 2–6 years: 0.1 mg/kg of body weight 3 times a day for starting dose. Starting dose not to exceed 2 mg (1 tsp) 3 times a day. If necessary dosage is sometimes increased to 0.2 mg/kg 3 times a day not to exceed 4 mg (2 tsp) 3 times a day
Nebulized liquid: Ready to use bottles or a solution prepared by mixing a 0.5% solution with normal saline solution	*Nebulized liquid: Adults and children over 12 years:* 1 ready to use bottle for nebulization, 3–4 times a day or a solution prepared by adding 2.5 ml of normal saline solution to 0.25 ml–10.5 ml of the 0.5% solution, nebulized 3–4 times daily

COMMERCIAL (GENERIC NAME)	DESCRIPTION	ACTION	INDICATIONS	ADVERSE REACTIONS	DOSAGE AND ADMINISTRATION	PRECAUTIONS, WARNINGS
					Children: (6–12 years): 2.5 ml of saline mixed with 0.25 ml of the 0.5% solution, nebulized 3–4 times daily *Children (4–6* years): 2.5 ml of saline solution mixed with 0.2 ml of the 0.5% solution, nebulized 3–4 times daily *Children (2–4* years): 2.5 ml of saline solution mixed with 0.15 ml of the 0.5% solution nebulized 3–4 times daily	
Quibron-T	Immediate release tablets each contain 300 mg anhydrous theophylline. Tablets are scored to deliver 100–300 mg in 50 mg increments	Bronchodilator	See Slo-Phyllin	See Slo-Phyllin	See Slo-Phyllin	See Slo-Phyllin

Quibron-TSR	300 mg anhydrous theophylline (sustained released) 300 mg can be divided into 100, 150, 200, and 300 mg sections	Bronchodilator	See Slo-Bid	See Slo-Bid	See Slo-Bid	See Slo-Bid
Slo-Bid	Bead-filled with sustained release capsules that contain 50 mg, 100 mg, 200 mg or 300 mg anhydrous theophylline (Long-acting)	Bronchodilator	Reversible Bronchospasm (not usually indicated in an acute attack)	GI distress, irritability, seizures, arrhythmias	*Adults and Children over 12 years:* (Starting dose): 8 mg/kg every 12 hours not to exceed 200 mg every 12 hours. Increase by 25% for 3 day intervals up to 800 mg in a 24-hour period (at that point a blood level is needed)	*Note: When used properly, most side effects do not occur, but you can see why we suggest measuring theophylline so carefully 1. Blood levels should always be obtained to make sure the appropriate amount of theophylline is being administered

COMMERCIAL (GENERIC NAME)	DESCRIPTION	ACTION	INDICATIONS	ADVERSE REACTIONS	DOSAGE AND ADMINISTRATION	PRECAUTIONS, WARNINGS
Slo-Phyllin SR Gyrocaps	*Gyrocaps:* 60 mg, 125 mg and 250 mg (bead-filled) (intermediate-acting)	Bronchodilator	Reversible Bronchospasm (usually used in an acute attack when patient is not taking theophylline)	Gastric irritation, nausea, vomiting, CNS (central nervous system) agitation, arrhythmias (irregular heartbeat)	(Starting dose) 2.4 mg per pound of body weight given every 8 hours, not to exceed 125 mg per dose or 375 mg per day. Higher doses are used in some patients (consult your physician)	2. Cimetidine, erythromycin, troleendomycin, influenza vaccine, acute viral illness, smoking, and marijuana can raise the level of theophylphylline in the blood resulting in toxicity 3. Use with caution in patients with congestive heart failure, liver disease, and peptic ulcers
Slo-Phyllin	100 mg and 200 mg tablets and 80 mg/15 ml anhydrous theophylline (Short-acting)	Bronchodilator	Reversible Bronchospasm (usually used in an acute attack when patient is not taking theophylline)	Gastric irritation, nausea, vomiting, CNS (central nervous system) agitation, arrhythmias (irregular heartbeat)	Starting dose: 1.8 mg /pound of body weight given every 4–6 hours, not to exceed 100 mg per dose or 400 mg per day. Higher doses can be used in some patients. (Consult your doctor)	4. Sustained release preparations must not be crushed. Some can be halved, but never quartered. Always check with your physician or PDR concerning handling of these pills or capsules

						5. Food can decrease absorption of sustained release preparations. High protein, low carbohydrate diets can reduce the level of theophylline significantly. The converse is also true 6. Too much theophylline can cause irregular heart rate which can be dangerous, nausea, vomiting, stomach irritation, and convulsions and death. This is why we suggest careful measurement of the theophylline level
Somophyllin	*Liquid:* 105 mg aminophylline per 5 ml. (Short-acting)	Bronchodilator	Reversible Bronchospasm	See Slo-Phyllin	See Slo-Phyllin	See Slo-Phyllin

COMMERCIAL (GENERIC NAME)	DESCRIPTION	ACTION	INDICATIONS	ADVERSE REACTIONS	DOSAGE AND ADMINISTRATION	PRECAUTIONS, WARNINGS
	DF: Dye Free, 105 mg aminophylline per 5 ml (Short-acting)					
	T-Capsules: 100 mg anhydrous theophylline (immediate release-Short-acting)					
SusPhrine	Each cc contains epinephrine 1:200	Bronchodilator	Reversible Bronchospasm (Long-acting)	Anxiety, restlessness, tremor, headache, dizziness, pallor, respiratory weakness, palpitations	*Parenteral:* *Adults:* 0.1 to 0.3 cc subcutaneously Dose in *Children* should not exceed 0.15 cc *Children 2–12 years:* 0.005 cc/kg s.c. Dosage should not be administered more frequently than Q 6H. Maximum dose should not exceed 0.15 cc	Contraindicated in cerebral arteriosclerosis, shock, organic heart disease. Administer with caution to patients with bronchial asthma of long standing

Tedral (Not recommended by me)	*Tablets or Suspension:* Contain 118 mg theophylline; 24 mg. ephedrine HCl and phenobarbital 8 mg per tablet or 10 ml *SA Tablets:* Sustained action tablets contain 180 mg theophylline, 48 mg ephedrine HCl and 25 mg phenobarbital *Tedral Elixir:* 88.5 mg theophylline, 18 mg ephedrine HCl and 6 mg phenobarbital in 15% ethanol per 15 ml	Bronchodilator	Reversible Bronchospasm	Drowsiness, mild epigastric distress, palpitation, tremulousness, insomnia, difficulty of micturition (urination), CNS (central nervous system) agitation	*Tablets or Suspension (Adults):* 1 or 2 tablets or 10–20 ml Q 4H *SA Tablets (Adults):* are tablet Q 12H *Elixir (Adults):* 15–30 ml Q 4H	Use with caution in presence of cardiovascular disease, severe hypertension, hyperthyroidism, prostrate hypertrophy (enlarged prostrate), glaucoma

COMMERCIAL (GENERIC NAME)	DESCRIPTION	ACTION	INDICATIONS	ADVERSE REACTIONS	DOSAGE AND ADMINISTRATION	PRECAUTIONS, WARNINGS
Theo-24	Each sustained release capsule contains 100 mg, 200 mg, or 300 mg anhydrous theophylline (ultra long-lasting)	Bronchodilator	Reversible Bronchospasm	See Slo-Bid	(Starting Dose) *Adults and children over 75 pounds:* 400 mg *Children 65 to 75 pounds:* 300 mg (Increase every three days after obtaining blood level. In both children and adults, if level is not adequate, the medication is usually increased in 100 mg increments	See Slo-Bid
Theobid	Each sustained release capsule contains 130 mg or 260 mg anhydrous theophylline long-acting	Bronchodilator	Reversible Bronchospasm	See Slo-Bid	See Slo-Bid	See Slo-Bid

Theo-Dur	*Sustained Release Tablets:* contain 100 mg, 200 mg, 300 mg and 450 mg anhydrous theophylline *Sustained Release Sprinkles:* contain 50 mg, 75 mg, 125 mg, and 200 mg anhydrous theophylline	Bronchodilator	Reversible Bronchospasm	See Slo-Bid	See Slo-Bid	See Slo-Bid
Theolair	*Tablets:* 125 mg or 250 mg anhydrous theophylline (short-acting) *Liquid:* 15 ml contains 80 mg anhydrous theophylline (short-acting)	Bronchodilator	Reversible Bronchospasm	See Slo-Phyllin	See Slo-Phyllin	See Slo-Phyllin

COMMERCIAL (GENERIC NAME)	DESCRIPTION	ACTION	INDICATIONS	ADVERSE REACTIONS	DOSAGE AND ADMINISTRATION	PRECAUTIONS, WARNINGS
	SR Tablets: Sustained release tablets which contain 200 mg, 250 mg, 300 mg or 500 mg anhydrous theophylline (intermediate-acting)			See Slo-Phyllin SR	See Slo-Phyllin SR	See Slo-Phyllin SR
Uniphyl	Each sustained release capsule contains 200 mg or 400 mg anhydrous theophylline (ultra long-lasting)	Bronchodilator	Reversible Bronchospasm	See Slo-Bid	(Starting Dose) *Adults and children over 75 pounds:* 400 mg *Children 65 to 75 pounds:* 300 mg (Increase every three days after obtaining blood level. In both children and adults if level is not adequate, the medication is usually increased in 100 mg increments. May	See Slo-Bid

					be useful when taken 1 hour before dinner in preventing early morning bronchospasm	
Vanceril (Beclomethaeone diproportionate)	Each inhalation delivers 42 mg beclamethaeone diproportionate	Corticosteroid	Patients who require corticosteroids to control bronchospasm	See Azmacort	See Azmacort	See Azmacort
Ventolin (by Glaxo) albuterol	Same as Proventil except for repetabs	Bronchodilator	See Proventil	See Proventil	See Proventil	See Proventil

7

CASE STUDIES: BASIC THERAPY APPROACHES IN ACTION

In the previous chapters of this book, I have presented the separate components of my approach to the treatment of an asthmatic patient. Sometimes the patient can be effectively managed by using only one component of the four that I have presented (environment control, drug therapy, immunotherapy, and diet). Typically, more than one component will be utilized. This chapter will present actual case studies to illustrate the application of these treatment approaches. This will help to bring it all together.

You should not expect to find your exact story in these case reports. But you may find certain characteristics that will be applicable to your condition.

I will discuss uncomplicated asthma. I will not discuss very young children or the elderly, nor will I include patients with severe heart disease, emphysema, or any other major medical complications. It would be inappropriate to generalize from these kinds of complicated and atypical cases.

The first meeting with any patient follows a fairly standard procedure that you read about in Chapter 2. To review briefly, a patient fills out a questionnaire designed to obtain a comprehensive medical history and detailed description of his problem. When I see the patient, we review the salient information from the questionnaire supplemented by additional questioning, as needed, to provide me with a complete picture. I then examine the patient, looking for signs of asthma, allergy, or other illnesses. I decide whether additional tests, such as chest X ray, pulmonary functions, RAST, or skin tests, should be ordered. At this point, I can formulate a treatment plan and discuss it with my patient. I will now present a series of cases.

Barbara Z. is a thirty-year-old homemaker who came to see me because she had developed a severe cough and wheezing after she did her laundry. She was perfectly well at other times. This had happened three times, and on the third time she ended up in the emergency room. Adrenalin was required to bring her under control. She cleared up and after a few days she was better. She was then referred to me. She had no allergic history as a child or any family history of allergies. Neither parents, sisters, brothers, nor her two children had any manifestations of allergies in any form. Her only illness was this sudden onset of asthma. Close questioning revealed that Barbara had started using an antiwrinkle substance that is placed in the dryer and gives the wash a refreshing fragrance. This is a great idea, but in rare cases can cause severe asthma. It was not necessary to do any allergy testing on Barbara. I did advise her to get a chest X ray just on the outside chance that something else was happening. I strongly suggested that she stop using that product or any related product. Barbara has been fine ever since. This case illustrates that in sporadic asthma, very often there is something in the environment that can cause the problem. Sometimes just giving a little thought to what you were doing right before your asthma attack gives you the answer to your problem.

Murray K. is a thirty-seven-year-old attorney who lives in New York City. He had spring and fall hay fever as a child and as a young man, but he outgrew it, with the exception of some nasal congestion. He also had some wheezing as a child, but it was never severe. He had allergy shots that appeared to control his symptoms. As an adolescent, these symptoms disappeared. In his late twenties, after completing law school and moving to the city, he noticed that he had difficulty with nasal congestion again, mainly in the spring and fall. Occasionally, if he had a bad cold, he would have some mild wheezing though it didn't bother him. He self-medicates with over-the-counter antihistamines that control his symptoms rather nicely.

Murray, like many city people, had a passion for jogging. Every morning before work he would jog a few miles around the reservoir in Central Park. He began to notice that after jogging he would become extremely short of breath and very uncomfortable. He bought an over-the-counter Adrenalin inhaler that we have already discussed (see Chapter 5). This made his heart race, helping one problem but creating another. Since it is no reward for a part-time athlete to get short of breath after a workout, Murray consulted me. He thought his problem was the shortness of breath, not the nasal congestion. The simplest thing would have been for me to tell Murray, "Well, stop running—try chess and exercise your mind instead." However, running was very important to Murray and I agree that exercise is very important for all of us.

I immediately recognized the phenomenon as exercise-induced dyspnea (shortness of breath) that occurs in certain asthmatic patients. It may occur alone or as part of a constellation of symptoms. It can also occur in a child with hay fever and no asthma symptoms at any other time. What happens is that you do not get short of breath progressively as you exercise, but at a certain point (usually five to eight minutes after exercising strenuously), you become very short of breath. This can be rather debilitating. I felt in Murray's case, since he was thirty-seven years of age, some tests should be done. I did a chest X ray, an EKG, and pulmonary functions, all of which were normal. This assured both of us that a full allergic evaluation was not necessary since the only symptom that was severe was the exercise-induced dyspnea. I gave Murray two alternatives: He could do short sprints or swim instead of jog. When you swim, you breathe in moist air and therefore, you will not get exercise-induced dyspnea that is caused by breathing cold, unhumidified air. I also encouraged him to breathe exclusively through his nose, which would also ease the dyspnea. Murray chose to continue jogging. I taught him how to use cromolyn sodium, which he used fifteen minutes before exercising. In most cases, this will completely block exercise-induced dyspnea providing it is used within two hours of exercising. I cautioned him not to use it once he began to exercise or if he was wheezing. This would make the situation worse. Murray is back jogging and using his medication and has developed no other symptoms. He sees me once a year and we check his pulmonary functions and his X rays. I imagine that he will be jogging well into his sixties.

Barbie L. is a thirty-nine-year-old homemaker who never had any allergies. Her husband was a nonallergic man, but two of their daughters had allergies. The seven-year-old girl had spring hay fever; the nine-year-old girl had intermittent attacks of bronchitis, mostly associated with infection. The third daughter had no problems. Barbie developed a cough that at first was very mild, however, it got progressively worse. At first, she attributed the coughing to being in air-conditioned places, but eventually the cough became more constant. A chest X ray was normal, but an examination of her chest did reveal wheezing. Her internist gave her 250 milligrams of Slo-Phyllin every eight hours, which made her quite nauseated. When the dose was cut to 125 milligrams every eight hours, she did well. Previously, she had been treated with antibiotics that did not help. She was maintained on the Slo-Phyllin for three or four weeks before it was discontinued. The condition disappeared.

Since the episode had lasted only one or two months, and the chest X ray was normal, I did not advise an allergic workup. Baseline pulmonary functions were obtained instead. Barbie was seen the next year during the same period of time and she was symptom-free; two years later she was still symptom-free. She has never had a recurrence of these symptoms. It is impossible to predict that she will never have a problem, but this case illustrates that it is possible to have sporadic asthma that may occur once every twenty or twenty-five years. Until the symptoms become continuous or debilitating, it is not advisable to do a full workup. Barbie should have her pulmonary functions monitored every few years just to make sure that there is no deterioration. She should also have a checkup and a chest X ray every five years. She may never have problems again.

Albert K. is a thirty-four-year-old accountant. Albert had mild ragweed hay fever almost all his life. He lived in the suburbs of New York, on Long Island, and had some problems that were controlled by antihistamines. This particular year he moved into Manhattan with his new bride. Not only did his hay fever become worse, but when the normal hay fever season ended, Albert was still having problems. Not only was he suffering with nasal congestion, but now he had significant wheezing as well. When I examined him, I could hear wheezing. I ordered a chest X ray to make sure there were no other problems like pneumonia. The chest X ray was normal. Pulmonary function tests showed significant breathing impairment caused by the asthma.

Albert admitted that his beloved wife had three cats and they lived in a small apartment. He, of course, felt that the cats were completely blameless, especially since they were his wife's cats. Actually, he was quite fond of them. In this case, I felt that an allergic workup was warranted and we did it. A RAST demonstrated significant reactions to ragweed and molds, which accounted for the hay fever symptoms. It was no surprise to me that his most extreme allergy was to cats. He was placed on 200 milligrams of Theo-Dur every twelve hours, but this did not relieve his symptoms. As we raised his theophylline dose to 300 milligrams every twelve hours, he became quite nauseated. The theophylline level was 9.7 at this dose and not in the therapeutic range (10–20). For Albert, theophylline was useless because he suffered side effects even before we reached a therapeutic level. Albert was started on cromolyn sodium that was much more helpful and he was more comfortable, although he refused to get rid of his cats. He was started on allergy injections to cat, ragweed, and molds and so far has done quite well. However, he needs injections to control his allergy to cats and medication

(Intal) on a regular basis to maintain himself. Although I did not feel that Albert made an appropriate decision, I could not force him to get rid of his cats. Therefore, I had to treat him in the most effective way possible to maintain his health. A sharp contrast can be noted with the next case.

Jim G., a thirty-one-year-old photographer, had mild rhinitis (nasal irritation) most of his life. He had been married for three years and lived in an upstate New York suburb. His wife's vocation was raising dogs. The dogs were kept outside the house, but as puppies they were kept inside. It was then that Jim's symptoms would get worse.

He began having rather significant wheezing and sought my consultation. His chest X ray was normal while pulmonary functions showed definite impairment with obstruction in the breathing pattern. An allergy workup, once again, showed significant allergies to many substances, including pollen, dust, and molds, but an extremely positive reaction to dogs. He was controlled with 400 milligrams of theophylline every twelve hours without significant side effects.

Finally, the dogs were given away and Jim's wife found a new vocation. As their reward, Jim slowly improved over a period of several months, which is the time it takes to dedander a home. I saw him six months after they removed the dogs and he was almost symptom-free. A year later, he was symptom-free with the exception of his mild hay fever. Because Jim removed the dogs, he did not require allergy shots.

What each of these cases has illustrated is that a careful search and removal of factors producing the asthmatic symptoms will very often eliminate the disease. In some cases, the causes are obvious and easy to deal with. When they are simply avoided or removed, it may obviate the need for a prolonged program of hyposensitization or the need for medication.

Sammy T., an eleven-year-old boy who had nasal congestion almost all of his life, is our next case. For the past two years, he had wheezing, mainly in the winter, sometimes associated with infection. His pediatrician controlled his symptoms with 300 milligrams of Theo-Dur every twelve hours. However, his mother was alarmed at the increasing frequency of attacks and the constant nasal congestion. When I first saw Sammy, his appearance was that of an allergic child. He had allergic shiners (dark rings under his eyes) and nasal congestion. His X ray was normal and his pulmonary functions were relatively normal with minimal obstruction in getting the air out. This was compatible with mild asthma.

Careful history revealed that Sammy was a "milkaholic." He loved milk; he consumed four or five glasses a day. In addition, ice cream and cheese were his favorite snacks. In fact, a good deal of his diet was milk and milk products. Therefore, before I did any detailed tests, I discussed with his mother and Sammy the idea of removing milk from Sammy's diet. Sammy was annoyed at first, but he was bright and agreed to give it a try. After two weeks of being off milk, his symptoms disappeared, as did his nasal congestion. His mother reported that Sammy was also less irritable and he began to improve in school. Sammy eliminated milk from his diet for two years, and at the present time he can have small amounts. He usually reserves this treat for ice cream and cheese. He was given a milk supplement, Neocalglucon, which provided him with the needed calcium for his diet. Here was a case in which very careful detective work led to an obvious solution. Once milk was removed, our friend did very well.

Elvira M., a forty-year-old woman, suffered from asthma for four or five years. She also had nasal congestion and a severe sinus disease. Elvira had been carefully evaluated by several allergists and had been well controlled with medication at the time. She was found to be allergic to dust, some molds, and animals. She removed the animals from her home and there was some relief, but more recently she had significant difficulty. When I saw her, she was clearly a woman with a severe sinus disease and with polyps and allergic asthma symptoms. Careful questioning revealed that Elvira took aspirin every day, whether she needed it or not. The aspirin helped to relieve the severe pain in her sinuses and in her teeth. As time went on, she needed more and more aspirin. I suggested that she stop taking aspirin and all aspirin-containing substances. After a few weeks, Elvira's sinus condition disappeared, her asthma markedly diminished and she was much healthier. Here is another case where good detective work to find an easy-to-remove allergen was very helpful.

Margaret T.'s case illustrated the effect of infections on allergic diseases. Margaret has had asthma for many years. She is highly allergic to ragweed, dust, and mold and has been on a treatment of allergy injections that has been helpful, as well as 20 milligrams of cromolyn sodium, four times a day to control her symptoms.

Once or twice a year, Margaret gets a cold. After she has had the cold for two or three days, she develops wheezing and shortness of breath that becomes rather severe. Originally, when this happened, Margaret was given cortisone in very high doses, both initially and for months after. When I observed her typical pattern, it became obvious that once the cold was gone, she was fine. She did not have persistent symptoms that would have required the long-term use of cortisone. Margaret has learned to contact me whenever she has a cold. I have instructed her to keep antibiotics and Prednisone in her home. When she gets a cold, she starts with 60 milligrams of Prednisone a day, every day, while she has the cold (which is for three or four days), and then stops it abruptly. She does not need Prednisone after the attack. She takes antibiotics for approximately a week and then goes back to her normal regimen, cromolyn sodium (Intal). Fortunately, she requires no cortisone. As you can see, an infection can be rather devastating to asthmatics, causing symptoms to appear in some patients and mild symptoms to flare up in other patients. Although Margaret requires cortisone in high doses to block the flare-up of asthma symptoms produced by an infection, there is no reason for her to take cortisone all the time.

John J. is a twenty-five-year-old man who very rarely has asthma attacks. However, when he gets it, it's usually after a cold. When

I did the history and physical examination, I found that he appeared perfectly normal. He reported four asthma attacks in his whole life. The last attack occurred a few weeks prior to his visit, precipitating his need to see me. There is no special time of the year that the attacks occur. Once the attack starts, it takes several weeks to clear up and it is usually associated with what appears to be a cold. Since coldlike symptoms can often mask an allergy attack, I felt that he should be evaluated. He had a previous chest X ray which was normal. I thought it was important in this case to evaluate pulmonary functions to get a baseline on this man's breathing pattern to see if any damage had been done to his lungs. There was none.

At the time I saw him, he was symptom-free. Both a careful review of his environmental situation at the time and an allergic evaluation revealed no obvious triggers for his reactions. I gave him Proventil spray and a fast-acting theophylline to take immediately at the first sign of an attack and instructed him to call me. He did not have an attack until the following year at which time he began to use the spray and the fast-acting theophylline with some benefits from both. He did not come to see me until his next attack. When I saw him, I suggested that he take antibiotics and cortisone. Consequently, his attack was much shorter, lasting only a few days. He was maintained on antibiotics and cortisone for a week, and kept on bronchodilators for three weeks. These medications were then discontinued and he was well until a year and a half later. Once again, he was treated in the same way and again did well. I then provided him with an antibiotic, theophylline, cortisone, and a sympathomimetic spray, all of which were kept at home to be utilized in the event of a future attack. This type of case is not uncommon and represents a syndrome manifested by sporadic attacks of asthma. Patients with this type of problem should be evaluated thoroughly to pinpoint factors that cause these attacks. If an obvious cause cannot be found, a regimen should be established so that the patient can know what medication to use when an attack occurs. If you have this type of problem, you should not wait and suffer. Once you and your doctor become familiar with your pattern, your doctor can provide you with medication to utilize when you have these types of symptoms.

Anna H. is a twenty-six-year-old woman who works as a secretary for a large corporation. For many years, she has had mild nasal allergic symptoms that start in April and end in October. As a child, she had allergy shots that helped. Her disease disappeared during adolescence and then recurred in her early twenties, this time with wheezing and tightness in her chest. She was completely evaluated and she was found to be highly allergic to trees, mold, ragweed, grass, and dust. When I first saw her, her wheezing and shortness of breath were making her feel acutely uncomfortable. I alleviated her symptoms with 350 milligrams of Theo-Dur every twelve hours. As long as she took the Theo-Dur, her symptoms were controlled. I felt that since she had a progressive increase in symptoms, and obvious allergies, she would do well on immunotherapy. Anna was started on allergy injections and the next year she had diminished symptoms. She still required Theo-Dur, but she found she could miss doses and not have any significant attacks. The following year, Anna was basically symptom-free. This illustrates that in certain cases of asthma, allergies can be very important and allergy injections can be very helpful. It is unusual to obtain complete relief, but in Anna's case, most of her symptoms disappeared. The therapeutic approach I used with Anna was to treat her with allergy injections on a weekly basis for approximately a year, then every two weeks for a few months, and then every four weeks. After she was symptom-free for two years, treatment was discontinued. Overall, she required treatment for approximately four years. I have just recently discontinued treating her. Chances are that she will remain symptom-free.

Nobody can tell you exactly when to discontinue immunotherapy, but most allergists agree that if a patient has done very well for two years while on maintenance therapy every three to four weeks, the shots should be discontinued. At that time, there is at least a 50 percent chance that the patient will not relapse immediately and perhaps will be symptom-free for many years, or indefinitely. Therefore, it is worth a try.

Jeffrey A. is a fifty-five-year-old printer who has had allergies most of his life. As a child, he suffered from nasal allergies and some severe wheezing attacks. He does not remember much about his childhood asthma, although he does know that he never had to be hospitalized. His symptoms disappeared for a while until he was in his early thirties. At that time, he began having mild nasal congestion that progressively worsened. Jeffrey developed sporadic colds that induced wheezing. Unless he took antibiotics, the wheezing would persist for weeks. He was seen by an allergist, and he was found to be allergic to various substances including pollen, dust, and mold. He was started on injection therapy that helped, and after a few years Jeffrey discontinued it and remained symptom-free for several years. When he reached age fifty, his symptoms became increasingly more severe with frequent asthma attacks.

I first saw Jeffrey when he was fifty-one. His chest X ray was normal and his pulmonary functions showed a typically asthmatic type of curve. His RAST indicated that he had a marked allergic reaction to various substances just as he had before. Since Jeffrey was a printer, my first thought was whether the constant exposure to various toxins and chemicals and other environmental pollutants had contributed to his illness. At this time there is no standard method to evaluate environmental sensitivities. One must utilize careful observation and obtain detailed information from the patient concerning his life-style. Since Jeffrey told me that even when he was on vacation and away from his business for as long as a month he still had significant difficulty, I was able, by deductive reasoning, to determine that the printing was not the cause of the problem.

I started Jeffrey on Theo-Dur and found the appropriate level for him was 550 milligrams every twelve hours. At this dose, his therapeutic level, he was reasonably comfortable. When he did have an attack, he used Proventil spray as needed. After a while, he was given Proventil spray to use on a regular basis and he was also started on Vanceril to be taken after the Proventil spray. This combination helped to some degree. Since Jeffrey was a highly allergic individual who had symptoms for many years that had responded to allergy shots before, I decided to start him on injection therapy again. Over a period of time, they again helped Jeffrey to some degree. He does well, then, on a regular program of bronchodilators in addition to Proventil and Vanceril sprays and immunotherapy. When he gets an infection, he still experiences difficulty, despite this medication, and requires antibiotics and cortisone for up to a week at a time. In general, his asthma is much more controlled than previously. He no longer wheezes all the time. I attribute this improvement to continuous rather than haphazard medication. Also, putting him on antibiotics and cortisone as soon as possible after getting a cold has cut down on weeks of suffering.

Susan S., a thirty-nine-year-old New Jersey teacher, mother, and homemaker, came to me with severe asthma. She began to have hay fever when she was thirteen. Her hay fever improved after she received allergy shots for a few years but she gradually developed moderately severe wheezing, initially associated with infection, and then at any time. Wheezing and coughing became chronic. She was on fast-acting theophylline, Brethine, Proventil, and Prednisone every other day when she first came to see me. She had tried cromolyn sodium several years before and it was not successful.

The first thing I did was put her on long-acting theophylline, of which she required 450 milligrams every twelve hours to reach therapeutic levels. A careful review of her case history revealed that although she was symptomatic almost all of the time, her worst episodes followed eating. However, there did not seem to be any food that she could pinpoint as the culprit. She had no favorite, nor did she report a craving for any one kind of food. I suggested that she try an elimination diet in which she would eat allegedly "nonallergic" foods for a week in as great a quantity as she wanted. Within a week's time, the results were startling.

Susan was breathing better than she had in years. She was not cured, but she was much improved.

We gradually introduced foods, one at a time, in order to single out her food allergies. The list of offenders included artificial colors, artificial flavors, preservatives, mustard and foods in the mustard family, and a host of other foods. We immediately changed all of her medications to brands that were white, rather than the more available colored tablets, a task that was not easy. When she gets an infection, she must take a white antibiotic or transfer the powder from the prefilled capsules to a clear gelatin capsule. Antibiotics, increased Prednisone for a short time, and her regular medications help her get through an infection without much difficulty.

Following this difficult diet, Susan has been able to significantly reduce her alternate-day dose of Prednisone. She uses the preferred Vanceril spray to minimize the amount of Prednisone she needs. We were even able to reintroduce Intal, which worked for her this time, demonstrating that it is sometimes worth the effort to try old medication again. Susan is now very well maintained on theophylline, Brethine, Vanceril, and Intal, as well as on her diet. She still is on low doses of Prednisone, every other day, looking to the day when she can eliminate the systemic corticosteroid permanently.

This treatment program, although fairly rigorous, allows Susan to lead a very active life, working full-time as a teacher at a community college, raising two sons, and managing a household, as well as being able to join me in writing this book.

Jacqueline Michaels: Jacqueline is a sixty-six-year-old housewife who developed severe asthma four years ago. She was highly allergic (unusual at her age) and was started on allergy injections. She was allergic to her dog and had gotten rid of him, but she was still having difficulty. I finally controlled her on Theo-Dur, albuterol, Intal, Atrovent, and Vanceril. Her thyroid gland which had been overactive in the past became overactive again. Her heart began to race and she was very nervous. Her asthma became severe and she required steroids to control her symptoms. I advised her to have her thyroid controlled as soon as possible and I kept in touch with her endocrinologist while this was being done. Once the thyroid was controlled, she no longer required steroids. This demonstrates that another illness not controlled, especially an endocrine one, can aggravate the asthma. That is why it is so important to assess general health when dealing with asthma.

Unfortunately, Jacqueline had more to teach us, because a year later she began to have severe attacks at night and I had to start her on steroids again. Close questioning made me realize that she had developed indigestion in the middle of the night. She had gastric reflux and when she learned to eat earlier and was placed on Ranitidine, the indigestion and the severe attacks stopped. See pages 154 for a full discussion of this problem.

Bonnie B., is a twenty-nine-year-old financial consultant for a large brokerage firm. She loves to jog in the morning before work and does two miles every weekday and four on weekends, holidays, and days off. As a child she had asthma, but it disappeared in her early teens. Naturally, she was panicked when she became short of breath while running early last year. She consulted me and after reviewing her story, I obtained a chest X ray and EKG. Once I knew they were normal and therefore there were no other complicating factors, I was sure she had developed exercise-induced asthma. I reassured Bonnie and gave her an albuterol spray with instructions to use it fifteen to thirty minutes before exercise. I didn't hear from her for a year. The next time she consulted me, it was for rather severe asthma attacks that occurred at night without any rhyme or reason. She had a feather pillow, so we got rid of that, with no improvement. I did a series of RASTs on her and although she was allergic, I couldn't correlate any specific allergen or irritant as a cause of her symptoms. I gave her a fast-acting theophylline to use in conjunction with her albuterol spray when she had the attacks at night, and this helped to control her symptoms. On close questioning I found out that the attacks only occurred on the days she did not use her albuterol spray prophylactically before running. She was getting so busy that on some days she could only run a mile. She found the wheezing associated with running a mile was minimal and went away easily. She did not like to use medication and therefore did not use it when she knew she would only run a mile. However, it was on those evenings she got the attack.

Some patients have both an immediate and a *delayed* response to exercise. If you prevent the early response you usually will not have the late response. Thus attacks of exertion-induced asthma, in addition to occurring while you run, can recur much more severely hours later. So Bonnie B. always uses her spray when she runs and no longer gets the nighttime attacks.

Jeffrey Wilford: Jeffrey is a forty-year-old owner of a shoe store who had asthma for many years. He is allergic and has done well on allergy injections. Prior to receiving allergy injections he would require ''bursts'' of steroids three or four times a year. He has improved since he has been getting allergy injections and he has not required steroids. He is well controlled on a regimen of Intal, Theo-Dur, albuterol, and Vanceril sprays. However, he still would cough and wheeze whenever he was exposed to a strong environmental stimulus, especially cigarette smoke. I increased his Vanceril to four puffs four times a day which helped, but when we added Atrovent, he became completely stabilized and could even be exposed to someone smoking in the same room with him. Atrovent sometimes will stabilize cough receptors.

Steven Hook: Steven was a twenty-seven-year-old designer who had mild asthma most of his life. His asthma was easily controlled, only requiring medication on an occasional basis. However, one year ago he developed influenza, and since that time his asthma symptoms are more severe. Although his attacks are still occasional, they have become severe enough to require steroids to control his symptoms. Once the attack was over, he would withdraw the steroid therapy. This worked and I thought he was well controlled, until six months ago when I got a call that he was in the intensive care unit of the hospital with which I'm affiliated. He had been at a concert where he developed severe wheezing and had gone into a respiratory arrest on the way to the hospital. Quick-acting paramedics resuscitated him and maintained him until he could be put on a respirator. Fortunately, he survived; and when he got out of the hospital and came in for an office visit, I very thoroughly investigated his medical and allergic problems.

I started him on allergy injections to whatever substances appeared relevant. I placed him on alternate-day steroids, but after one month he appeared to be well, so we were able to withdraw the steroids. He was also taking Slo-Bid, Atrovent, Intal, and albuterol and doing well.

One day while I was at a concert, I got a call that he had arrived at the hospital in respiratory arrest. Once again we pulled him through, and this time I realized that Steven was one of those patients who does not really know when he is getting sick. It is not a case of psychologically denying his illness. He truly does not sense when his breathing is worsening. Thus, his asthma can progress to a very dangerous level before he realizes that he is ill and goes into severe respiratory collapse. I now have him monitor his peak flows using a peak flow meter (see page 29), and if it drops below a certain level, we have a regimen to increase his medication. If it goes down further, he calls me. Now both of us have been able to go to concerts without any emergencies.

Thus, in summary, my method consists of

1. careful analysis of the problem
2. whenever possible, controlling (optimally removing) offending allergens including foods
3. allergy injections, if warranted
4. medication if necessary, initiating treatment with the drugs that have the least side effects:
    a. Proventil
    b. Intal
    c. Theophylline
    d. Atrovent
    e. Vanceril, Beclovent, or Azmacort
    f. Corticosteroids, when all else fails

Anything that is designed to suit an individual has to be custom-made, sometimes requiring several fittings and frequent alterations to produce the perfect fit. While I have presented the "pattern" I work from in asthma care, it must be tailor-made for you. This process may take time. Have patience. There must be open lines of communication between you and your doctor so that you both can agree upon what works for you. If there are changes in you, the design may have to be altered. If you are not satisfied with the finished product, you may have to go back to the drawing board, perhaps even with a new designer.

Treating asthma can be complicated, demanding the consideration of many potentially crucial variables. When all are considered and patient and doctor work intelligently with each other, I maintain an optimistic view that asthma can be controlled.

8

PSYCHOLOGICAL ASPECTS OF ASTHMA AND STRESS-REDUCTION THERAPIES

Let me start this chapter by stating very emphatically that asthma is not a psychological illness; it is a physical illness. The physiology and pharmacology that we have learned in this century clearly indicate that asthma is an enzyme deficiency that renders the asthmatic more sensitive to, and overly reactive to, allergens, environmental factors, and the body's own mediators. Without this deficiency, all the stress or neurotic conflicts in the world will not induce an asthma attack. It simply does not work this way.

The myth that asthma is "all in your head" is based on old theories that we now know are inaccurate. From the turn of the century until the 1940s, it was felt that asthma was purely a psychological condition. The "wheeze" of the asthmatic was seen as a suppressed cry for the mother or anger against the parent. In short, the parents were to blame for the child's asthma. In fact, the therapeutic "solution" to this problem was a "parent-ectomy," removing the child from the parent. The literature even reports some miraculous results, but for the wrong reasons. Along with the parent-ectomy was a very significant change in environment. The child was being moved from New York or California to Denver and into a clean hospital setting and this is why his asthma symptoms were relieved. While we no longer consider this psychological approach to be valid, the sensationalism of these stories is remembered, and the old-fashioned, wrong ideas continue to haunt us.

The long-lasting effects of these old views can easily be seen in some books, television shows, or plays. It is not uncommon for a weak or nervous person to be depicted as having asthma. In some dramas, when the parents divorce, the child is left wheezing on the doorstep, making the parents feel guilty and reinforcing the idea that asthma is psychosomatic. The audience believes it, and the myth lives on! Unfortunately, we do not have to look only to fiction for such examples. Many of my patients tell me that even their own physicians have often suggested that if they relax and stop worrying, their asthma will go away. A purely psychological approach to asthma is not only wrong, but dangerous. It may make the patient feel guilty and helpless and prevent him from actively taking the steps needed to improve his condition.

When it became obvious that this psychological approach was wrong, the pendulum swung 180 degrees, and then many believed that asthma was purely an immunological disease or an allergic illness. This extreme view was not appropriate either.

Where does the truth lie? As I have said at the start, asthma is a physiological disorder. It is an enzyme deficiency that renders the asthmatic overly reactive to the environment, to allergens, and to his own mediators. Asthma can be triggered by several things, including allergens, infections, exercise, changes in air flow (laughing or crying), and environmental irritants. Certainly, one very important trigger is stress. Since the underlying dysfunction in asthma lies in the autonomic nervous system, and stress plays a role in this system, stress can cause an increase in the frequency and the severity of an asthma attack. An important caveat: It is quite rare for stress to be the sole precipitator of asthma symptoms. Since the human organism is a complex interaction of mind and body, it should not be surprising that stress or severe psychological problems can certainly make an already existing condition worse. We must be aware of the possibility that stress is a triggering factor in asthma and incorporate some techniques for stress reduction into our total treatment program. However, stress is only one of many variables. The risk is in getting carried away with the psyche as the total cause and ignoring the basic physiological problem.

Does Asthma Cause Stress?

While stress can trigger asthma, asthma can trigger stress. As you have seen throughout this book, asthma has the potential to be quite disruptive to the asthmatic and his family. At its best, asthma may result in a variety of life-style restrictions and require special handling at times. At its worst, it is an unpredictable intruder with symptoms that can appear quite suddenly, further demonstrating the anxiety-producing ability of the disease. You really cannot "get used to" asthma. It is really quite understandable that a child who has been forced to watch his friends have relay races rather than participate in them himself is under stress. It is also understandable that a parent who is awakened three times a night feeling helpless as she watches her asthmatic child fight for breath is under a great deal of stress. It is equally understandable that an individual who has to watch what he eats; watch the clock so that he takes his pills on time; watch that he avoids smoke, perfumes, and animals; and watch his own body's reactions to the air he breathes is under a great deal of stress. Stress, then, is an end product of asthma that may require attention in and of itself.

While it is now clear that stress can aggravate asthma or stem from asthma, it is necessary for me to make one more point. You do not really want to eliminate stress altogether. You would not want to be so placid and passive that you would not even respond appropriately to fight an asthma attack. Some stress is good; it makes you want to face and deal with your problem. What you are aiming for is a happy medium. If your body tenses when under stress, or when you are in the midst of an asthma attack, or if having asthma adds a great deal of stress to your life, some help may be needed.

Psychological Support Services

As I see it, then, there are three reasons why you should seek psychological support services, two of which relate directly to your asthma. First, psychological therapy may be designed to help one cope with the potential stress of normal living in an attempt to reduce the effects of stress as a trigger in asthma. Second, therapy may be aimed at helping the asthmatic deal with the understandable stress that asthma creates. In both of these cases, I feel that psychoanalysis is less effective than behavioral approaches. I will elaborate later.

Third, a person may have a psychological problem unrelated to his asthma that may be alleviated by some type of psychological intervention. The treatment program must deal with the psychological problem—whatever it is—but must also be set up so that there are no negative interactions with the asthma program. When in treatment always be aware of your asthma if medications are prescribed, or if exercise or any other change in life-style is recommended: It may affect your asthma.

If you feel that your coping mechanisms are strained to the limit because of your asthma, I do not feel that you should sign yourself up for five years of Freudian analysis. There are several things you can do to help yourself. Two types of approaches that I find helpful in asthma-induced or asthma-related stress problems are a problem-oriented psychological approach and stress-reducing techniques that must be learned and practiced, such as autohypnosis, relaxation techniques, biofeedback, or any combination of these. These types of approaches are directed at the basic problem and they enable you to help yourself.

Problem-Oriented Psychological Therapy

It is perfectly understandable that after a long period of time, living with a chronic limiting disease can shake your self-confidence. If you cannot trust your body to work all the time, you may become overly cautious and hesitant to commit yourself to a task or to a time schedule. If this goes on long enough, whole new personalities can develop. Some patients might choose to speak to a psychiatrist or psychologist or social worker, or some may "vent" to a family member or close friend.

It is essential that you find a reputable practitioner to deal with your problem. I strongly suggest that you consult your internist, pediatrician, allergist, religious counselor, or the department of psychiatry of a major hospital in making your choice. If you seek individual therapy, your goal is to find a therapist who can give you support and specific suggestions for coping with your asthma and its ramifications. You need strategies for stress reduction and stress management that you can use to deal with your asthma when it affects only you or when it affects your relations with others. One-to-one therapy can be viewed as a helpful luxury, a time for thrashing out the many aspects of your asthma, how you affect it, and how it affects you.

You may opt for group therapy, sharing and learning with others in the same situation (either other asthmatics or parents of asthmatic children). It is very important for someone with asthma to find out that he is not the only one who is coping with the disease. Too often you feel that the difficulties you are encountering are unique and insurmountable. In fact, there are millions of asthmatics who are dealing with the same problems every day.

Meeting other asthmatics helps you to appreciate your strengths and weaknesses. It also helps you to see that asthma affects all kinds of people and that an asthmatic is not merely a stereotype. Since asthma can be such a misunderstood phenomenon, just talking about your own frustrations to someone else who understands is comforting. We know how frustrating asthma can be and how frustrating it is when no one seems to understand you. You might find yourself becoming defensive when in fact you are simply in need of an exchange of ideas. Seeking out other asthmatics, or any good listener who understands your problem, is beneficial and, I feel, crucial. You might be surprised to find that your nearby hospital has group therapy sessions for asthmatics. If there is no group in your area, perhaps you might consider starting one. I am sure you might entice many asthmatics to join, maybe even a few "closet asthmatics." Whether you seek psychological intervention to reduce stress that you feel might be aggravating your symptoms or to reduce the stress your symptoms cause, this problem-solving approach might be considered.

The Typical Vicious Cycle

Sometimes the normal stresses in life can aggravate asthma. Then the asthma itself becomes an added burden that feeds stress back into the cycle until things get entirely out-of-hand unless someone intervenes. At this point, you need a helpful outsider to see how locked into the cycle you are. One interesting case was a patient I treated several years ago.

Phoebe G. was a forty-two-year-old asthmatic who had a six-year-old daughter. There had been a great deal of conflict in the family, and the little girl would act up constantly to get attention. She resented her mother's illness. The acting up became so disruptive that neither parent knew how to handle the child. They hovered over her and gave in to everything that she wanted. The more the child acted up, the more they indulged her and the sicker Phoebe became.

I recognized this "vicious cycle" and sent Phoebe to a behaviorally oriented psychiatrist who evaluated the situation. He suggested various techniques to be used by the parents to gain control over their daughter. The vicious cycle was finally broken. The daughter's behavior improved and Phoebe had much less stress in her life to deal with. She still has asthma, but she has fewer attacks.

In this case, psychiatric intervention was very important. The psychiatrist didn't think emotion was the cause of Phoebe's asthma, yet he was attuned to the conflicts and problems that were occurring in her life, and the asthma improved.

This story highlights the main messages of this chapter. Asthma can clearly add stress to one's life, and stress can sometimes trigger a flare-up of symptoms. Asthma can also exist in an individual with poor coping mechanisms. But most of the time, asthma adds another factor to the complexities of everyday living. Since various types of people have asthma, various types of therapies can be helpful on many levels. My belief is that attention must be paid to modifying their immediate response to stress. Whether stress is a cause or an effect, it must be managed and reduced. Suggestions for doing this can come from individual, group, psychological, psychiatric, formal, or informal therapy. Some specific stress-reduction approaches, which you can do on your own almost immediately, are presented next.

Stress Reduction: Relaxation Techniques and Hypnosis

Stress is not unique to asthmatics. We live and work in a fast-paced, tension-producing world. As a consequence, we are all under stress. Certainly, limited stress can be positive, and we need to be prepared for it. But too much stress can be counterproductive. Therefore, the reduction of excess stress is a goal toward which most people try to strive. For the asthmatic, the reduction of stress can help to control another one of the factors that can increase the frequency and severity of his asthma.

There are many ways to relax. Just walk into your local bookstore and you will see no end of guides for stress reduction and relaxation. Some are more spiritually based and others are more scientific. Some appear to be fads and others have been more long-lasting. Some are traditional and others are quite nontraditional. As techniques to achieve inner peace and a relaxed bodily state, Transcendental Meditation (TM), yoga, Zen, autogenics (the repeating of certain phrases), and Biofeedback Training (BFT) have had a wide following. Those who have benefited from these approaches sing their praises.

Biofeedback Training has achieved considerable popularity as a more physiologically based, "establishment-sanctioned" process of achieving control of one's body's functions. Using sophisticated equipment, the patient is trained by a technician to monitor, evaluate, and alter a specific body process previously believed to be beyond conscious control. Biofeedback is a systematic trial and error process that establishes a strategy to control such body functions as pulse rate, temperature, blood pressure, and muscular tension. Biofeedback advocates suggest that when it is used with other therapies, the asthmatic can learn to relax (and even widen) constricted bronchi.

I am not an expert or a strong advocate of TM or yoga or BFT. I support all efforts to reduce muscular tension and reduce stress; but in my practice, when the patient and I have decided to address the issue of stress reduction directly, I have had the most success with some simple relaxation techniques and/or self-hypnosis. Neither approach is difficult, but both require some initial training. Depending upon the patient's preference, I have taught many patients self-hypnosis or relaxation with some good results.

RELAXATION TECHNIQUES: PROGRESSIVE RELAXATION

While there are many relaxation techniques, I have become very comfortable with an approach that focuses on training the patient to selectively monitor and control muscle groups. Progressive relaxation, as first described by Dr. Edmund Jacobson in 1922, has been a widely used relaxation approach, with excellent results in many different kinds of tension-filled conditions. The basic principle is that the body responds to environmental anxiety with tension that manifests itself in muscle spasms. If the patient can be trained to have a keen sense of when a particular muscle group is tense, which one it is, and how to impose deep muscular relaxation on it, then tension will be reduced and anxiety will be minimized.

Progressive relaxation can be done either lying down or sitting in a chair, as long as the patient is comfortable and his body is well supported. ''Progressing'' from head to toe, each muscle or muscle group is tensed for five to seven seconds and then relaxed for twenty to thirty seconds. The principle of this procedure is to concentrate on perceptions of tension and relaxation and the vast difference between the two. Thus, essentially what you do is tense one of your muscles to feel and remember what that muscle is like when it is tense. Then you relax one of your muscles to feel and remember what it is like when it is relaxed. You are learning to feel relaxation, and control it. The entire procedure can take about fifteen minutes and should be done twice a day as part of "basic training."

The standard progression involves the tensing and relaxing of the muscles in and around the following areas:

1. fist, hand, and forearm (first one side and then the other)
2. elbows, biceps, and forehead (using tight wrinkles for tension)
3. eyes (squinting for tension)
4. jaw, lips, and head (backward rolling for tension)
5. neck, shoulders, and chest (holding your breath for tension and then feeling the air hiss out in a continuous, relaxed, steady stream)
6. stomach (breathing deeply and watching your stomach expand and relax)
7. lower back, buttocks, thighs, legs, calves, knees, shins, ankles, and toes

You have progressively left each area in a deeply relaxed state. Reflect upon it and feel the absence of tension.

Once you achieve a degree of competence with the relaxation therapy, it should be used several times a day. The regimen I suggest for my patients is to use the technique twice a day and whenever else they feel it is appropriate. The technique is quite useful to reduce general stress. That in itself would be sufficient! However, it appears that in some patients the overall reduction of stress has a "secondary gain," the overall reduction in the amount and severity of asthma attacks. I usually recommend using this technique in any patient who suffers from stress in general or who feels that stress exacerbates his asthma.

For reasons that will become obvious to you when you read the following section on hypnosis, relaxation techniques should not be used in an acute attack unless certain precautionary measures are observed. When it is utilized, it is important for the patient not to pursue it unless it very rapidly produces relief; otherwise, I instruct my patient to follow a previously worked out scheme utilizing medication. If the technique fails to achieve its objective, I suggest to the patient that he utilize the relaxation technique on a regular basis, but only as a prophylactic measure. I do find relaxation techniques to be very helpful as an adjunct to the overall approach to the treatment of asthma.

HYPNOSIS

I have also found hypnosis to be a very helpful modality in the treatment of asthma since it induces a very powerful state of relaxation in any subject. In addition, the subject can exert some degree of control over his autonomic nervous system.

What is hypnosis? Most simply, hypnosis is a trance state or a natural state of consciousness manifested by heightened awareness and increased concentration.

Hypnosis, like asthma, is often surrounded by many myths that lead to serious misunderstandings. I would like to dispel some of the most frequently heard myths about hypnosis. First, hypnosis is not sleep. Quite the contrary, as I have indicated it is heightened awareness. Second, the hypnotist does not inflict an energy source onto the patient.

Third, it is untrue that only weak or unstable people can be hypnotized. As a matter of fact, you must have a fairly well integrated personality to be hypnotizable. Schizophrenic individuals and those with severe mental disorders cannot be hypnotized. Women are not more hypnotizable than men.

Fourth, it is also untrue that the doctor controls the trance state. The doctor may set the stage, but he is not in complete control. There is also a belief that when one symptom is removed, it will be replaced by another; for example, if I get rid of your asthma, you will start to have migraine headaches. This isn't so. It is also untrue that hypnosis can be dangerous. It is not and it can be used frequently.

A fifth concern for hypnotism is the question of what would happen if, while hypnotized, the hypnotist leaves. Can you ever be "pulled out" of the trance? Of course you can. If I were hypnotizing you and I was whisked off the face of the earth while you were in a trance, you would fall asleep and wake up in a few minutes. We would not have to fly in a superhypnotist from Timbuktu to get you out of the trance. The last myth that I'd like to debunk is that the hypnotist has to be charismatic, unique, or even weird. The fact is that most hypnotists are professional, responsible individuals and there is nothing about hypnotism that requires charisma or mysticism.

The trance state is a natural state. The normal person goes in and out of it, almost like daydreaming. Just think back to when you watched a play that captured your imagination. You may have become so engrossed in the drama's action that, when it ended, it took you a few seconds to become reoriented. This is a trance state.

Now that I have explained what a hypnotist is and is not, I will discuss how I use hypnotism as an adjunct in the treatment of asthma. If my patient and I have decided to attempt stress reduction through hypnosis, I first determine how hypnotizable he is. There are several methods that can be utilized to give a relatively objective hypnotizability index. The one that I have found most useful was developed by Herbert Spiegel at Columbia University in New York. It is called the Hypnotic Induction Profile and measures several aspects of hypnotizability including the eye roll.

The first step in this method is to measure the biological capacity of the patient to be hypnotized. This capacity is manifested by the eye roll. I instruct the patient to look up to the top of his head. While he does this he is instructed to close his eyes slowly. I can then measure the space between the pupil and the lower lid margin. In effect, I am measuring the amount of sclera (white of the eye) that is visible. If you stop and think about it, whenever you see a movie of an Indian fakir in a trance, you see that his eyes are completely rolled up. Indeed it is true, the higher the eye is rolled up, the greater the potential hypnotizability of the patient. However, the eye roll only measures your natural ability to be hypnotized.

The next aspect of the test measures your motivation and

attitude toward hypnosis. Through a series of programmed instructions you are encouraged to raise your arm. In effect, in this portion of the test, you are hypnotized into raising your arm in such a manner that the amount of instruction required and the time it takes for you to respond can be quantified. The less instruction required and the faster you respond, the more hypnotizable you are. The whole test takes less than ten minutes to perform. The test itself is actually the method I use to hypnotize the patient. This is a very convenient, simple, and effective method to both quantify hypnotizability and to effectuate it.

Once I have determined that my patient is hypnotizable, and that the patient is agreeable and involved in the process, I hypnotize him and then train him to hypnotize himself. One important caveat: Work with your physician on this. Do not attempt to do these procedures without professional advice.

In the basic training process, the patient engages in hypnosis every morning and every evening as a precautionary measure against asthma attacks. As the patient improves, I reduce his medication very slowly.

Hypnosis, like progressive relaxation, should be used with caution during an acute attack. Most patients who can utilize hypnosis find that when they use it during an attack, they feel markedly improved. However, not all patients have an actual change in their pulmonary functions. They just feel better. This is a potentially dangerous state of affairs, and the patients who have improved must be separated from those who have not. All patients who wish to use hypnosis during an acute attack should be checked with a peak flow meter to ascertain in an objective manner whether or not they have indeed improved. The patients who have improved are encouraged to use hypnosis during an acute attack. The patients who have not improved should not use it during an acute attack. When hypnosis is used during an acute attack, but fails to improve breathing, the patient is instructed to use a previously set up regimen to get him out of trouble. In most cases, however, hypnosis has its application (as does progressive relaxation) as a general approach to reducing the stress and muscular tension that can play a role in "setting up" the asthmatic for more severe or frequent symptoms.

Hypnotism works well with exercise-induced dyspnea, but its efficiency must be monitored. It also has been used well with children, but I tend not to use this before age twelve or thirteen. Even then, I actively involve the parent to insure mature judgment on when and how to use hypnosis.

Hypnosis, as I utilize it, is not a psychological tool. I do not take my patient back in time to look for the fight with his mother that occurred three hours before the first attack and attempt to undo that conflict. Hypnosis is a powerful physiological tool with which the patient can exert control over his autonomic nervous system. He can get his bronchi to constrict or open and close to some degree. He can induce a state of deep relaxation and thereby reduce the stress that may be exacerbating his asthma. He can gain self-control.

If you feel that you would like to attempt stress reduction through hypnosis, consult your doctor. Do not wander into a hypnotism clinic and decide to have your asthma cured. Hypnosis, like everything else in this section of my book, must be integrated into a total program of asthma management. Work with your doctor. You do not need a hypnotist. It is an easily learned skill that many doctors, psychologists, and psychiatrists use and teach well.

Whether you meditate; repeat your mantra several hundred times; spend an hour in the lotus position; train your bronchi to relax and widen through progressive relaxation; or think about cool, moist, pure, healing air during a hypnotic trance, if you remove stress from the list of possible triggers of your asthma, you have spent your time wisely. Stress reduction can be an important supplement in asthma management.

9

A PHYSICAL THERAPY APPROACH TO ASTHMA

Physical therapy is a branch of rehabilitation medicine the purpose of which is to train or retrain muscles to function optimally. In this way, the individual can function to his highest potential. There are several mechanical problems created by asthma that physical therapy techniques can be designed to solve or compensate for. These mechanical problems result from chronically impaired breathing patterns and may occur and contribute to the acuteness of an asthma attack. Therefore, physical therapy techniques are applicable for the chronic asthmatic and some of these techniques may be beneficial if used as emergency measures during an acute attack. This chapter will present those physical therapy techniques applicable to asthma.

The Mechanical Problems Asthma Creates

During the normal respiratory cycle, the diaphragm is the most important muscle. It has a dome shape at rest, separating the thoracic cavity (chest) from the abdominal cavity. During normal inhalation, the diaphragm descends, considerably enlarging the thoracic cavity, allowing air to flow in. During exhalation, the diaphragm returns to its normal position, pushing the air out of the thorax, via the respiratory passages (lungs, alveoli, bronchioles, bronchi, trachea, larynx, pharynx, nose, and mouth). The elasticity of the lung allows it to move up, out of the way of the diaphragm. The diaphragm's work accounts for approximately 65 percent of the needed activity during breathing. Supplementary chest muscles aid in inhalation and some supplementary abdominal muscles aid in exhalation. But basically, the diaphragm is the "prime mover."

As asthma becomes chronic, the lungs lose some elasticity and therefore do not contract and empty sufficiently to allow the diaphragm to rise to its normal position. The diaphragm becomes weak and because it cannot rise very much, it makes exhalation less efficient. Because it does not descend very much (since it is already lower than it normally should be), it makes inhalation less efficient. Instead of doing 65 percent of the work, the diaphragm may do as little as 30 percent. Supplementary muscles are called upon and breathing becomes labored and shallow. Because of the reduced efficiency, the asthmatic has to breathe more frequently. This all results in rapid, shallow breathing. The overuse of the neck, shoulder, and upper chest muscles creates the stereotypical barrel-chested appearance of the severe asthmatic. The physical therapy solution for these problems consists of breathing exercises to strengthen the diaphragm.

Another mechanical problem of asthma which physical therapy can address is the obstruction of the airways caused by excessive mucus production. The mucus can become so thick and sticky that it gets caught in the smaller respiratory passageways, obstructing breathing. This can become dangerous when the mucus plugging occurs in so many of the passageways that not enough air can get down into the lungs and not enough air can push its way out. The physical therapy solution for this problem is a program known as postural drainage, which is detailed thoroughly on pp. 240–45.

Still another problem is the rigid, tense posture that so many asthmatics assume. Whether this posture is due to the constant struggling for air, or due to the anxiety and fear of not being able to breathe, the resulting rigidity of the respiratory passageways and musculature can become a real physiological problem. We know that tense bronchospasm is a typical characteristic of asthma. If there is bronchospasm on top of tension or tension on top of

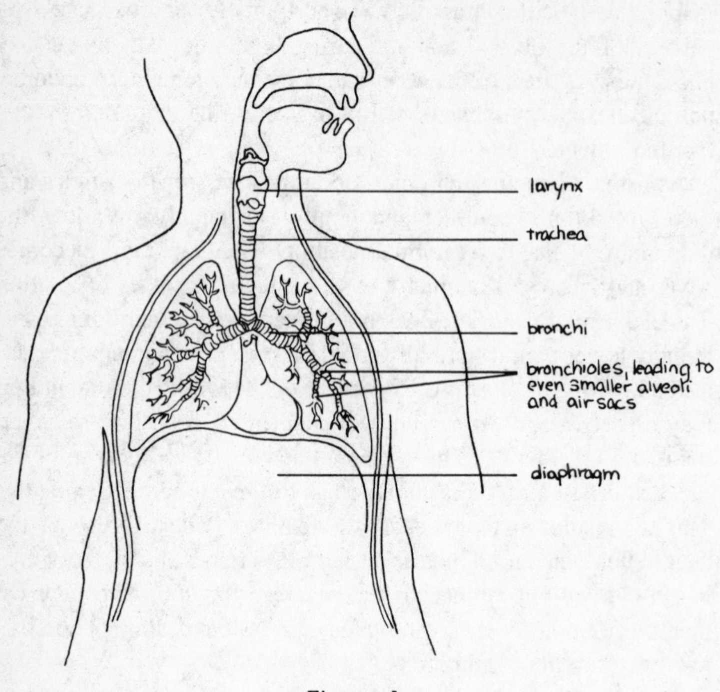

Figure 1

bronchospasm, the result is the same. The airways become more constricted and breathing becomes more difficult. The physical therapy solution for this problem consists of relaxation techniques.

The fourth problem associated with asthma involves the general lack of physical fitness on the part of the asthmatic. Everyone, of course, should be physically fit and too many of us are not. But asthmatics may actively avoid physical activities because they are afraid physical exertion may induce their symptoms. Chronic asthma restricts one's physical abilities, and some asthma medications (for instance, corticosteroids) may result in a less physically fit individual. Most asthmatics, however, can benefit from a graduated program of physical fitness, individualized according to their abilities.

Who's a Good Candidate for Physical Therapy?

Physical therapy is more appropriate for some patients than for others. If your breathing is rapid and shallow and if you use your neck, shoulder, and upper chest muscles to help you breathe better, you probably are a good candidate for physical therapy. This inefficient breathing pattern is much more prevalent among patients whose asthma is chronic and of long duration.

Another group of patients who might benefit from physical therapy are those who secrete an excess amount of mucus. Whether your asthma is mild, moderate, or severe, if excess mucus characterizes your symptoms, postural drainage may be helpful. Especially in instances where infection is a frequent precipitator of asthmatic symptoms, getting rid of mucus (which can be a breeding ground for infection) is important and can be somewhat difficult. Postural drainage can help loosen mucus so that it can be coughed up.

While breathing exercises and postural drainage procedures are applicable to certain types of asthmatics, the relaxation exercises that physical therapy advocates appear to be more widely applicable. No matter how severe your symptoms are, air passages can be more open and breathing more efficient if muscles are more relaxed. Tense muscles and body postures work against the asthmatic.

Physical therapy also advocates general physical fitness. This, of course, applies to everyone. Whether the asthmatic is in fact less physically fit because of the ill effects of his condition or his medication, or whether he is less physically fit because of a habitual avoidance of physical exertion, a program to increase fitness is appropriate.

Another ingredient in determining candidacy for any physical therapy techniques is one's level of motivation and commitment. These recommendations are for therapy programs, not just stopgap measures; they require long-term involvement. Changing one's breathing pattern is no easy task. Postural drainage necessitates time and helpers. If the type and severity of your asthma makes you a good candidate for physical therapy, add your commitment and you'll stand a better chance of benefiting. It should also be made clear that your candidacy for any therapy program must ultimately be determined in consultation with your doctor.

The following procedure is also applicable to children. See Chapter 11, Asthma In Children.

Breathing Exercises

Breathing exercises can accomplish three things for the asthmatic.

1. Control and coordinate the rate of breathing (our aim is for slower and deeper breathing).
2. Increase the air supply entering and leaving the alveoli (the small air sacs in the lungs) to maintain a normal exchange of gases.
3. Maximize the functioning of the diaphragm to minimize the energy required in breathing and reduce the strain placed on the upper chest and other helping muscles that try to compensate for the weakened diaphragm.

There are two major components of breathing exercises designed to achieve these goals. One is abdominal breathing and the other is pursed-lip breathing. These must be practiced together in order to be effective; separately they won't do much for you.

Abdominal breathing means using the abdominal muscles rather than the upper chest muscles during respiration. To improve your skill, lie on your back, place one hand on your upper chest and place the other hand on your stomach. As you inhale, deeply breathe in through your nose for two counts. You should feel your stomach rising if you are breathing correctly. Exhalation, which should be slow and to a count of four, should push the abdomen down. This long exhalation must be accompanied by the second component of the exercise, pursed-lip breathing. Purse your lips during the exhalation, giving you a slow, more efficient exhalation of air. (See Figure 2.)

This breathing exercise is not very strenuous and after you get used to it, it should be practiced in a variety of positions (for instance, reclining, sitting, standing, and walking).

In order to increase your muscular strength, it is also recommended that the exercise, when practiced in a supine position (lying on the back), be done with a weight ranging from four to twenty pounds, placed on the abdomen to add resistance to the movements. This new breathing pattern should be gradually introduced into your daily routines until it becomes natural.

There is some evidence that there is another application for these breathing exercises. They can also serve as a means of achieving relaxation during acute attacks. Especially in the case of children, breathing exercises can lessen the feeling of helplessness; in this way, they gain some control over the uncoordinated breathing pattern that occurs during an acute asthma attack.

Figure 2
Breathing Exercises

Position 1.
Lie flat on your back with your head lower than your body (use pillows if the bed cannot be adjusted).
Instructions: Placing the left hand on the upper chest and the right hand on the abdomen, inhale deeply through the nose while pushing outward with the stomach so that the right hand can feel the abdomen rise. Try not to move the left hand while inhaling: in other words, breathe in with your stomach muscles, not with your chest. Purse your lips and exhale slowly, pushing the abdomen

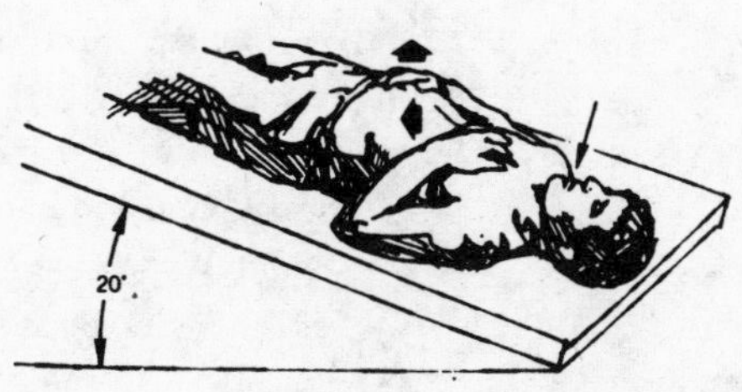

inward and upward toward the ribs with your right hand as you do so. Try to exhale as long as you can before inhaling again the same way as before.

Position 2.
Sit up, leaning back slightly, in a completely relaxed position.
Instructions: Same as for Exercise 1.

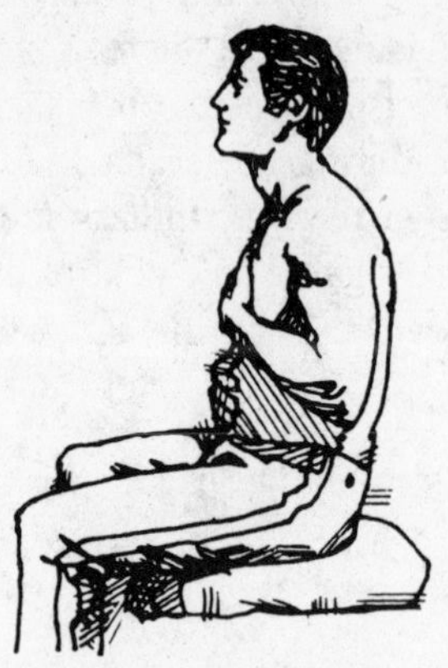

Position 3.
Stand in a relaxed position.
Instructions: Same as for Exercise 1.

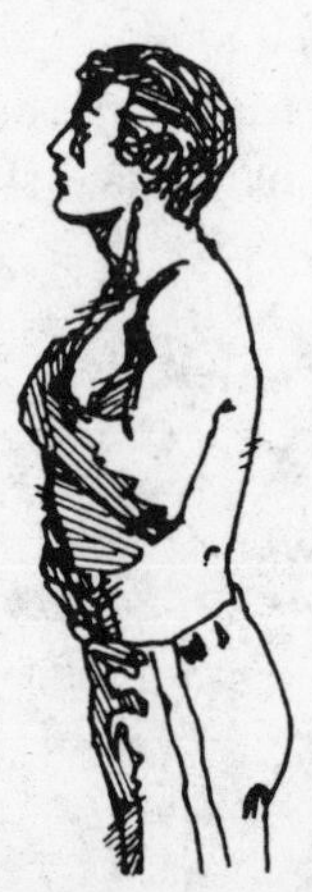

Position 4.
Walking.
Instructions: Same as for Exercise 1. Walk slowly. Try to time one step with an inhalation and the next with an exhalation.

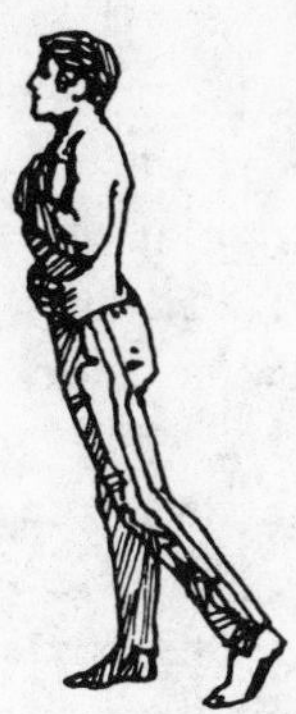

Position 5.
Walking up stairs.
Instructions: Same as for Exercise 1.

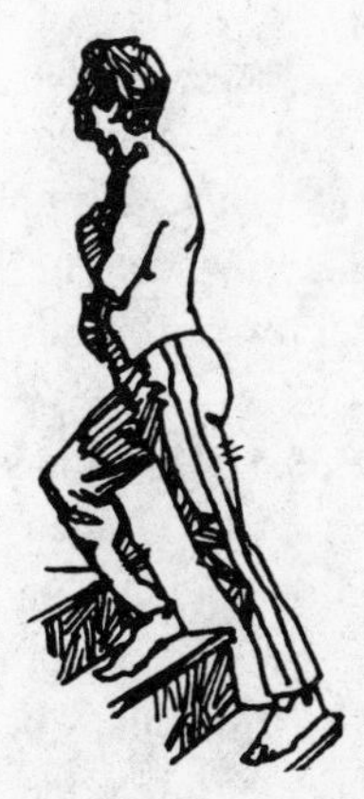

Postural Drainage

Postural drainage, a mechanical technique to help loosen and eliminate mucus and mucus plugs, is sometimes known as back-clapping, percussion, or pulmonary toilet. Excess mucus makes already narrowed passages narrower and often creates a breeding ground for bacteria. This makes the asthmatic's lungs a potential site for the growth of infections. These mucus plugs can be dangerous during an acute attack. I've had patients tell me that they would give anything to have their lungs vacuumed. Postural drainage is the next best thing to Roto-Rooter. Postural draining is a simple and logical procedure. By placing a patient in different positions, slants, and angles, the force of gravity can be used to guide the excess mucus out. This mucus first has to be loosened. This is done by "clapping" or gently pounding and then vibrating a specific area of the patient's chest or back.

Although postural drainage can be performed professionally by nurses, physical and respiratory therapists, it is a method that can also be learned easily by family members (even children) or friends who are willing to lend a "helping hand" quite literally. I would suggest, however, that the techniques be demonstrated by professionals at least the first time. You might want to contact the local Visiting Nurse Association that employs nurses and physical therapists who are trained in postural drainage and prepared to make home visits. Watching an experienced therapist may make a difference. Make sure that the family member who will be doing the therapy with you is there for the demonstration lesson.

Before beginning postural drainage, if your doctor thinks it is advisable, it is also a good idea to "lubricate" yourself by drinking a great deal of liquid. This is always a good practice for asthmatics, but is especially helpful in creating a medium for bringing up the loosened mucus. The use of bronchodilators, such as Proventil spray, is also effective, so that the air passages can be as open as possible to allow the mucus to pass. In these ways, you can set up a mechanical advantage so that postural drainage can work well. Never do postural drainage when you are having significant respiratory distress. Postural drainage can intensify the distress.

POSITIONING

Since there are a variety of angles in the bronchial tree, the patient is placed in a variety of positions during this therapy. These positions are designed to take advantage of gravity to drain the lungs along each of these different angles. There are eight positions. Each is assumed for two to three minutes. Some physicians recommend only doing Positions 5 and 6 that drain the lower lobes (or areas) of the lungs that are the most important ones in asthma. Discuss this with your physician.

Each area of the chest cavity is rapidly "clapped" with a cupped hand. With the palm of the hand cupped and the wrist loose, you should move your arm from the elbow. Clap the area for approximately one minute. If you are doing this correctly, the sound should be like the hollow sound of a horse's hoof. This shakes and loosens the mucus. After the clapping, the area is vibrated by shaking the hand rapidly over the area in the direction of gravity. This begins to move the mucus. Vibration should continue until the patient has exhaled five times. Sometimes the patient can cough up mucus immediately. Sometimes the mucus comes up after a while. Most of the time, people do postural drainage with their hands, but there are some mechanical devices available. Consult your doctor before using postural drainage. Here are the positions:

Position No. 1

Sit on a chair and lean back against a pillow. The patient should be clapped on both sides (right and left), just above the collarbones, between the neck and the shoulders.

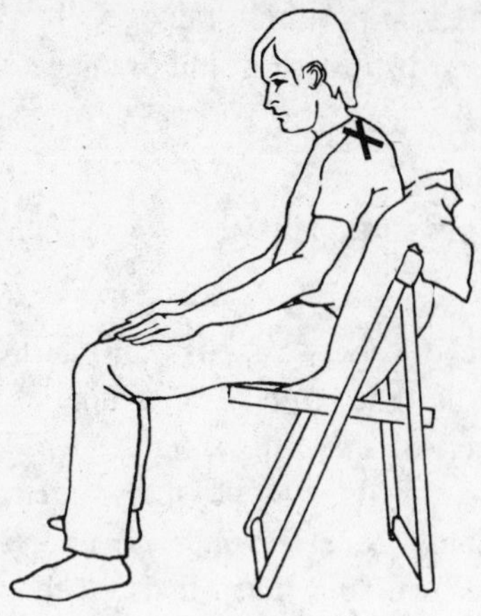

Position 1

Position No. 2

Sit in a chair and lean forward onto a pillow. The patient should be clapped on both sides of his back, above the shoulder blades. The fingers usually go over the shoulder a bit.

For the remaining positions, the patient will have to be placed on a sloping surface. Slant tables are excellent, but if you do not have one, use several pillows to achieve the angles that I'll specify.

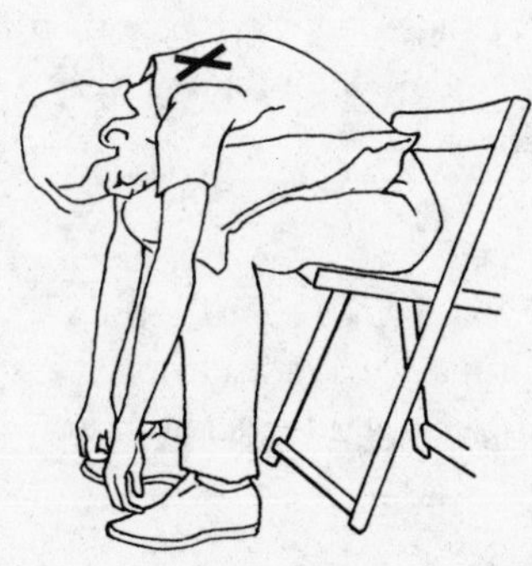

Position 2

Position No. 3

The patient should be placed so that his feet are approximately 18–20 inches above his head. Lying on his left side with knees bent, clap the lower ribs.

Position No. 4

This is the same as Position No. 3, with the patient lying on his right side.

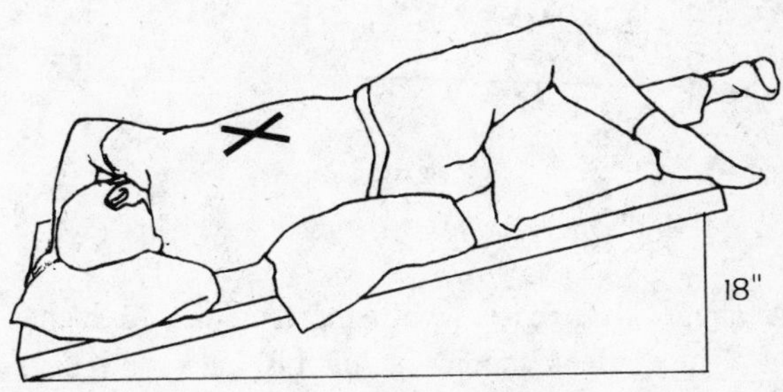

Positions 3–4

Position No. 5

Still in the same position, with his head down and feet up (18–20 inches) the patient should lie on his stomach with a pillow placed under his hips. The lower ribs should be clapped on both sides.

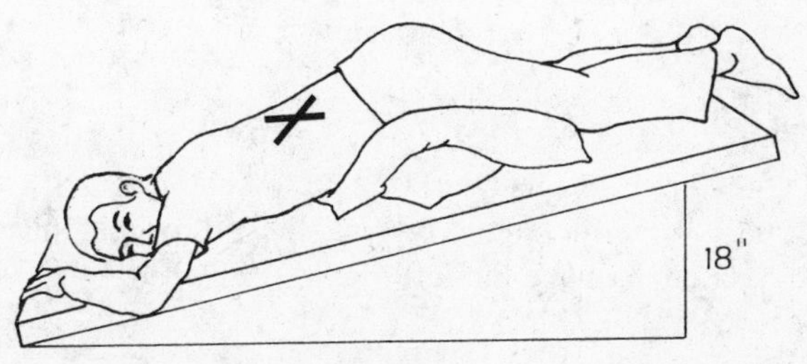

Position 5

Position No. 6

Using the same angle as Positions 3–5, lie on your back and place the pillow under your knees. The lower ribs should be clapped on both sides.

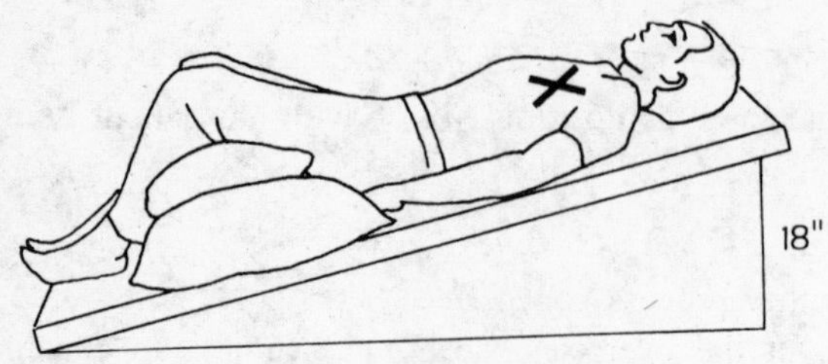

Position 6

Position No. 7

Now the angle is decreased, with the feet just 14 inches above the head. The patient should lie on his back and then take a quarter turn to the left, placing a pillow behind his back for support. Clap the area above the right nipple.

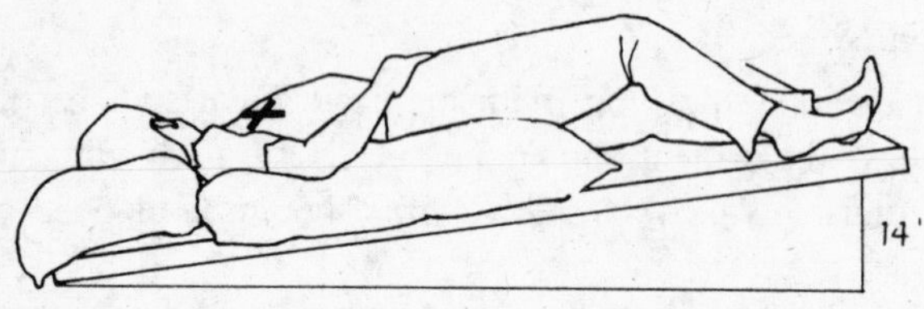

Position 7

Position No. 8

This position is the same as Position No. 7 except that the quarter turn is to the right, placing the pillow behind you for support. The area above the left nipple is clapped.

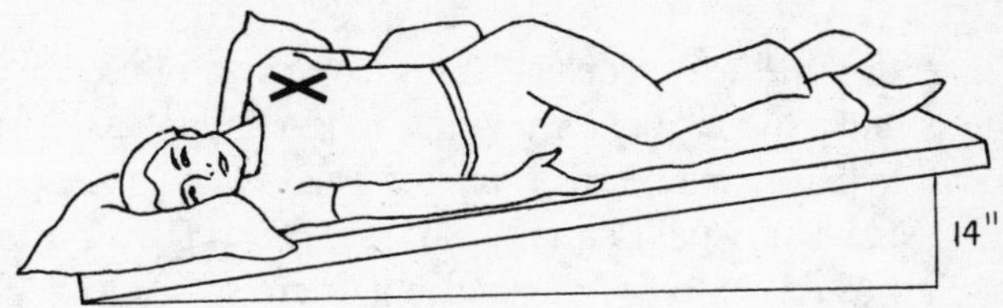

Position 8

The entire process can be repeated two or three times a day. Throughout the exercises the patient should be encouraged to cough as much as possible.

There may be some changes parents may want to make in positioning their small child. Improvising is fine, as long as the specified angles remain essentially the same. A small child may be uncomfortable or frightened when placed on a steep, sloping surface. Leaning the child across your lap or over a pile of pillows, or over an inverted little chair, may do the same thing, allowing the child to feel more secure. You know your child well, so use your imagination and judgment, but follow the guidelines as stated.

Relaxation Exercises

It makes sense that rigid body positioning and tense musculature reduce efficiency of movement. When this occurs in the breathing process, muscular tension works against the asthmatic. It follows, then, that any program of tension reduction can be beneficial for the asthmatic. Many such programs exist, including progressive relaxation, biofeedback, hypnosis, yoga, and meditation. The application of these techniques can be to reduce bodily tensions or the specific tensions induced by, and accompanying, an asthma attack. A review of these various techniques can be found in Chapter 8, Psychological Aspects of Asthma and Stress-Reduction Therapies.

Physical Fitness

It is easy for me to understand why so many of my patients tend to avoid physical activity since it is common for asthma symptoms to be precipitated by exercise. This is known as exercise-induced asthma. It would be very easy for me to tell all asthmatics to play chess and checkers and not exercise. However, this easy way out is in fact exactly the wrong thing to suggest. Physical fitness is important for everyone, asthmatics included.

There are three things you can do to make exercise possible as well as enjoyable. First, there are some medications that work especially well to reduce the possibility of asthma symptoms after exercise. Intal, Proventil, and Ventolin have worked very well when used before exercising (see Chapter 6).

Second, symptoms can also be reduced or avoided by choosing the correct type of exercise. Asthmatics can usually handle short periods of activity, rather than long, continuous exertion.

The third thing that asthmatics can do to prepare themselves for physical activity is to begin a program whereby they gradually increase their activity level to improve their physical fitness. Under their doctor's direction, they may design a program that begins with short walks that can be increased in a planned and graduated sequence. They might consider joining a health club. With moderation as the guiding principle, the asthmatic can and should become physically fit. If you happen to have a friend who is also asthmatic, the moral support and encouragement you can give each other can make achieving physical fitness fun!

Special attention should be paid to the physical fitness of children. Again, while it is perfectly understandable that a parent would become so concerned about allowing an asthmatic child to participate in sports that she might take steps to prevent it, it is physically, psychologically, and socially damaging to the child to do so. Swimming, which is an excellent exercise by any standard, has been very successful with asthmatic children. Consult your doctor. Then you must discuss any limitations with your child. Classroom teachers, physical education teachers, coaches, babysitters, family, and friends must also be involved and aware. Again, planning and moderation are good guiding principles.

Conclusion

As you read this book, it becomes obvious that asthma is a very complex disease that often requires a wide range of therapeutic approaches. Even though physical therapy is a less common treatment approach and applicable primarily to the chronic asthmatic population, some aspects of the program are important for every asthmatic to know. Too often we rely on the doctor or other significant others to do the work of treating us. Physical therapy is something the asthmatic patient can actively do for himself.

10

ASTHMA AND PREGNANCY

The decision to have a baby is a personal and often difficult one. The presence of asthma in the family complicates this decision. There are many concerns an asthmatic woman may have that a nonasthmatic would never dream of. She may be concerned about whether

1. her baby will be asthmatic
2. pregnancy will make her own asthma worse
3. her asthma will affect the development of the fetus
4. her asthma medications will affect the baby
5. she will be able to go through labor, delivery, and breastfeeding in a normal way

These are, indeed, weighty concerns and for some of you, this may be the most important chapter in the book. It is full of information you will need to ease your concerns and help pave the way for a happy pregnancy and delivery.

Is Asthma Inherited?

In general, the answer is yes. A susceptibility to asthma appears to be passed on genetically. Whether or not a person who has inherited the predisposition actually becomes asthmatic depends on many things, including the body's characteristics, the environment's characteristics, and how the individual interacts with the environment. When I talk about asthma being inherited, I am speaking more about the inheritance of a tendency that could lead to asthma rather than the inheritance of the symptoms themselves.

The exact mechanisms of the genetic transmission of asthma are unclear. Many of the key studies on the subject offer conflicting data. There really are no good statistics. What follows are rules of thumb to guide you:

A. When neither parent is asthmatic and neither has a family history of asthma or allergies, there is a very slight chance of having a baby with a tendency to develop asthma.
B. If neither parent is so afflicted, but one parent has a family history of asthma, then the chance of having a child with asthma is less than 10 percent.
C. If both parents have a family history of asthma, but do not themselves have the condition, their chances of having an asthmatic child exceed that of the general population and are greater than 10 percent.
D. If one parent is asthmatic, the chances of having an asthmatic child increase.
E. The chances of having an asthmatic child are greater when both mother and father are asthmatic.

We have been talking about inheritance probabilities based on the characteristics of the mother and father—and for good reason. The presence of asthma in immediate family relatives (mother, father, sisters, and brothers) is more important than the presence of asthma in a distant relative.

The probability of having an asthmatic child has even been studied in relation to the time and place of conception. One such study concluded that the highest incidence of asthma in England occurred in children who were born in the autumn. Other studies have claimed that there was a higher incidence of asthma in developed rather than in underdeveloped countries.

These results are not accepted as facts, so I do not advise you to pack your bags for a fall safari in the deepest jungles of Africa to have your baby.

Is There More Risk to the Baby When the Mother Is Asthmatic?

Older studies showed that an asthmatic mother had a higher probability of having more complications during her pregnancy and of giving birth to an underweight infant with more problems than the average newborn. Recent studies are much more encouraging. They show that the risk of unnecessary complications in mother and child can be cut significantly when proper medical care is taken during pregnancy under the careful eye of a competent doctor. The pregnant woman need not have an increased incidence of complications, nor need the baby experience any more problems than if born to a nonasthmatic woman.

I think the crucial difference between the older and newer studies lies in the importance placed on the need for careful monitoring of the asthmatic by her doctor or doctors. When you decide whether or not to become pregnant, include in your plan the need for continued close contact with both your allergist and your obstetrician. I will elaborate considerably later.

IS THERE MORE RISK TO THE ASTHMATIC MOTHER-TO-BE?

Many of the studies that relate to this question are contradictory, but there are some general conclusions I can offer you. Statistically during pregnancy one third of asthmatic pregnant women will get worse, one third will get better, and one third will remain the same, as far as their asthma symptoms are concerned. If you have moderate to severe asthma, you may remain as severe or possibly get worse; if you have mild asthma, you might remain unchanged or perhaps improve.

If you were pregnant previously, and if your asthma got worse, the previous problem may reoccur. If you got better, then perhaps you can look forward to improvement again. This is not always predictable; many women have very different experiences with each pregnancy. Whatever the change in asthma symptoms during pregnancy, you will often return to prepregnancy severity levels after your pregnancy is over.

Fortunately, it is rare for a nonasthmatic to become asthmatic during pregnancy. When it does happen, the asthma will usually disappear when the baby appears.

THE FINAL DECISION

Certainly I hope it is clear to you that the presence of asthma in either parent should not automatically preclude a couple from having a baby. Except for the very severe case, where pregnancy may create a life-threatening situation, the majority of pregnancies among asthmatics are manageable, if you want to manage them. But, again, this is a very personal decision that depends upon your desire to have a child, the severity of your asthma, your experience with asthma, your experience with pregnancy, your values, your life-style, and your determination to work things through. In my practice, I have helped manage many asthmatic pregnant women and I am glad to say that the results have been very rewarding.

THE DECISION IS MADE

Assuming that you have decided to become pregnant, there are some facts you need to know immediately. You are becoming a "special case" in asthma and you need special attention.

During the time before you actually conceive, you must make every effort to get yourself in the best physical shape possible. You and the doctor managing your asthma must meet and decide upon a plan. I will soon present my philosophy and plan for treating a pregnant asthmatic, but you and your doctor should decide upon a course of treatment enabling you to use the least medication for optimal breathing. As you will soon see, some medications are not recommended while others are recommended freely.

If you do not have an obstetrician, seek one out now. Perhaps your allergist can help you with your choice. The choice of a doctor is always an important one, but for the pregnant asthmatic it is even more important and complicated. You cannot assume that your allergist will know everything about pregnancy, and you cannot assume that your obstetrician will know everything about asthma.

To a great extent, pregnancy in an asthmatic woman requires a team approach. Remember, you, the patient, will be playing an active part in this team effort. You may have to be the liaison, insuring that each doctor knows the status of your pregnancy, your asthma, and your medication.

As you try to reach as low a level of medication as possible, without increasing the risk of becoming more symptomatic (and thereby creating the need for increased medication), you must be very careful to avoid potentially adverse conditions. As much as possible, avoid any agents that trigger your symptoms. This is a good time to aggressively pamper yourself.

Our discussion of the preparations for conception has focused only on the female partner. What about the father-to-be? Well, aside from the inheritance factors that I have already explained, the male asthmatic does not have any precautions to take. The medications he is taking for his asthma, even on the day of conception, do not pass via the sperm into the egg to create any problems for the fetus.

TOP PRIORITY

It is clear that the health of the woman just prior to conception and throughout her pregnancy bears directly on the health of the newborn. It is also clear that women who are about to conceive or who are pregnant should strive to take the least amount of medication possible. This is easy enough for anyone who does not have a chronic problem, but for the asthmatic, it is not so simple. She will have to choose medications carefully, considering the effects of her medications on the baby. While I will discuss at length the specific medications, there is a guiding principle that must be understood. The top priority goes to the maintenance of good breathing in the mother-to-be.

When you are pregnant, your blood supply is for both you and the baby and, therefore, your blood oxygen supply is for both you and the baby. You must keep the blood oxygen in good supply. Low oxygen (hypoxemia) to the baby must be avoided. It can be more harmful to the baby than any of the medications' side effects. So do not avoid or delay taking your medications for fear that the medications will harm the baby. The avoidance or the delay may be worse! Remember, you are not working alone. Consult your doctor.

Consider the example of Debra Z., a thirty-three-year-old woman who has asthma, severe enough to require steroids at certain times. When she first saw me, I knew that she was trying to conceive. Because theophylline is a safe drug to use during pregnancy, I placed her on this medication to control her symptoms. Every once in a while, she had acute attacks that required supplemental medication. Knowing that she might be pregnant at any time, she did not use the additional medication she was supposed to during one acute attack. Her attack worsened considerably, and by the time she finally decided to contact me, she was experiencing significant breathing difficulties. Had she been pregnant, she could have been placing the baby in jeopardy.

The point this case history makes is the need to maintain open communication between you and your doctor(s) both before and during your pregnancy so that you will know what to do and when to do it. You and your doctor(s) must design a plan that you can follow during a variety of situations. You must feel comfortable with the doctor(s) you have chosen. If not, change doctors.

Asthma Medications and Pregnancy

The most ideal situation would be to have your asthma symptoms under control with no medications at all. Depending upon the severity of your asthma and the effects of pregnancy on your asthma, this may or may not be plausible. For most of you, however, you will need to use some asthma medications during your pregnancy.

In fact, the time to start dealing with your medications is before you are actually pregnant. During the weeks or months before conception, follow the general rule of trying to reduce your medications to the lowest level while maintaining symptom control. Medications stay in your bloodstream for a while, so reduce their levels as much as possible before your pregnancy begins.

Because it is such a well-known standard policy to eliminate drugs during pregnancy, you might think that you should throw out all your pills and sprays the moment you discover that you are pregnant. This is the wrong thing to do for both you and your baby. In fact, beware of any doctor who tells you to suddenly stop taking all of your medications. Some medications should be stopped, but others can (and should) be continued.

DRUGS THAT MUST BE ELIMINATED DURING PREGNANCY

The following drugs should not be taken during or immediately preceding pregnancy: hydroxyzine hydrochloride (Vistaril, Atarax, and Marax) that may cause abnormalities in the fetus, potassium iodide (SSKI) or any iodinated medication since this can cause a goiter in the fetus, and tetracycline or its derivatives (Vibramycin, Achromycin, and Terramycin) that cause staining of the baby's teeth and malformation of the skeletal system.

In the third trimester of pregnancy, avoid aspirin and sulfas, which can cause jaundice in the infant. As a matter of fact, avoid aspirin throughout pregnancy.

Only when absolutely necessary will I prescribe any of the oral (tablet) preparations of the beta sympathomimetic drugs: metaproterenol (Alupent or Metaprel), albuterol (Ventolin or Proventil), and terbutaline sulfate (Brethine or Bricanyl). Besides having a substantial inhibitory effect on labor, these drugs have been found to cause other complications as well.

DRUGS THAT CAN BE TAKEN (IF NEEDED) DURING PREGNANCY

In the best of all possible worlds, no medications would be needed during pregnancy. But in the best of all possible worlds, you would not have asthma. It is of supreme importance to keep the mother-to-be healthy and breathing well so the fetus will breathe well also. As a general guiding principle, a pregnant woman who needs asthma medication should use as many inhaled medications (Brethaire, Alupent, Metaprel, Vanceril, Beclovent, Azmacort, and Intal) as possible because they are minimally absorbed and reduce the amount of systemic medications (pills). This principle includes the use of nasal sprays (Nasalcrom, Vancenase, and Beconase—but NOT Decadron Turbinaire, since it is absorbable) as the drugs of choice over antihistamines for the treatment of nasal congestion (rhinitis). The following is a list of drugs which have not been shown clinically to be associated with any complication during pregnancy or birth defects. But remember, during pregnancy always discuss any drugs with your physician prior to using them.

Theophylline. There have been no specific problems documented about the use of any of these drugs (short-, intermediate-, or long-acting theophylline). A theophylline blood level should be taken at least once each trimester during your pregnancy. Pregnant women have significant changes in weight and theophylline metabolism because of the baby and initially require more theophylline. However, in the last trimester therapeutic dosages may have to be decreased, and theophylline levels may have to be checked as often as once a month.

Adrenalin-like Drugs (Sympathomimetic). As I have already mentioned, the tablet form of these sympathomimetic (Adrenalin-like) drugs is not cleared by the FDA for use during pregnancy. If it is absolutely necessary to use a drug in this class, one may use ephedrine, although it is no longer widely used.

Sympathomimetic Sprays. Terbutaline (Brethaire), metaproterenol (Metaprel, Alupent), albuterol (Proventil, Ventolin). At the present time, terbutaline is used as the primary inhaled sympathomimetic spray for pregnant asthmatic women. This is because studies have shown that it is the safest inhalant medication to use. If terbutaline is ineffective (a not uncommon occurrence), I then try metaproterenol. Usually one of these drugs is effective. In patients who are not pregnant, I prefer albuterol, which in my experience is the most effective sympathomimetic drug with the least side effects. There have been no reports of fetal malformations secondary to the use of albuterol, but it is teratogenic (damaging to the fetus) in mice, and since there are no studies to show its safety in humans, allergists prefer not to prescribe it for their pregnant patients. In rare circumstances when all else fails, I will use albuterol, but only after discussing all possible side effects with my patient. When inhaled terbutaline and metaproterenol are effective in my pregnant patients, I utilize these drugs in the same fashion as for nonpregnant patients. (See pages 159–161.)

Injectable Adrenalin or epinephrine must be used judiciously, but can be used. They have been known to increase uterine contractions, but their effectiveness in relieving acute attacks is substantial enough to justify their use. The hypoxemia (low oxygen in the blood) that may result from an acute asthma attack can do much more harm than the Adrenalin.

Cromolyn Sodium (Intal). Intal appears to be a good, safe drug for use in pregnancy. There have been virtually no birth defects reported that could be linked to the use of Intal. As is always true, keep in touch with your doctor who will have the latest information on all medications.

Antibiotics. Ampicillin, amoxicillin, erythromycin, penicillin, and cephalosporin are safe during pregnancy. Tetracycline is not.

Corticosteroids. Cortisone does not appear to have adverse effects on the human fetus. Although I would not prescribe cortisone if it could be avoided, it does not appear to be harmful. When other therapies are not as successful, the oral form of corticosteroids can be used effectively to manage moderate to severe asthma in pregnant women. However, I would always recommend the nonabsorbable spray form of this medication (beclomethasone, available as Vanceril or Beclovent) first. This may all sound contradictory to what you may have heard, but after years of study, the use of corticosteroids during pregnancy appears to be justified when absolutely necessary to control the asthma.

Over-the-Counter Medications. In general, I would not recommend over-the-counter drugs because their use implies that you are not consulting your doctor. This is crucial—now that you are pregnant, more than ever. Second, these are usually combination drugs, containing ephedrine and theophylline and usually phenobarbitol. Phenobarbitol should not be used during pregnancy.

Immunotherapy (Allergy Shots). For pregnant patients who have been receiving immunotherapy and are doing well (no systemic reactions), I would certainly recommend that they continue getting their allergy injections. The effects of immunotherapy have been carefully studied, and there is no evidence of harm to the fetus. If the allergy shots are working well, it would seem unwise to stop and risk increasing your asthma symptoms. If immunotherapy is not helping, or if it causes a great many adverse reactions, it should be stopped.

I do not start immunotherapy for allergies during pregnancy. The reason is that patients just beginning immunotherapy have an unknown propensity to systemic reactions. I have no way of knowing what their reactivity would be, and systemic reactions can cause a miscarriage. I also will not administer skin tests to patients when they are pregnant. I prefer to do a RAST, which is not invasive and will not cause any problem.

RHINITIS IN PREGNANCY

Rhinitis (chronically congested nose) is very common in pregnancy, occurring in approximately 30 percent of women. Rhinitis can also bring on some swelling of the respiratory passages. Therefore, the presence of rhinitis in the pregnant asthmatic can be particularly problematic. *I prefer not to use any medications to treat rhinitis during the first trimester of pregnancy*. If the patient is very uncomfortable, I prescribe normal saline spray. If there is no alternative, I would try Nasalcrom, and if there is no relief, I would try Afrin intermittently (remember not to use Afrin for more than three days in a row as it can damage mucus membranes). In severe cases, if there has not been any relief from saline spray, Nasalcrom or intermittent use of Afrin, I might prescribe intranasal beclomethasone (Vancenase or Beconase), which is a nonabsorbable steroid spray. I make sure to tell my patients that this is a cortisone spray, and since nasal congestion is not nearly as dangerous as asthma, the spray should only be used if all else has failed. Usually one of the sprays handles the problem. If this isn't the case, then I would try Pyribenzamine.

MANAGING DIFFERENT TYPES OF CASES

Now that I've reviewed the individual drugs, let's look at some typical cases. Even though each patient is different, there are some general procedures I follow with different severity levels.

The most obvious case is the pregnant asthmatic who has no symptoms. Therefore, she requires no medication. When symptoms are intermittent and mild, I would not give any medication during symptom-free periods.

When symptoms occur, assuming there is no infection, I presently prescribe Brethaire (terbutaline). If this does not work well, I would switch the patient to metaproterenol (Alupent or Metaprel) on an as-needed basis. If future evidence shows that Proventil and Ventolin are safe for use in pregnancy, I will prescribe one of them as the drug of choice over Brethaire, Alupent, or Metaprel, since they are more effective.

If the symptoms persist, I would use short-acting theophylline tablets as needed. If the symptoms become more continuous, I would place the patient on long-acting theophylline at the lowest therapeutic level. Remember, theophylline blood levels should be measured more frequently during pregnancy than is generally necessary during the nonpregnant state.

If the theophylline does not work in combination with an inhaled sympathomimetic spray (Brethaire, Alupent, Metaprel) but the symptoms are relatively mild, I would introduce Intal.

When I am managing a patient with severe and continuous wheezing, I recommend corticosteroids in the doses needed to control the asthma. As always, I would strive to discontinue the use of the corticosteroids as quickly as possible. When the use of corticosteroid medicine is necessary it is prescribed in alternate-day doses whenever possible. However, I usually prefer to prescribe the inhaled nonabsorbed steroid spray if prolonged steroid therapy is needed.

Whether I see a patient before or during her pregnancy, the general procedure is to keep the patient's symptoms under control by using the least amount of the least absorbed forms of the required medications.

THE ACUTE ATTACK IN THE PREGNANT ASTHMATIC

If an acute attack develops during pregnancy, I treat it almost the same way I treat it in a nonpregnant woman, except that I encourage closer communication between the patient and physician. Rather than allow the patient to treat herself at home, I might encourage more liberal use of a hospital emergency room where it is easier to administer oxygen, fluids, and an inhalant sympathomimetic bronchodilator (terbutaline or metaproterenol) via a nebulizer. Terbutaline is preferable to epinephrine by injection. Terbutaline can be administered, if necessary, and depending upon the amount of theophylline taken previously, I would prescribe aminophylline intravenously. Certainly, I would add steroids if required.

If it is found that your acute attack may have been triggered by an infection, an antibiotic may be prescribed. Remember, as far as the pregnancy is concerned, you can safely use ampicillin, amoxicillin, erythromycin, penicillin, or cephalosporin, but not tetracycline.

GETTING READY FOR THE BIG DAY

During the last months of your pregnancy, you must begin to plan for your hospital stay. You and your obstetrician must discuss the possible use of anesthetics, the management and availability of your medications on the maternity ward, and the availability of other professionals if necessary (particularly an allergist, pediatrician, and possibly a respiratory therapist). While the imminent onset of labor means hospitalization, bringing with it a feeling of security in being in a medical setting and relief that "others" can now manage your medications, do not be misled. While you may be surrounded by doctors and nurses, you may still be the only one able to understand, predict, and manage your own asthma. Make sure you can! Make certain that your doctor clearly indicates your medication regimen on your chart and that he instructs others to listen to you. The doctors and nurses around you are often "programmed" by their daily experiences to think almost exclusively about the baby, or delivery emergencies. The staff on a maternity ward is accustomed to dealing with well patients most of the time. They may not be as tuned in to a mother with chronic asthma. Especially in the labor and delivery rooms, hospital staff doctors and nurses may not even be aware of your problem, since your own doctor will not be there all of the time. Protect yourself.

Once your baby is born you are relieved of the anxiety, but not of the asthma! This persists and must be managed as usual (or more aggressively). Your medication must be administered in accordance with the usual pattern. Unless you are planning to breast-feed (an issue that we will discuss), you might want to generously fortify yourself with medication following delivery so that you may enjoy yourself and your new baby. The crucial point I am making here is the need for careful planning ahead of time. If, for example, you sleep best on three pillows, request them or have your husband bring them. I know some patients who were very comforted by being allowed to bring an inhalant spray, such as Brethaire or Alupent, with them to the delivery room. Discuss the use of these medications with your physician. Do not use them unless your physician knows about them. Make sure that your schedule for medication is not forgotten. Do not let anyone confiscate your medication until you know it will be replaced at the request of your physician. *Plan!*

NATURAL CHILDBIRTH

You might want to discuss the possibility of natural or near-natural childbirth with your doctor. Depending upon the severity of your asthma, there does not seem to be any data that would argue against an asthmatic woman using a method such as the Lamaze. Many of my patients have been able to participate in the exercises and breathing patterns involved. Certainly it can have a relaxing effect, which is always to your benefit. It may also reduce the amount of anesthetic that you would require during labor. General anesthesia always increases the risk in surgery; unfortunately even more so in the asthmatic. Obviously, when you need general anesthesia, you must have it. Therefore, anything that would help obviate the need for general anesthesia is helpful to the asthmatic and nonasthmatic alike.

MEDICATIONS AS YOU APPROACH LABOR

With the onset of labor, or when a cesarean section is scheduled, measures must be taken to insure that the patient receives her regular medication and any supplementary medication needed. In the case of cesarean section, if the patient has been taking oral theophylline, she must be given this medication intravenously. If the patient is on corticosteroid medication or has been on it in the past for a significant duration (see page 169) and is scheduled to have a surgical delivery, then she should receive oral steroids from one to three days prior to surgery, the duration and dose dependent on the severity of her asthma (her physician's decision). Just prior to surgery she should receive intramuscular steroids; and during surgery she should be given intravenous steroids. Postsurgery she will also need intravenous and/or intramuscular steroids and, as soon as possible, oral steroids (the duration and dose once again dependent on the severity of her illness).

In a normal vaginal delivery, theophylline must be maintained either orally or intravenously depending on the condition of the patient. Sprays should be continued if possible. For patients on corticosteroids at the time of delivery, or who have required them for a significant amount of time in the past to suppress their adrenal gland, steroids should be administered as described above. Once again the duration and dose of the steroids to be given will be dependent on the severity of her illness, which is a judgment call by her physician.

DELIVERY

During delivery there is a need for a good anesthesiologist. If possible, consult with the anesthesiologist prior to delivery. Although local anesthetics are preferred, Halothane, a gas, is the preferred general anesthetic when necessary.

If you are delivering by cesarean section, as I have just mentioned, intravenous or injectable theophylline and cortisone might be in order. You will be told not to take any medications for nine to twelve hours before surgery. Ask your doctor what you can do during this time period if your asthma becomes a problem. Can you use a spray? What medications are least prohibited? Again, the key word is *plan* for all contingencies.

IMMEDIATELY AFTER DELIVERY

After the delivery of a healthy baby, everyone should be tremendously relieved and joyous. That is, if the asthma has been managed well. As I have said, this can be a time to increase medication, free of the concerns of the baby. The mother should be made very comfortable now so she can enjoy motherhood. If the situation is not managed well, needless difficulties can ensue, as the following case study will demonstrate. A patient who came to me after her healthy son had been born told this story.

She had had a cesarean section for reasons unrelated to her moderately severe asthma. She had not taken any medication for the nine hours before her surgery. Seven hours after delivery she awoke quite groggy and asked for her regular set of pills. The intern told her to go back to sleep and that she was just imagining her breathing difficulties. Twelve hours later (after twenty-eight hours without medication), she awoke with severe symptoms. Her physical condition after the surgery absolutely prevented her from getting out of bed to get her pills. The nurses not only refused to give the medications to her, but also refused to telephone her doctor or even to give her the phone to call him herself. The mistake that had been made was the agreement between doctor and patient that she was the best one to manage her own medications. She was—but only when she was physically able to do so. After a cesarean, she was not! She was denied credibility as a patient, which put her in a potentially dangerous situation. She complained enough to get some Adrenalin that helped only temporarily. Three hours later (now morning) her doctor arrived, became furious with the staff, and ordered the intravenous aminophylline that should have been started over thirty-one hours before. Her symptoms were soon controlled, but the needless physical and emotional drain spoiled the first few days of motherhood for her.

Another point to be made about this postdelivery period concerns coughing, which is often painful after childbirth, especially after a cesarean section. Since asthmatics need to be able to cough often, this pain can become a problem. A binder around the abdomen or a folded pillow pressed to the stomach helps to serve as a shock absorber. If medications are used appropriately at this time, problems with coughing can often be minimized. However, if you intend to breast-feed your baby, then the amount and type of medication you take has to be modified.

BREAST-FEEDING

When breast-feeding, with the exception of iodides and tetracycline, almost all the other antiasthmatic drugs that a pregnant woman takes are allowable. Discuss your medication regimen with your pediatrician who will be the final arbiter for you concerning breast-feeding. If you are breast-feeding while taking theophylline, the baby must be watched for signs of jitteriness or irritability. If the baby becomes slightly irritable, the pediatrician may request that the baby's theophylline level be checked. The chances are that sufficient theophylline will not be secreted through the breast milk to cause a problem.

Similarly, the use of the sympathomimetic drugs and even corticosteroids do not normally preclude breast-feeding although I typically suggest that patients on oral steroids not breast-feed. Patients on low to moderate doses may want to discuss the pros and cons of their own situation with their own physician.

Antihistamines and decongestants do not generally present a problem for the baby, although drowsiness or irritability may develop. Cromolyn sodium is no problem during breast-feeding.

I usually recommend that allergic or asthmatic mothers breast-feed their infants because I think it will reduce the degree of allergic sensitization of the newborn, and this is the most important preventive measure one can take to reduce a child's allergic potential. Some observers note that if the breast-feeding mother eats allergenic foods such as milk, chocolate, eggs, corn, or wheat, the baby might develop allergic symptoms. The data here is very controversial, and in each instance, the approach should be individualized. A nutritious diet is recommended for the breast-feeding mother. In fact, I feel that babies should be breast-fed for as long as possible, withholding solid food and multiple or combination foods.

We have covered a great deal of territory in this chapter so far, from preconception days all the way to breast-feeding your healthy baby. There is a great deal to consider and manage for the asthmatic pregnant woman, but I am optimistic that all can be taken into consideration and managed successfully. My general message focuses on two points. First, pregnancy in the asthmatic patient requires a team effort, obliging the patient and doctor (or doctors) to keep the lines of communication open. Changes in asthma may influence changes in pregnancy care, and vice versa. All involved must be informed.

Second, the mother's health is crucial. It reflects directly on the health of the fetus. Therefore, the number one priority is to keep the mother healthy and breathing well. This will keep the baby "breathing" well too. Pregnancy is always exciting, but in the asthmatic patient it is both exciting and challenging!

Now it is time to consider how asthma affects the growing child.

11

ASTHMA IN CHILDREN

The Statistics

The following statistics and trends are true of childhood asthma:

- Asthma is more common in children than in adults.
- Asthma affects nearly 10 percent of all children in the United States.
- Approximately half of childhood asthma begins before the age of three.
- Until puberty, males are affected twice as frequently as females.
- During the teens and early adulthood, there are more female asthmatics than males.
- Asthma represents one of the leading causes of child mortality.
- Asthma is one of the leading causes of school absenteeism.
- Approximately two thirds of children who have asthma will outgrow it. The earlier the onset and the more severe it is, the less likely one is to outgrow it.
- There are frequent remissions of asthma during puberty, with recurrences in adulthood.
- If asthma symptoms occur before the age of six months, symptoms often tend to be severe and long-lasting.
- If asthma symptoms continue or begin during puberty, symptoms often tend to be severe and long-lasting.
- Immunotherapy tends to be more effective with children and young adults than with adults aged fifty or greater.

- If asthma begins after the age of two (up to approximately thirty-five years of age), there is a good possibility that it has an allergic basis.

Asthma in children differs from asthma in adults. The similarities include its causes, signs and symptoms, and treatment programs (environmental control, immunotherapy, diet, and medication). Differences arise because we are dealing with someone who has a great deal of growing to do, both physically, socially, and emotionally. The doctor and the parents have the responsibility of making sure that as little as possible gets in the way of this growth.

As a parent you may feel helpless, but you are not. The treatment of asthma in children is couched in considerable optimism. You will not be working alone, but as part of a group effort. The group may include the patient, parents, doctors (pediatrician and allergist), school nurses, teachers, camp counselors, coaches, grandparents, and friends. With some knowledge and aggressive involvement on your part added to all of the modalities and techniques now available to us in asthma care, you can look forward to having your child's asthma under control. With the exception of a few very severe cases, the majority of asthmatic children lead normal to near-normal lives and some (as you will see) may even outgrow their problem.

Our optimism is further encouraged when we understand that asthma in children need not lead to emphysema or permanent heart disease—misconceptions I often hear spoken of. Nor does asthma necessarily result in permanent lung scarring or other damage. Since the effects of asthma in children are reversible, whatever abuse the heart and lungs endure during an asthma attack is not permanent.

SIGNS AND SYMPTOMS

The symptoms of asthma in the child are generally the same as in the adult. They can include wheezing, coughing, shortness of breath, complaints of chest congestion, tight chest, exercise intolerance, recurrent bronchitis, or recurrent pneumonia. Very often asthma begins with coughing and no wheezing, especially in conjunction with a cold or during the pollen season.

One difference between asthma symptoms in the child and in the adult is the speed with which symptoms can occur. There are differences in anatomy between the lungs of a child and the lungs of the adult. In the child, the airways are small and can close quickly. Mucus plugs can more easily block passages in the child's lungs. These differences place the child with respiratory disease at a distinct disadvantage. Breathing problems may very rapidly become severe. Therefore, prompt medical attention is required.

Is It Really Asthma?

Before I describe how I handle an asthmatic child, I will first discuss the diagnosis of asthma in children. The differential diagnosis of asthma in a small child is not always easy. Breathing problems can be symptomatic of many ailments in children. Respiratory difficulty can be dangerous and, therefore, early recognition, proper diagnosis, and treatment of those conditions that require prompt medical help are essential.

Refusal of an infant to suck (or in an older child to eat), fussiness, rapid or labored breathing, or continuous coughing may herald significant respiratory tract diseases. As a parent, you can also recognize breathing problems when your child's nostrils flare or if there are retractions (sucking in of the skin under the rib cage, in between the ribs, or just above the breastbone) sometimes causing the head to bob because of increased respiratory efforts.

In children, other major causes of breathing difficulty that are not asthma include bronchiolitis and croup.

BRONCHIOLITIS

The most common cause of wheezing in the first year of life is bronchiolitis. This usually occurs in the winter and is caused by a virus. Bronchiolitis may produce a great deal of difficulty in breathing with shortness of breath, wheezing, and loss of appetite. Most of the time, this disease can be handled outside the hospital. Bronchiolitis may be a forerunner of asthma. If it occurs during an epidemic in the winter and if there is no family history of allergies, the chances of it being a forerunner of asthma are slight. When it occurs in a child with a family history of asthma or allergies and does not occur during a winter epidemic, then there is a greater likelihood that asthma will subsequently develop. If the latter pattern of bronchiolitis recurs, then the development of asthma becomes a likely possibility.

CROUP

Croup is usually a viral, but occasionally a bacterial, infectious disease most commonly found in children aged three months to three years. There is difficulty in getting air into the lungs because the tissues of the larynx and/or trachea become swollen. With asthma, by contrast, initially there may be difficulty getting air out of the lungs because of an obstruction in the airway lower down beyond the larynx and trachea. Croup is characteristically accompanied by hoarseness, a barking cough, and a low-grade fever. Croup can begin as an upper respiratory tract infection that spreads to involve the larynx. To everyone's chagrin, croup symptoms usually become most severe at ten or eleven o'clock at night. The child becomes short of breath, air hungry, and anxious. He may start to cry and become agitated, thereby increasing his respiratory difficulty. Croup is usually an acute illness and it is sometimes treated with antibiotics, decongestants (not antihistamines), and steam. Croup can be dangerous, and close contact with your physician is important.

While bronchiolitis and croup are the most frequent mimickers of asthma symptoms, there are others. Though they may be rare, they are worth mentioning so that we have a complete picture of breathing problems in children.

EPIGLOTTITIS

Epiglottitis is an inflammation of the epiglottis (the cap that closes off the trachea when you swallow, thus keeping food out of your respiratory passageway). The onset might be quite sudden, often within one to two hours. The child usually has a fever of 102–104 degrees, appears sickly and anxious, is lethargic, breathes hesitantly, and complains of pain in the throat. If the pain becomes severe enough, the child will drool rather than swallow. This must be recognized as an emergency situation. An airtube or *tracheotomy* may be necessary to open the airways.

FOREIGN-BODY OBSTRUCTION

Children often accidentally swallow objects that they have put into their mouths. Sometimes such foreign bodies are inhaled into the trachea or lungs. When this happens, the child may cough explosively and repeatedly; wheezing will also accompany this attack. Very often, a child will swallow or inhale a foreign body and apparently recover without telling his parents. The foreign body may then produce wheezing that may be intermittent and mimic asthma. A chest X ray is often used to diagnose a patient with asthmalike symptoms to look for evidence of a foreign body present in the airways or lungs.

PNEUMONIA

Pneumonia, an inflammation of the lungs, characterized by fever and a frequent cough, can also be confused with asthma. It is diagnosed by X rays, and treated with antibiotics. When pneumonia is recurrent, an evaluation for asthma and perhaps other diseases is probably in order.

CYSTIC FIBROSIS

Cystic fibrosis is a progressive disease that affects the lungs in children and is characterized by recurrent bronchial infections, wheezing, harsh coughing, other nonrespiratory symptoms, and generally poor growth. I routinely do a differential diagnostic test called a sweat test on children with severe asthma to rule out cystic fibrosis.

HEART DISEASE

Heart disease may also account for breathing difficulty in children. It is sometimes accompanied by poor growth and poor oxygenation of the blood or cyanosis, giving the child a "blue" look.

CONGENITAL ANOMALIES

Birth defects can block either the trachea or the bronchi, causing difficulty in breathing. One such anomaly, a vascular ring, occurs when a blood vessel such as the aorta circles around the trachea instead of being in its usual position in front of the trachea. In such situations, a diagnostic clue is the observation that changing the position of the head often helps breathing.

HYPERVENTILATION SYNDROME

This syndrome of overbreathing (too deeply or too rapidly) occurs primarily in adolescents and adults. It may be mistaken for asthma or it may coexist with it. The patient is anxious and is having difficulty getting his breath. There may be complaints of headaches, tingling in the fingers and toes, stomach and chest pain, dizziness, and a fainting sensation. Despite these reports, the patient appears to be breathing well without wheezing and has normal pulmonary function studies. Very often, patients with hyperventilation syndrome will refuse to perform pulmonary function tests because they are afraid of smothering.

MITRAL VALVE PROLAPSE

The *mitral valve* is one of the major valves of the heart. If it is not set perfectly in place, it can cause minor dysfunctions of the heart. The disorder, mitral valve prolapse, is usually seen in slender adolescents and adults and is much more common in females than in males. These patients complain of chest pain during or following strenuous exercise. Therefore, this can be confused with exercise-induced asthma. On physical examination, a doctor can usually hear a clicking sound, and an echocardiogram will establish the diagnosis.

In addition to these specific syndromes, there are more generalized problems, the symptoms of which may have asthmalike characteristics. For example, chest pain might indicate a rib fracture or heart disease. Shortness of breath may indicate anemia or heart failure. All that wheezes is not asthma, and some of these other diseases can be quite serious. Consult your doctor!

WHAT WILL THE DOCTOR DO?

As you can see, the differential diagnosis of asthma can be complicated, sophisticated, and tricky. When you bring your symptomatic child to the pediatrician, his job is to bring the acute symptoms under control as well as to reach a correct diagnosis. Expect him to ask you questions about your child's symptoms and health history, your family's health history, and your home environment. He will probably request some laboratory tests such as a chest X ray, sweat test, pulmonary function, and blood count (see Chapter 3). It is with this information that your doctor will be able to confirm a diagnosis of asthma.

Managing Asthma in a Child

YOUR CHILD HAS ASTHMA

Don't panic! While this is not the happiest news you have ever heard, there is a great deal that can be done to enable your child to lead a normal or as near to normal life as possible. Your child may have to learn to cope with a few restrictions and a few medications, but he should adjust and adjust well, probably better than you. The best thing you can do is to become a supportive and knowledgeable parent. As I said before, asthma is a problem that includes not only the patient but a list of significant others (family members, friends, teachers, coaches, and so forth). While this chapter will present the information you will need to have about your child's asthma, it is based on the assumption that you have an understanding of the information presented in previous chapters.

CHOOSING THE DOCTOR

As I have indicated, caring for a child with asthma requires team effort that includes the patient, the parent, and the doctor. Probably the single most important decision that has to be made is the choice of a doctor, either a pediatrician, an allergist, or a pulmonary specialist. He must be knowledgeable and considerate and must be willing to spend a good deal of time with you and your child explaining his philosophy of the management of asthma and the role you are to play. Since asthma in children can be treated very successfully, the doctor's plan must be an aggressive one with normal or near-normal functioning as its goal. He must be available to you when you need him, especially in the event of an acute attack. He must be willing to take the time to speak with your child's teacher, school nurse, coach, and camp counselors when the need arises. Choose carefully!

Initially, you may have been working with your child's pediatrician. He may refer you to an allergist for consultation, possibly for allergy testing, or to take over the management of your child's asthma. Although many physicians are involved, only one physician should make the decisions regarding treatment approaches and priorities. Do not allow yourself and your child to get caught between varying opinions, philosophies, and instructions.

As important members of the team, you and your child have the responsibility of keeping your doctor informed about everything relevant to your child's asthma. You must keep the lines of communication open and honest. Ask questions. Make sure you understand what the doctor tells you. Be prepared to follow through on all recommendations and instructions. The success of the treatment program depends not only on the doctor, but you and your child as well.

ENVIRONMENTAL FACTORS

Based on the results of the evaluation (case history, physical examination, and laboratory tests), the doctor may first attempt to help you eliminate or control any offending allergens or irritants in the child's environment. As I described in Chapter 3, let the severity of your child's symptoms dictate the degree of involvement you need in environmental control. Controlling one's environment can be an endless task. If your child's symptoms are mild and intermittent, you need not replace your home's heating and air-conditioning systems, throw out all of his toys, remove his carpeting, cancel his trip to the circus, and prevent him from going to summer camp. If your child's symptoms are severe, with acute attacks occurring frequently, you probably should go to great lengths to control those allergens or irritants that have been shown to trigger his symptoms. For a complete discussion of possible environmental factors that may cause asthma symptoms, see Chapter 3.

FOOD

Another method to be used in the control of asthma symptoms in children focuses on their diet. Since allergy testing for food sensitivities is not as reliable as it is for airborne irritants, I rely on the parents' or the child's reports of food reactions. First, you should consider the possibility of foods that he eats most often; these can be allergenic foods. In general, there are certain foods such as milk, wheat, eggs, and corn that often present problems for children. Diets to omit these foods might be tried. Sometimes food is suspected, but no one food is an obvious problem. If you feel strongly that foods are a problem for your child, you may want to attempt an elimination diet. This may be quite rigorous. For a complete discussion of dietary factors in asthma, see Chapter 4.

PHARMACOLOGICAL MANAGEMENT OF ASTHMA IN CHILDREN

Several new devices and forms of medications which have recently become available have made great differences in increasing the number of effective and low side effect producing drugs that can now be used by children (even infants).

Spacing devices are now used extensively, enabling children three years and older to use some of the inhaled medications. Inspirease and Aerochamber are the most commonly used. Children have difficulty with the hand-held metered dose sprays because they lack the ability to coordinate taking a deep breath and pressing the spray at the appropriate time. In a spacing device such as Inspirease, the spray container is attached to a flexible accordion-type tube that is then attached to a mouthpiece. The medication to be inhaled is sprayed into the tube and the child may then breathe at his or her own pace, inhaling the medication until it is all used. In this way, the breathing and the spraying need not be synchronized. Even three-year-old children would be able to use this device.

For younger children another device called a nebulizer may be used. A nebulizer is a machine that changes a liquid medication into a mist. The medication is put into the nebulizer and the child wears a small mask through which he or she can just breathe normally while inhaling the medication. Nebulizers have been used with older children or adults during emergency situations for years. What is new is the fact that some drugs that are excellent for children now come in a liquid form and can be nebulized. For example, cromolyn sodium (Intal), an excellent drug, was previously unavailable to children. Since it can now be administered in a nebulizer, children six months and older can use it. Sympathomimetic medications (metaproterenol or albuterol) may also be nebulized.

When the inhalant drugs are not sufficient, I often use a combination of inhalants and systemic (oral) medications to control the patient.

The sections that follow will present a general discussion of the procedures I use in the management of medication in children. For a detailed discussion of each medication, refer to Chapter 6. Pay close attention to the instructions on how to use the devices that administer the various medications. Especially for the child who is to use a spray on his/her own, there are definite rights and wrongs in the use of sprays. Read this carefully with your child.

Also be aware that all inhaled sympathomimetic products (Alupent, Metaprel, Proventil, Ventolin) are not recommended by their manufacturers for use by children less than twelve years of age. However, all physicians who deal with respiratory problems use this medication in any age group. All of these medications are safe and very effective even in small children. I use them for all of my patients, and I have given you suggested doses for your child. Of course, your physician will be the final arbiter as to whether you should use these medications for your child.

MILD TO MODERATE ASTHMA

For the child who has mild asthma with occasional attacks, I usually prescribe albuterol (Proventil or Ventolin) on an as-needed basis. If the child is between the ages of three and six, I would administer albuterol with an Inspirease (the spacing device described above). For younger children, I would use the nebulized medication (Alupent or albuterol, sympathomimetic drugs). If the family doesn't want to use a nebulizer, I might prescribe a liquid sympathomimetic medication such as metaproterenol or albuterol or a liquid theophylline. I prefer the short-acting theophylline in this situation. If the symptoms occur every day, I would prescribe the liquid albuterol on a regular basis rather than on the as-needed basis. If this does the trick, I would try to go back to the as-needed basis after a while. Sometimes I use Intal prior to trying theophylline, and if the Intal does not work, I use theophylline together with Intal.

When occasional acute attacks occur, I prescribe a short-acting theophylline. If these attacks become more regular, an intermediate or long-acting theophylline would be in order. Children who are too young to swallow a pill can be given liquid theophylline. Alternatively, I may suggest removing the time-released granules in Slo-Bid and placing them in a food such as applesauce. Here is an important warning, however, about giving medications in this manner. Be sure to give the medication immediately or else it will dissolve in the applesauce, releasing its entire contents, in which case the child will get too large a dose. Also, and for the same reason, the child must not chew the time-released granules.

If the above regimen does not yield good results, I would add Intal by inhalation, i.e., assuming I have not already added it. I would use the nebulized form for children up to the age of three and Inspirease for children three to six years of age. The hand-held Intal spray would probably be fine for children ages six and over. They must be mature enough to follow the dosage carefully. Too often, hand-held sprays are not viewed as serious medications. They are! Make sure your child is using them appropriately and only as prescribed. If the Intal controls the symptoms, then continue the Intal on a regular basis indefinitely. I usually watch pulmonary functions and eventually try to withdraw the drug. The drug can be completely withdrawn after a year if no symptoms recur.

If what we've tried so far is not sufficient, a new medication, Atrovent, is available and should be added to the regimen. Although this drug is not approved for use by children younger than twelve years of age in this country, Atrovent has been used safely worldwide with children younger than twelve. Check with your physician. If Atrovent does not help significantly, and very often it does *not,* I discontinue it and add one of the inhaled corticosteroid medications (Vanceril, Beclovent, or Azmacort). Once again, the child between the ages of three and six would need to use the Inspirease device to facilitate taking these medications. A patient who uses the inhaled steroid sprays on a regular basis is characterized as a moderate asthmatic.

SEVERE ASTHMA

I categorize any patient who requires systemic corticosteroids such as Prednisone, either intermittently or regularly, as a severe asthmatic. This patient is one who cannot be controlled with a combination of theophylline, cromolyn sodium, or the sympathomimetic sprays. If attacks are intermittent, I give corticosteroids intermittently. However, when I find that I am giving intermittent corticosteroids on a regular basis, I usually try to use steroid sprays, often inhaled following the use of a sympathomimetic spray such as Proventil. In a child, I will use two to four sprays four times a day of a steroid spray. If this is not sufficient to control his symptoms, I will add Prednisone given every other morning or, as a last resort, Prednisone every day. Fortunately, this is rarely necessary.

THE SEVERE ATTACK AT HOME

Although an acute attack at home can be frightening for the child and the parents, the best you can offer your child is the knowledge of what to do and the ability to do it calmly and promptly. You should work out a regimen with your physician as to how to handle the acute attack, including guidelines as to when he should be called for advice in treating the child at home. If your child appears to be seriously ill, prompt medical attention is necessary. Use whatever community resources are available, including physicians, emergency treatment facilities, and local rescue squads and paramedical personnel. If necessary, the child should be admitted to the hospital.

Previously it was difficult to administer the most appropriate medications to a child in the midst of an acute attack. Now with the availability of the nebulizer and Inspirease, the appropriate medications can be administered easily, and the management of the acute attack at home can also be handled more effectively and easily. I recommend the use of albuterol sprays (Proventil and Ventolin). I describe how these should be used in Chapter 12, The Acute Attack.

For the trained parent, I recommend that Adrenalin be available at home for use in emergency situations. I recommend EpiPen, a gadget that releases a set amount of Adrenalin without having to take the time to carefully fill a syringe. Although it was originally designed for those who are allergic to bee stings, its ready availability makes it convenient for use during an acute attack. There are two concentrations: EpiPen Sr., 0.3 mg Adrenalin for children aged nine or older (60 lb or greater) and EpiPen Jr., 0.15 mg Adrenalin for children aged three to nine years. For children less than 33 lb, this device may not be suitable. Check with your doctor. Giving your child some warm liquids (water, tea, or broth) while helping him to relax may help to ease the bronchospasm and bring up mucus.

ASTHMA AND INFECTION

It is very common for the asthma symptoms to occur or worsen when there is an infection. The best way to avoid this is to avoid infections. It is difficult to keep your child away from other children with runny noses, but at least give it a try. Certainly, if other family members have colds, I would try to keep them away from the asthmatic child's room, food, and toys. If your child does get a cold, you should have a preplanned approach that has been worked out by your doctor. The doses of the child's medications may have to be increased or decreased. Decisions concerning the need for antibiotics have to be made. Consult your doctor.

ALLERGY SHOTS

Telling your five-year-old that he has to get an allergy shot every week may not be easy. However, the fact is that allergy shots do work well for asthmatic children. Patients should receive allergy injections when (1) their asthma is not easily controllable by medications, (2) they have severe attacks frequently, and (3) they have a demonstrable allergy to substances that they cannot easily avoid (for instance, pollen, dust, mold, and mites). A more complete description of immunotherapy can be found in Chapter 5.

Helping the Child to Cope with Asthma

In order for your child to be a good member of the team, he must be made aware of the nature of his problem. As he gets old enough to understand, he must know what is happening to him and how he can help himself. Above all, he must learn to know and respect his limitations. Doctors and parents have set specific guidelines, and the child must follow them. He must develop judgment that will allow him to coexist comfortably with the limitations of his illness. The child growing up with asthma must know himself well enough to make the appropriate decisions on his own behalf.

CAN THE ASTHMATIC CHILD EXERCISE?

In previous summer Olympics, five gold medalists in swimming events were asthmatics. The answer to the question, Can the asthmatic child exercise? then is yes. Exercise is as important to an asthmatic child as it is to any child. Some precautions may need to be taken, but eliminating all activity is wrong.

Almost all children who have asthma have some degree of bronchoconstriction when they exercise. Their exercise-induced dyspnea (shortness of breath), occurs *after* the exercise begins, approximately six to eight minutes into the exercise. Therefore, we can be smart and select those exercises that allow some respite; that is, those that do not require constant physical exertion. Good sports with intermittent activity include baseball, bowling, doubles in tennis, golf, volleyball, and short sprints. Soccer, racquetball, singles in tennis, and marathon running would be difficult. Swimming, which is done in very humidified air, is a very good sport. Any activity done in cold air is a problem. In this situation, the child should try to breathe more through his nose than his mouth. The use of a ski mask or cold air mask is helpful when the air is cold. One brand that is useful is a Spenco cold air mask.

In addition to the proper selection of a sport activity, premedication can also be considered. Sports are so important to children that I feel it worthwhile to use medication if necessary to enable the child to participate. The drug of choice here may be cromolyn sodium, usually given fifteen to thirty minutes before exercise begins. It is not taken once the exercise has induced wheezing, as this will usually aggravate the asthma. Albuterol (Proventil or Ventolin) taken before exercise may also be helpful, but I prefer cromolyn sodium because it has fewer side effects.

Whatever decisions you make regarding your child's physical activities, you must inform the physical education teacher. He must know what your child can and cannot do, and know how to handle your child's medications and physical limitations.

SCHOOL

Asthma is one of the leading causes of absenteeism in schools. Time lost leads to poor grades, poor retention of material, and feelings of hopelessness and inferiority. In the case of a child with significant asthma, there should be a meeting (or conference call) of the parents, teachers, school nurse, and doctor to discuss the child's asthma. This group should concern itself with the severity of the asthma; the type, dosage, side effects, and administration of the child's medications; emergency procedures; and activity restrictions. Under specially arranged and carefully monitored circumstances, the child may be able to take his medication in school. In general, there should be open lines of communication about problems and progress. The teacher has to know that certain medications can cause side effects (hyperactivity, drowsiness, headaches, stomachaches, loss of memory, and personality changes) and the parents have to know if these possible side effects occur and adversely affect school performance. There may then have to be some alteration in the medication program, if possible. Teachers may also have to explain to the asthmatic child's classmates what asthma is and why the child needs his medications.

The teacher needs to be aware of those allergens that trigger the child's symptoms. For example, the asthmatic child should not be in charge of the chalkboard, nor should the asthmatic child tend to the pet gerbils. In fact, the gerbils should be removed, if possible. A thoughtful teacher could avoid wearing heavy perfumes and she might keep a watchful eye on the foods that the child eats in school.

DISCIPLINE

My entire treatment approach to the asthmatic child has as its goal normal functioning. This applies to discipline as well. ''Upsetting'' your child by appropriate discipline will not precipitate an asthma attack. Your child must be treated normally. Even if there is a relationship between discipline and wheezing (there usually is not), the detrimental effects of a lack of discipline far outweigh the detrimental effects of a little wheezing. One of course must be vigilant to insure that a child is not using his asthma symptoms to achieve his goals.

Psychological Effects of Asthma on the Child and His Family

The extent of the psychological effects of asthma on the child and his family will probably be in proportion to the severity of the asthma. A mild, well-controlled asthmatic child will probably have very few, if any, adjustments to make. The child who has to endure frequent acute attacks, be on a continuous regimen of medication, live with life-style restrictions, and be faced with the possibility of frequent hospitalization is understandably under an emotional strain that spreads to his family. Since the entire family is involved, the ability to deal effectively with other stresses and problems may be lessened. Tensions in the home may rise quickly; this is understandable and should be addressed as a family problem. If the team of supportive people I have been describing in this chapter works well together, then hopefully they can control the child's asthma and minimize his feelings of anger, fear, inferiority, and depression. There are parent and family groups that discuss the problems of coping with asthma. (Check with your asthma specialist, local hospital, or Lung Association chapter.) There may often be a legitimate need for individual or family counseling to find some outside support for the difficulties associated with asthma.

My experience with asthmatic children and their families brings me to the optimistic conclusion that often asthma can be handled very successfully, minimizing its effects and achieving near-normal living.

The following is a list of summer camps that are designed to meet the unique needs of the asthmatic child:

Asthma Camps

Arizona

Friendly Pines
Senator Rd.
Prescott, AZ 86301
(602) 445-2125

Arkansas

Alders Gate Camp
2000 Alders Gate Road
Little Rock, AR 72205
(501) 225-1444

California

Boys Club
Running Springs, CA 92382
(714) 867-2155

Breathe Easy Day Camp (Local residents)
295 27th Street
Oakland, CA 94612
(415) 893-5474

Sierra Asthma Camp
234 N. Broadway
Fresno, CA 93701
(209) 233-6125

Scamp Camp
3861 Front Street
San Diego, CA 92103
(619) 297-3901

Colorado

Champ Camp
119 W. 6th #100
Pueblo, CO 81003
(303) 545-5864

Georgia

Camp Breathe Easy
723 Piedmont Avenue, NE
Atlanta, GA 30365
(404) 872-9653

Idaho
Camp Easter Seal East
Worley, ID 83876
(206) 284-5706

Indiana
Julia Jameson Health Camp for Children, Inc.
201 S. Bridgeport Road
Indianapolis, IN 46231
(317) 923-3925

Camp Superkids
615 N. Alabama St., Ste. 335
Indianapolis, IN 46204
(317) 634-5864

Iowa
Camp Superkids
1321 Walnut
Des Moines, IA 50309
(515) 243-1225

Kentucky
Camp Green Shores
Star Route One, Box 261
McDaniels, KY 40152
(502) 257-2508

Michigan
Camp Michi-Mac
8578 Canton Center Road
Canton, MI 48187
(313) 453-2661

Minnesota
Camp Superkids
YMCA Camp Induhopi
Loretto, MN 55337
(612) 871-7332

Montana
Camp Huff-n-Puff
825 Helena Avenue
Helena, MT 59601
(406) 442-6556

Nebraska
Camp Superkids
8901 Indian Hills Drive, Ste. 107
Omaha, NE 68114
(402) 393-2222

New Hampshire
Camp Superkids
456 Beech St.
P.O. Box 1014
Manchester, NH 03105
(603) 669-2411

New York
Hidden Valley Camp
Sharpe Reservation
Route 3
Fishkill, NY 12524
(914) 897-9860

Wagon Road Camp
Chappaqua, NY 10514
(914) 238-8106
(914) 238-4761

Camp Superkids
23 South Street
Utica, NY 13501
(315) 735-9225

North Dakota
Dakota Superkids
212 2nd Street
Box 5004
Bismark, ND 58502
(701) 223-5613

Ohio
Camp Allyn
Amelia Olive Branch Rd.
Batavia, OH 45103
(513) 732-0240

Stepping Stones
5650 Given Rd.
Cincinnati, OH 45243
(513) 831-4660

Oklahoma
Camp Green Country
5553 S. Peoria
Tulsa, OK 74105
(918) 747-3441

West Virginia
Broncho Junction
R.D. No. 1
Red House, WV 25168
(304) 755-7621

12

THE ACUTE ATTACK

If you ever have had an asthma attack, or if you have ever witnessed one, you certainly know that it is always alarming, often frightening, and never convenient. There is never a good time to have an acute asthma attack. How do we define an acute attack? *Acute* means something that happens suddenly and is usually of short duration. *Attack* is some sort of an assault, and in this case it is an assault on one's lungs. So, by the acute attack we mean some deleterious factors that rapidly change the status quo of the lungs.

The important part of the definition is the change in the status quo. One patient may be well stabilized on high doses of theophylline and steroids and be quite comfortable. When he develops difficulty in breathing, this is his acute attack. Another patient may be on no medication at all. Somewhere along the way he develops shortness of breath and difficulty in breathing; this is his acute attack.

In a previous chapter about drugs, I outlined the most appropriate medication therapy program to maintain the asthmatic patient's lungs at their highest level of function. When the status quo changes during an attack, action must be taken. When one begins breathing with difficulty, breathing more quickly, starting to wheeze, becoming short of breath, or having difficulty getting air in, this is when the patient should take action. This will certainly vary for each individual, but most patients know when their breathing ability is deteriorating.

Some patients, however, do not know when the going is getting a bit more rough. They either cannot self-monitor (because they are too young or old, for example) or they do not self-monitor (because they are not sensitive to their own body's changes). For these patients and for any other patient who wants an easy-to-use objective measure of breathing deficiency, I recommend a device called a peak flow meter. This gadget helps you measure your lung capacity and tells you when your breathing ability is changing enough to warrant action. It is a handy little device that many patients find helpful.

The peak flow meter is a thin tube about six inches long that looks something like a small flute. When you blow into it as hard and as fast as you can, you can measure pulmonary capacity (breathing velocity) in liters per minute. While this is only one phase of one's pulmonary capacity, it does change in asthma. Some patients never reach "normal" capacity, but they have a usual range in which they "normally" blow. Therefore, when it begins to drop by more than 15 or 20 percent, they know they are in trouble. The peak flow meter can be an early warning signal telling you it's time to take some action. When an attack occurs, there are many measures that you can take to help yourself.

Some of you may have to call your doctor immediately, take medication, or supplement the medication you are already taking. Some may have to go to an emergency room for quick treatment. Whatever the appropriate course of action, there is one thing that is inappropriate—panic. Do not panic! Panic reactions will cause a reflex that makes the attack worse, regardless of its cause. Panic is useless and can be counterproductive. Keep a clear head and follow the guidelines you have learned, either from your doctor or from this chapter.

By the way, the most appropriate time to read this chapter is *before* an asthma attack strikes you—not during—so that you can be better prepared. This chapter will give you the facts necessary to proceed in a purposeful direction to either help yourself eliminate the attack or know where to go for help with the attack or, more important, to know when to call for help.

Self-help is fine only when it is appropriate; it can be dangerous otherwise. As I said in the chapter on the use of drugs, the information presented here is to be used in conjunction with your doctor, not instead of your doctor. Some instances can be handled directly by the patient, and some cannot. Some patients should not be working independently at all. Certainly you should call your doctor if you are

1. pregnant and having an attack (see Chapter 1)
2. having your first attack
3. dealing with an infant with breathing difficulties, or a child with a high fever (greater than 101 degrees) and asthma symptoms
4. asthmatic and coping with diabetes, hypertension, cardiovascular diseases, emphysema, or hemoptysis (spitting up blood)
5. an adult with fever, severe chest pain, or an infection along with the asthma symptoms

These situations or conditions all require relatively immediate medical attention. If you are pregnant or have other medical problems, only your doctor can take all the factors into consideration and coordinate the proper treatment suggestions. If this is your first attack, or if an infant is demonstrating breathing difficulties, you really do not know what is happening. Only your doctor can diagnose the situation. If you have fever or an infection, your doctor may want to prescribe an antibiotic in addition to the medications you may be familiar with. Infection, by the way, can be particularly troublesome (a "trigger") for asthmatics. Older patients, who tend to develop bacterial infections, may very well benefit from antibiotics while younger patients, who tend to develop viral infections, may not require antibiotics. You can often tell if you have an infection by the color of your mucus (yellow with green or brown), or a temperature of greater than 101 degrees. Needless to say, your doctor must be consulted in any of these cases.

It is a good idea to work out a careful plan with your doctor—describing what to do when an attack strikes. If he gives you a few prescriptions, fill them and have the medications on hand when you need them. A prescription in your wallet will not relieve asthma symptoms. Be prepared and knowledgeable. In the instances that I have listed, there may be too many complicating factors for you to consider on the spot. If you have not been told what to do, then call your doctor. If you are following his directions and they don't seem to be helping your asthma, call him. If you can't reach him (or his covering physician) then go to an emergency room immediately.

Everyone should know where emergency medical aid can be obtained. Ask around to find out which emergency room is best equipped to care for asthma patients. This is the preferable place to go when you need help. If you are in a small community and have no choice, know where the hospital is and go there, armed with the knowledge you will gain later in this chapter when I discuss what to do in the emergency room.

It is impossible for me to know whether you, the reader, are asthmatic, and if your condition is severe, and if you're taking medications. Knowing these facts would enable me to give you specific advice. I am left, then, with no alternative but to advise you in a general way, taking several typical levels of severity into consideration.

Intermittent Attacks with No Medication on a Regular Basis

If you are a patient who has intermittent attacks of asthma and are not on any medication in between these episodes, then you should probably discuss with your physician what medication you can start if you experience tightness, shortness of breath, or difficulty in breathing. He has probably advised you on one of two things.

First, he has probably prescribed one of the sympathomimetic spray medications, most likely Proventil or Ventolin. I usually prescribe two sprays every four hours for wheezing. Of course, if this provides you with little or no relief, then get in touch with your doctor. There are many patients who do very well with no medication most of the time and a Proventil or Ventolin spray on occasion. It is very important to remember not to fall into the trap of overdosing on any asthma sprays, since you might get a rebound or paradoxical effect. In that case, rather than serving as a bronchodilator, the spray actually gives you bronchospasm. Just because it is a spray doesn't mean that it can't be overused.

In a rebound effect the asthma spray, through a mechanism not clearly understood, causes your air tubes to clamp down and become narrow (bronchospasm), thus slowing the flow of air through the air tubes. Instead of helping you to breathe, the overuse of the spray actually makes breathing more difficult. If you get relief after one or two sprays, but then you find yourself reaching for the canister more often than every four hours, call your doctor.

Second, your doctor might advise you to start a fast-acting theophylline medication such as Elixophyllin, Somophyllin-T, or Slo-Phyllin. He will specify the dose according to your weight and age. These drugs are normally taken every six hours. In conjunction with the Proventil or Ventolin, theophylline can be very helpful during an attack. If you have immediate relief, you might be able to discontinue the medication. However, if you are continuing to have difficulty, then call your doctor.

THE MILD ASTHMATIC

If you require albuterol spray on a regular basis (three or four times a day), you are classified as a mild asthmatic. If you have an attack in between sprays, your doctor probably advised you to increase the sprays to every four hours, up to twelve sprays a day. In special situations your doctor might suggest more than two sprays, or a dosing interval of less than every four hours. Discuss this with your physician. If increasing the frequency of the sprays does not work, then your doctor might advise you to start a fast-acting theophylline medication, as described in the previous section.

The Moderate Asthmatic Who Is on Some Form of Medication

If you require medication (usually theophylline or cromolyn sodium) on a regular basis to control your asthma symptoms, then you are classified as a moderate asthmatic. If the medication you are taking is theophylline, then your dose should be adjusted by your doctor. This technique is called theophyllinization. Although we have discussed it in previous chapters, it is important enough to warrant repeating. Theophyllinization is done by measuring the level of theophylline in your bloodstream and increasing the amount that you are taking until the level is appropriate, so that you are not suffering from intolerable side effects and your symptoms are diminished or gone.

When you are theophyllinized, you can either be maintained at a high or low therapeutic blood level of theophylline, depending on many factors that are beyond the scope of this book. If your blood theophylline level is maintained at a high level, and if you have an acute attack, you must use a medication other than theophylline to control your symptoms; adding increased theophylline to your regimen with an already high blood level of theophylline can lead to very severe side effects. On the other hand, if your theophylline dose is maintained at a lower level, and if you have an acute attack, you may take additional doses. This should be predetermined by your physician. It is certainly preferable, when this option is open for you, to know the dose of additional theophylline that you can take before the attack occurs. Therefore, work this out with your physician in advance.

This theophylline-level business is tricky, and as you may recall from the chapter on drug management, theophylline is not always metabolized the same way in every situation. You should be aware that if you have a viral infection with fever, your capacity to excrete theophylline is reduced. Your doctor must be aware so that he will adjust the level of theophylline intake down by 10 to 25 percent, depending on your level. It is very important to have this all worked out before an attack stops you in your tracks.

So if you are controlled with only theophylline, and if you cannot increase it during an attack, you will probably be advised to use one of the sympathomimetic sprays, such as Proventil or Ventolin. These are usually prescribed in dosages of one to two sprays every four hours. If the spray relieves you, then you can continue using it every four hours and get in touch with your physician.

If the spray gives you no relief at all, and if you appear to be getting worse, this may be the time to either call your doctor or go to the emergency room. When you are having an attack, you may be given the oral (pill) forms of the following sympathomimetic drugs in a dosage prescribed by your physician: metaproterenol (Alupent or Metaprel), terbutaline sulfate (Brethine or Bricanyl), or albuterol (Proventil or Ventolin).

If your primary drug is cromolyn sodium, and if you have an acute attack, then your first option is to add a fast- or intermediate-acting theophylline to your regimen. If this is your first attack, you should be advised, and preferably were advised by your physician prior to the occurrence of the acute attack, to add an amount of theophylline compatible with your age and weight. On the other hand, if you are unfortunately an old pro at this, then you will have already worked out the appropriate dose to add. If adding theophylline does not work, then I usually advise my patients to proceed to the other steps that are outlined in the previous section for those patients who are taking theophylline. In addition, I very often advise my patients who are on cromolyn sodium as their primary drug to take a sympathomimetic spray such as Proventil as their first option, then to add theophylline if the spray is not that helpful. Cromolyn in the inhaler form may have to be stopped in an acute attack, since it can irritate the airways and worsen the attack. Discuss this with your physician, as this varies from patient to patient. For the patient who is on an oral sympathomimetic drug such as terbutaline sulfate or Proventil (or Ventolin) as their primary drug, I usually suggest adding theophylline as the first measure and then proceeding to the other steps that are outlined in the previous section for those patients who are taking theophylline. Obviously, this group will omit the instructions about adding an oral sympathomimetic drug as they are already taking one.

If you are running a fever, having chest pains, bringing up colored sputum, or feeling particularly achy, let your doctor know so that he may consider prescribing an antibiotic for you. These are symptoms of viral or bacterial infections.

The Moderately Severe Asthmatic Who Is on a Regular Regimen of Medications

Patients who have been theophyllinized and who also require an oral or inhaled sympathomimetic drug on a regular basis are classified as moderately severe asthmatics. During an attack this patient may take an extra dose of the inhaled sympathomimetic drug Proventil or Ventolin, as it is permissible to take up to twelve sprays a day. For this patient, the doctor may prescribe an antibiotic and/or cortisone (Prednisone), depending on the circumstances. Most physicians will use a ''burst'' of cortisone with high doses of Prednisone (20 to 60 milligrams or sometimes higher) or its equivalent, for three or four days or longer. (The dosage in children is 1–2 milligrams/kilogram per pound of body weight or 0.5–1 milligram per pound up to 60 milligrams.) This will usually break the attack. This may be done with or without an antibiotic depending upon whether the patient has an infection. The doctor is the best judge of this.

Severe Asthmatics Who Are on Steroids

I classify any patient with asthma on steroids as a severe asthmatic. Thus, these patients are usually adequately theophyllinized, taking one of the sympathomimetic drugs and steroids on a regular basis. Steroids may be taken every day or on alternate days or preferably as a spray.

First, let's consider the situation of a mild attack. A mild attack is characterized by wheezing or coughing that is easily controlled by the addition of one or two sprays of a sympathomimetic bronchodilator. This, of course, is always the first line of defense for almost all asthmatics who have mild bronchospasm and who have not taken the bronchodilator spray within the last hour. I would then advise them to increase the number of steroid sprays that they are taking from two sprays four times a day to four sprays four times a day. If they are taking four sprays four times a day, I would increase it to five sprays four times a day, which in my experience is about the maximum that you can really take before the benefits to side effects ratio is reversed.

The next situation is a moderate to severe attack. A moderate attack is one that is only partially helped by the use of sympathomimetic sprays and a severe attack is not helped at all by the use of these sprays.

In the moderate or severe attack there is a large amount of mucus on the lining of the bronchi and lungs, thereby preventing the absorption of the steroid sprays. In these situations it may be necessary to utilize systemic (oral or injectable) steroids. When a severe attack is unresponsive to bronchodilator sprays and to other measures, a call to the physician or a trip to the emergency room is in order; that will be discussed a little later on.

In a moderate attack if there is some response to the bronchodilator sprays, and if the patient is not severely short of breath, then the addition of oral steroids would be indicated. I make it a practice to tell my patient what dosage of the oral steroid I would want him/her to take in the event of an acute attack. This is discussed beforehand and the dosage is dependent upon the patient's age, weight, and symptoms. For the patient who is on steroids on an every-other-day-basis, I would advise him to take an additional dose of steroids on the nonscheduled cortisone day if he is having trouble or to double the dose on the scheduled cortisone day if the attack occurs at that time. Patients who take cortisone every day would be advised to increase the level of their dose. If the cortisone that the patient is taking is in a spray form (Vanceril or Beclovent), the addition of oral steroids (pill form) may be indicated.

As you recall from the chapter on drugs, Prednisone and the

other steroids are very effective, but at a high cost in terms of possible side effects. Because of the high degree of effectiveness of steroids, patients (and some doctors) are tempted to use them freely. Please understand that steroids are not the drug of choice. They are the last drug to be used and the first one to be removed. If you find yourself taking Prednisone on an everyday basis for several days every other week or so, you are getting into a bad habit. This is the time to discuss a change in your medication schedule with your physician.

Extraordinary Measures for Extraordinary Times

NEBULIZERS

A small percentage of my patients have attacks that can become difficult enough to require the use of some extraordinary procedures at home. If these patients are capable and willing (or have a family member who is capable and willing) to handle simple equipment at home, I recommend their use.

One device is a nebulizer (air compressor) that delivers an aerosolized mist of a sympathomimetic drug (usually Metaprel, Alupent, or albuterol) and saline to the patient. (See drug chart at end of drug chapter for dosages.) With this method the aerosolized mist can be administered gradually over a four- to five-minute period. This method is much more effective than a canister spray. The medicated mist produced by the air compressor penetrates deeply and continuously into the lungs for a long period of time. (An increasing number of my patients, especially the very young or very old, find the nebulizer a convenient and often indispensable way to administer their medication on a regular basis.)

The same caution about overusing spray forms of medication applies when nebulizers are used. If you do not get excellent results from the nebulizer, contact your physician. He may want you to go to the emergency room. The nebulizer is used in conjunction with all of the other medications and instructions we have been talking about. Anyone using a nebulizer must be well trained. It should be standard procedure for the doctor who is prescribing the use of the nebulizer at home to give the patient adequate training in its use. Depending upon the model you have, there are specific procedures to follow regarding filling, breathing, and cleaning. Each machine comes with its own instructions. (Refer to page 158 for recommended use of a nebulizer.) Don't get this device confused with positive-pressure machines—these are rarely needed.

ADRENALIN

The use of Adrenalin at home is another extraordinary measure that can be employed by a patient with significant asthma during a stubborn attack. Adrenalin is used when the going is very rough. If you lived next door to the emergency room, that would be the ideal situation. Since you probably do not live next door to the emergency room, Adrenalin can be used at home at those times when you wish that you lived next door to an emergency room!

Adrenalin is injected. Therefore, you must be trained in the exact method of administration. Your doctor must train you for there are very specific steps to be followed (for instance, taking your pulse, drawing up the drug, inserting the needle, and injecting the drug). Whoever administers the injection must be fully trained in the skills of drawing up the appropriate dose and administering the injection correctly.

The dose of Adrenalin is calculated on body weight; the dose is 0.01 milligrams per kilogram, or 0.022 milligrams per pound. A small two- to three-year-old child would receive 0.05 milligrams, and an adult would receive 0.3 milligrams; 0.5 milligrams is the absolute maximum. The drug (usually aqueous Adrenalin 1:1000) is given subcutaneously with a syringe (usually a 26- to 27-gauge disposable tuberculin syringe).

Adrenalin can be very useful in breaking up an acute attack. It works very quickly, usually within three minutes. If this does *not* work, go immediately to the nearest emergency room—you are in trouble! If you cannot get yourself to the emergency room, call the rescue squad or a neighbor.

If Adrenalin works well, some physicians recommend a longer-acting substance called Sus-Phrine, which is Adrenalin in an oil base that is absorbed slowly, and works for several hours. This will keep you breathing for a while. The dose for this is 0.005 milligrams per kilogram, or 0.011 milligrams per pound, which in a small baby would be about 0.05 milligrams, in a large child 0.15 milligrams, and in an adult would be as much as 0.1 to 0.3 milligrams. Since there is some immediate benefit from Sus-Phrine, some doctors use it as the recommended form of Adrenalin for their patients to use. This is a matter of preference. I opt for the short-acting Adrenalin, which gives me greater freedom to use other medications if it does not work. When the longer-acting Sus-Phrine does not work, you are restricted in your choices because the drug is still in the patient's system over a longer period of time.

Many of my patients feel that it would be difficult for them to administer an injection to themselves during an attack, and another person may not be available to them at any given time to administer the injection. For those who still wish to inject Adrenalin under those circumstances, I recommend EpiPen, a ready-to-go Adrenalin shot administered simply by pressing it against the thigh. This releases the premeasured amount of Adrenalin. It is used as an emergency kit for those allergic to bee stings and is also applicable in asthma attacks. EpiPen is available in two sizes, children (0.15 mg) and adults (0.30 mg). Check with your doctor for advice concerning the appropriate size for you and for all Adrenalin doses. (EpiPen is my preferred method of administering Adrenalin at home.) Your own physician will know what dose is best for you.

WHAT TO DO WHILE YOU ARE WAITING

While you are waiting for the drugs you have just taken to work, or to decide if you need medication, or waiting for your spouse to fill the syringe with Adrenalin, or for the rescue squad to come, or for the emergency room procedures to work, there is something that you can do besides waiting. Relaxation may seem like the least likely thing you can do, but it may be within your control. As I have said, panic is useless and may make things worse. Tight, constricted airways are the opposite of relaxed, open passages. It will help to try and relax. The chapter on stress reduction outlines some specific steps you can take to gain control over your body's tension at this time.

I believe this outlines all that can be done by a patient at home. This information (to be used only in conjunction with your doctor) will hopefully keep you out of the emergency room. There are times, however, when you have no choice and you must get medical attention at an emergency room.

THE EMERGENCY ROOM

Whenever possible, go to the emergency room of the hospital with which your doctor is affiliated. You should either have a prior arrangement with him to contact him before you go to the emergency facility or to notify him when you are there. Some emergency rooms function better and treat you better if they expect you. Call ahead if you can, or call your doctor and have him call ahead to discuss your case with the doctor who will be taking care of you. Most emergency rooms will contact your doctor for you if you request it. If you are not in a great deal of difficulty, the emergency room can usually handle you with little difficulty. If you are having significant problems, and if you think your doctor could be of help, insist on his being called. They must do this for you. They do not have the right to refuse to call your doctor and if they do, this is unacceptable behavior that can place them in legal jeopardy if complications should arise. Stand up for your rights. Of course, if you are with a companion, he or she can contact the doctor from an outside phone, if necessary.

When you enter the emergency room, your first encounter will usually be in the triage area. A registered nurse is usually in charge of this operation. When you arrive state exactly what your problem is. Do not try to be considerate; if you are very uncomfortable, announce that you are having breathing difficulty. Emergency rooms are run on a first come-first served basis—unless you are an emergency. Asthma is usually an emergency and they should take you quickly. Do not be embarrassed to state that you are an asthmatic. Although some necessary paperwork will have to be done, if you are very ill, your companion or family member can do this while the staff rushes you through.

Usually in the next step you will meet another nurse, either in the triage area or in the treatment area, who will want to know exactly what medication you are taking and something about your history. Give a very concise history. It is helpful for her to know that you have had asthma for five years (or whatever applies to you), that you are possibly on cortisone, that you are taking medications (and their specific names and dosages), that you took medication that day, and what specific medications you took since your attack began. These facts are crucial. Also tell her whether this is an unusual situation. Tell her if you have any signs of infection (colored mucus) or fever. This should not take more than a minute. This is not the time to go into the whole history of your disease over the past twenty-five years. More details may be required later, but right now, emergency information is all that is needed so that the doctor can come on the scene and make a decision as to what to do.

Next the doctor will examine you, listening carefully to your lungs and heart, among other things. The doctor's function at this point is to ascertain how much trouble you are in so as to quickly evaluate your general health status. He or she may use a peak flow meter. For milder attacks, the physical examination and the information obtained from the peak flow meter usually provide sufficient information for the doctor to proceed with treatment. However, in patients with very severe difficulty or those patients who do not respond to simpler therapeutic measures (Adrenalin and intravenous Aminophylline), it may be necessary to measure blood gases. This procedure is the measurement of the actual amount of oxygen and carbon dioxide in the blood. The oxygen level is called the PO_2 and the carbon dioxide level is called the PCO_2. When your lungs are not functioning well, such as in bronchial asthma, your blood oxygen level drops and your blood carbon dioxide level rises. This happens because the lungs are so congested that the blood cannot come in contact with enough oxygen to oxygenate (blood combining with oxygen) itself properly and it cannot get rid of its carbon dioxide. These measurements are not something the doctor can determine merely by looking at you. This is an unpleasant and painful procedure because a small, thin needle has to penetrate deeply to get at the artery rather than the vein. Since this is painful, usually the doctor will use lidocaine to numb the area so that you will not be too uncomfortable.

In reading this section it may seem as if you will be in the emergency room for hours before they do anything. However, all of the previously mentioned procedures are usually done with very rapid dispatch. As a rule, most emergency room personnel act efficiently, and they can take care of you quite readily. If they are letting you sit for an hour, gasping for breath without any medication, then you are in the wrong place!

If you have not been given Adrenalin in the previous hour or two either by yourself or by your physician, the emergency room staff will probably try Adrenalin first (unless you have a cardiovascular problem). In addition to Adrenalin, most emergency room staff will attempt to help you by administering a solution of Metaprel via a nebulizer, a device that breaks up liquid into tiny particles that can be inhaled deeply into the lungs. If you do not respond to Adrenalin and/or inhaled Metaprel, or if you have been given several shots of Adrenalin already, the emergency staff may want to start an IV. The IV (intravenous) will usually contain Aminophylline. This is why it is very important for the physician to know if you are taking a long-acting preparation of theophylline. The IV dose of Aminophylline is completely dependent on what type and how much theophylline you have taken in the last twenty-four hours. The doctor may order a theophylline test to determine the amount of theophylline in your blood. However, this test takes several hours to perform. More rapid methods, which take less than thirty minutes to perform are now available in some emergency facilities. Therefore, the physician must utilize the information that you have given concerning your theophylline status. The doctor is not a magician. You *must* know and you *must* tell him what medications you have taken, your status (how severe your attack), and the general progression of your illness (how fast you are getting worse) in the last few hours.

At this point, depending on your response to medication, several possible situations can occur. If you respond well to Adrenalin, the doctor may send you home as soon as your chest sounds clear. If you do not respond well to Adrenalin or need IV Aminophylline, you probably will have to be hospitalized or placed in a holding area so that further medications can be given to you.

LEAVING THE EMERGENCY ROOM

Assuming that you are now ready to leave the emergency room, several combinations of events may have occurred. One, this is either your first attack or one of infrequent attacks. You responded to the Adrenalin and no other measures were required to control your attack. Now the emergency room physician is sending you home. Under no circumstances should you leave without specific instructions and/or medications. Normally, if you have not been on theophylline, you will be given theophylline medication to take until you contact your doctor. You may also be given some sympathomimetic drugs such as Metaprel or Proventil tablets. These are effective alternatives. It is a good idea to take this theophylline or the sympathomimetic drug for at least several days as long as they do not produce side effects. After an attack, your lungs are in a "twitchy" state and the bronchodilator and/or sympathomimetic drug will stabilize your lungs. If the doctors feel that an infection may have triggered the attack, they may give you an antibiotic.

The next possibility is that you were already on bronchodilators and/or sympathomimetics before the acute attack. You had this attack, you went to the emergency room, and the Adrenalin worked. You are now about to be sent out of the emergency room. If you have done well, the emergency room physician may advise you just to continue your regular medication, perhaps suggesting that you use your spray more frequently (but not to exceed twelve sprays per day). In addition, if the emergency room physician thinks you have an infection, he or she will probably recommend that you take antibiotics. If you responded to the Adrenalin without any difficulty, then this is usually the appropriate treatment. If it had been a more rigorous attack, and if you were in the emergency room for hours before you improved, then in addition to the previously discussed measures, you may also require steroids. This is a decision that the doctor must make, but you should be aware of this option.

The third possibility is that you were in the emergency room, you did not respond easily, you are already on bronchodilators, and you might have an infection. If you have an infection, you will be started on antibiotics. You may also be started on steroids. Your doctor should also be contacted for advice on the management of your medication during the next few days, after you have left the emergency room.

If you are on steroids already (on an alternate-day basis) and you have an attack, you will probably be told to take the steroids every day for a few days. If you are on Vanceril, you may be told to take cortisone in tablet form (Prednisone) anywhere from 20 to 60 milligrams a day for a few days. In addition, you may be given antibiotics and told to contact your physician.

HOSPITALIZATION

Now we get to the less happy situation. You have not responded to Adrenalin, oxygen, or any similar measures. At this point, you will probably be started on intravenous therapy and be given oxygen. In the IV you will probably be given Aminophylline in an amount determined by your previous doses of theophylline. As I said, it is your obligation to know what medication you are taking, your previous doses, and how much difficulty you have been having recently. It is the doctor's obligation to ask you these questions. Make sure the doctor is aware of what medications you have taken, even if he does not ask you! Fortunately, I think you will find that most doctors will ask you these questions.

Most hospitals will admit you when you need IV Aminophylline and oxygen. Some may place you in a twelve-hour holding area which is really like being in the hospital. In any event, most hospitals are well equipped to handle severe attacks of asthma and this kind of treatment is usually helpful. If you are hospitalized, your doctor will be involved, and you are probably in very capable hands.

Now that you have read about the rigors of an asthma attack, I hope you will know what to do if you are involved in one. Attacks should be the exception to the rule. If your attacks are becoming more frequent and/or severe, this might be a good time to reevaluate your total asthma treatment program.

Review this chapter every once in a while. Determine which type of asthmatic you are and be prepared to act appropriately. Keep the required medications available and fresh. Let your family or friends know the procedure. (It may be helpful to have a summary of the relevant emergency information handy, for example.) An asthma attack can be a lonely, frightening experience. Get help and help yourself! Try not to panic and remember what to do!

Here's an example of the kind of relevant information you should have with you at the time of an emergency.

Doctor's Name ___John Jones___

Doctor's Telephone No.: ___1-208-555-1212___

Emergency Room Telephone No.: ___(123) 456-7890___

Rescue Squad's Telephone No.: ___(987) 654-3210___

Current Medications	Dosages
1. Theo-Dur	200 mg 2 × day
2. Proventil	2 sprays 4 × day
3. Intal Inhaler	2 sprays 4 × day
4. Prednisone	10 mg every other day

Things to Do

1. Take the medication you and your doctor have agreed upon.
2. Call your physician.
3. Alert other family members or neighbors if necessary.
4. Try any relaxation techniques you know.

Things Not to Do

1. Panic
2. Overdose

13

SURGERY

I'm sure we are all aware of the wonders that medical science can accomplish through surgery these days. The asthmatic, like anyone else, may have to undergo a surgical procedure for any one of a dozen reasons unrelated to their asthmatic condition and may require some extra special care.

First of all, there are two types of surgery: elective and emergency. In elective surgery the patient and doctor have time to make plans. Emergency surgery does not allow for this luxury. Since there are definite things to prepare for when dealing with the asthmatic undergoing surgery, the asthmatic can be at a real disadvantage in emergency situations. I'll talk more about this later.

As is well known, there are always risks in surgery. According to statistics, the risks are greater for the asthmatic, in proportion to the severity of his condition, but the risks can be lessened if the proper precautionary measures are taken. Nevertheless, I would counsel the asthmatic to think twice before undergoing surgery that might not be necessary.

When one of my asthmatic patients tells me that he is going to have surgery, I want to know and I want him to be aware of the following things:

1. Is he a mild asthmatic or a chronic asthmatic?
2. Is he currently symptomatic?

3. What are the current pulmonary functions of the patient? Certain pulmonary functions would indicate that surgery should be postponed, if at all possible.
4. What drugs is he currently taking?
   a. Is he taking theophylline? If so, at what level? It is very important to get a theophylline level on a patient just prior to surgery. The theophylline level must be at a therapeutic level at this time. Just before surgery your theophylline in pill form will be discontinued, and an IV solution will be administered. Your doctor will not take the risk of subjecting you to an asthma attack during surgery because of too low a theophylline level.
   b. Is the patient on cortisone on a regular basis or has the patient taken cortisone in significant doses for more than five consecutive days in the last twelve months? You are considered steroid dependent if you are currently taking cortisone or even if you have taken it for a total of ten separate days or for five consecutive days within the last twelve months.

      Steroid dependency means that your adrenal system is suppressed. You need to supplement this suppressed system with additional cortisone in preparation for surgery. This is true whether the surgery is to bypass a clogged coronary artery, set a broken leg, or pull a loose tooth. If you have been on steroids in the last eighteen months, and if you are no longer on them now, your physician will probably give you cortisone, usually starting two days prior to surgery. Six to twelve hours before surgery, when you are not allowed any oral medication, the cortisone will be added to your IV; and shortly after surgery, it will be discontinued. If you are on steroids on a regular basis, the dosage will be increased just prior to surgery; you will be given steroids during surgery as described above; afterward the dosage will be reduced as quickly as possible to your initial dose.

   c. Is he taking any other medications? The patient should be returned to his normal medication routine as soon after surgery as possible.
5. What is the extent of the surgery? How complicated will it be? How long will it last?
6. What anesthetics are going to be used? How will it be administered? What other drugs may be needed? It is not unreasonable to expect the asthma specialist to contact the surgeon or anesthesiologist to answer some of these questions. The surgeon and anesthesiologist must know that you are asthmatic so they won't be surprised if you start to wheeze during surgery. As a rule of thumb, local anesthesia is preferable to general anesthesia, when possible.
7. Does the patient have any other complicating disorders?
8. Is the patient a smoker? If the patient is smoking, he must stop at least one week before surgery—longer if possible—forever would be best.

I make it a practice to see all of my patients one week prior to their surgery. I do a general assessment and, most important, pulmonary functions. I then adjust their medications accordingly. Then I see them one day prior to admission and recheck everything at that time. Presurgical visits are important.

Once the proper precautions are taken, your management becomes no different than any other patient's. You should be hospitalized in order to be stabilized a day or two in advance. Be sure to tell the appropriate personnel about any foods you cannot have. Bring some extra pillows if you do better with your head elevated when sleeping. In some cases, I tend to be a bit more liberal than usual with the medications I prescribe so that the patient's postoperative recovery can proceed undisturbed by symptoms.

It is not unusual for patients to have some difficulty bringing up mucus and secretions after surgery. The asthmatic may have more difficulty than the nonasthmatic. Coughing may be quite painful after surgery, and asthmatics need to cough. It is especially important for the asthmatic to get up and around as soon as possible to help break up any mucus congestion in his lungs.

These patients need a supportive companion during this somewhat difficult time. A private nurse; a family member who can remain with the patient for much of the day; or a compassionate respiratory therapist can be a great help in coaxing the patient to withstand the discomfort, move around, and cough up the excess mucus.

DENTAL SURGERY

It is generally agreed that nitrous oxide, a general anesthetic used in dentistry, is permissible with asthmatic patients, as long as the patient's pulmonary functions are good. Local anesthetics are always preferable. You will have to check with your physician and undergo some pulmonary function tests to determine your candidacy for nitrous oxide. Both you and your physician will have to decide. Remember, an asthmatic needs special handling. Make sure to take the necessary steps to insure that you get it. Your asthma specialist and your dentist *must* coordinate your treatment whenever a dental procedure is prolonged and/or requires more than a local anesthetic. Steroid dependent patients may require additional steroids. Always check with your physician.

WHEN YOU ARE NOT IN CONTROL

Emergencies happen, unfortunately. If you are conscious, let the doctor who is going to take care of you know that you are an asthmatic. Tell him what medications you are taking and whether you have been on cortisone in the last eighteen months. With this information, the doctor is much better able to care for you appropriately.

If you are not conscious, there is no way you can tell the attending physician what he needs to know, unless you are wearing a Medic-Alert bracelet. (See Glossary for address.) It will have your doctor's name, telephone number, your medications (especially cortisone information), and doses. I strongly recommend this to my patients, especially those who take medications on a regular basis or who have serious food or drug allergies. A card should also be kept in your wallet that states your present medications and doses, the use of cortisone within the last eighteen months, drug allergies, and your doctor's name and telephone number.

To a certain extent it is the patient's responsibility to prepare himself for proper treatment prior to, during, and after surgery. If the surgery is elective, make sure that all involved are well informed. If the surgery is an emergency, plan now for that unfortunate possibility by wearing the Medic-Alert bracelet and keeping it up-to-date. By taking these steps, you help to eliminate asthma symptoms as a possible complicating variable.

14

ASTHMA CENTERS AND CLINICS

Fortunately, most of those suffering from asthma can be controlled by using a combination of the treatments I've discussed throughout the book by working closely with their physician and becoming knowledgeable about their disease. However, there is a small percent of the asthma population for whom the symptoms are severe, medication can't be stabilized, the physical condition is deteriorating, depression caused by chronic illness won't cease and, in general, the asthma threatens to run away with the patient's life. It is at this time when a specialty treatment center may be the best solution. There are several such centers. The one which I have recommended to many of my patients with excellent results is the National Jewish Center for Immunology and Respiratory Medicine in Denver, Colorado.

National Jewish Center for Immunology and Respiratory Medicine

The National Jewish Center for Immunology and Respiratory Medicine is the world's largest treatment and research center for adult and childhood asthma. Each year patients are accepted from every state and even from many foreign countries. The center is a nonprofit and nonsectarian institute that accepts coverage by Medicare, Medicaid, and most private insurance programs. In some cases financial assistance is available.

The National Jewish Center for Immunology and Respiratory Medicine offers treatment programs that embody an intensive "whole-person" approach, providing psychological as well as medical support. Its doctors and nurses are specialists in respiratory and allergic diseases and immune system disorders. Because so many hard-to-manage cases are referred to the center, they've seen nearly all of the special problems that patients might have. If after much experimentation you feel that your current status is unacceptable, it would be a good idea to discuss such a center with your physician.

The primary goal of treatment at National Jewish is to bring patients' asthma under control and then to pinpoint their highest level of respiratory functioning while using the least amount of medication possible. Through training in asthma self-care, the center prepares patients to live with minimal medical supervision after discharge.

Central to adult asthma evaluation and treatment at National Jewish is the PRIDE Program (Progressive Rehabilitation through Individual Development and Education). It incorporates medical management, education, a variety of therapies, and nutritional counseling in a package that is customized for each patient. Some of the classes offered in the PRIDE Program are Understanding the Physiology and Mechanisms of Asthma, Asthma Management at Home, Nutrition and Asthma, and many others. Family members are encouraged to attend classes with patients so they learn how to better participate in managing their loved one's asthma.

Pediatric programs at the center stress health and well-being rather than sickness. Their message is, "You're basically healthy and happen to have asthma." Even toddlers learn self-care skills. Parents are very involved and are encouraged to stay throughout their child's hospitalization. Preschool is augmented with play groups that familiarize youngsters with medical tools of asthma management, such as stethoscopes, needles, monitoring devices, "doctors" in white coats, etc.

The living units for children six and older encourage friendships and peer support by grouping dorm rooms around shared recreation, laundry, and dining facilities.

Pediatric patients stay, on the average, one month and attend school on the center's campus. Special education teachers help them keep up or catch up with their classmates at home. The accredited K–12 school maintains close contact with each child's home school.

There is a special program at National Jewish for youngsters and adolescents whose serious medical conditions are complicated by psychological or mental adjustment problems. Professional counselors, working in partnership with medical personnel, play a key role in this long-term unit, helping their young patients develop greater emotional stability and self-reliance. Some patients attend the center as outpatients, getting the same diagnostic, treatment, and educational opportunities as those who stay at the hospital.

Communication between National Jewish and each patient's referring physician is ongoing throughout his or her stay. Upon discharge, a final treatment summary and report is sent to the physician, insuring consistency and continuity of care as well as facilitating a smooth transition back to the individual's home life-style.

A very valuable service offered by National Jewish is the toll-free LUNG LINE. This free telephone information service is staffed by specially trained nurses who answer questions about asthma and other respiratory diseases, provide free literature, and give information about patient care programs at the center. LUNG LINE nurses take calls on weekdays between 8:00 A.M. and 5:00 P.M. (Mountain Standard Time). The number is 1-800-222-LUNG.

The center is an excellent resource that provides the intensity and duration of care needed in some especially severe, multifaceted cases. I refer to the center with confidence.

A list of asthmatic centers and clinics throughout the country follows:

Asthma Centers and Clinics

Arkansas

University of Arkansas Medical Center
4301 W. Markham St.
Little Rock, AR
(501) 661-5000

California

Scripps Clinic and Research Foundation
476 Prospect St.
La Jolla, CA 92037
(714) 455-9100

Los Angeles-USC Medical Center
1200 N. State St.
Los Angeles, CA 90033
(213) 226-6503

UCLA Hospital
10833 Le Conte Ave.
Los Angeles, CA 90024
(213) 825-6481

University of California
Irvine Medical Center
101 City Dr. S.
Orange, CA 92668
(714) 634-6011

Children's Hospital at Stanford
520 Willow Rd.
Palo Alto, CA 94304
(415) 327-4800

University Hospital
University of California Medical Center
225 W. Dickinson St.
San Diego, CA 92103
(714) 294-6222

Kaiser Foundation Hospital
2200 O'Farrell
San Francisco, CA 94115
(415) 929-4000

University of California Hospitals and Clinics
513 Parnassus Ave.
San Francisco, CA 94143
(415) 497-2300

Harbor General Hospital
1000 W. Carson St.
Torrance, CA 90509
(213) 533-2104

Sunair Home and Hospital for Asthmatic Children
P.O. Box 338
Tujunga, CA 91042
(213) 352-1461

Colorado

Fitzsimons Army Medical Center
Peoria and Colfax Sts.
Denver, CO 80240
(303) 341-8281

National Jewish Center for Immunology and Respiratory Medicine
3800 E. Colfax Ave.
Denver, CO 80206
(303) 388-4461

University of Colorado Medical Center
4200 Ninth Ave.
Denver, CO 80262
(303) 394-7601

Connecticut
Yale-New Haven Medical Center
333 Cedar St.
New Haven, CT 06510
(203) 436-8060

District of Columbia
Children's Hospital National Medical Center
111 Michigan Ave.
Washington, DC 20010
(202) 745-5000

Georgetown University Hospital
3800 Reservoir Rd. N.W.
Washington, DC 20007
(202) 625-7001

Howard University Hospital
2041 Georgia Ave. N.W.
Washington, DC 20060
(202) 745-1596

Hospital for Sick Children
1731 Bunker Hill Rd.
Washington, DC 20017
(202) 832-4400

Florida
William A. Shands Teaching Hospital and Clinics
University of Florida
Gainesville, FL 32610
(904) 392-3771

Asthmatic Children's Foundation
Residential Treatment Center
1800 N.E. 168 St.
North Miami Beach, FL 33160
(305) 947-3445

Illinois
Institute of Allergy and Clinical Immunology
Grant Hospital of Chicago
550 W. Webster Ave.
Chicago, IL 60614
(312) 883-2000

Michael Reese Hospital and Medical Center
508 E. 29th St.
Chicago, IL 60616
(312) 791-2000

Northwestern University Memorial Hospital
Superior St. and Fairbanks Ct.
Chicago, IL 60611
(312) 649-8624

La Rabida Children's Hospital and Research Center
65th St. at Lake Michigan
Chicago, IL 60649
(312) 363-6700

Rush-Presbyterian-St. Luke's Medical Center
1753 W. Congress Parkway
Chicago, IL 60612
(312) 942-5000

University of Illinois Hospital
1919 W. Taylor St.
Chicago, IL 60612
(312) 996-7000

Iowa
University of Iowa Hospitals and Clinics
650 Newton Rd.
Iowa City, IA 52242
(319) 356-1616

Kansas
University of Kansas College of Health Sciences and Bell Memorial Hospital
39th St. and Rainbow Blvd.
Kansas City, KS 66103
(913) 588-6008

Louisiana
Tulane University School of Medicine
Allergy Clinic
1430 Tulane Ave.
New Orleans, LA 70112
(504) 588-5578

Maryland
Good Samaritan Hospital
5601 Loch Raven Blvd.
Baltimore, MD 21239
(301) 323-2200

Johns Hopkins Hospital
601 N. Broadway
Baltimore, MD 21205
(301) 955-5000

Mount Washington Pediatric Hospital
1708 West Rogers Ave.
Baltimore, MD 21209
(301) 578-8600

Massachusetts
Children's Hospital Medical Center
300 Longwood Ave.
Boston, MA 02115
(617) 734-6000

Massachusetts General Hospital
Clinical Immunology and Allergy Unit
Fruit St.
Boston, MA 02114
(617) 726-2000

Robert B. Brigham Hospital
125 Parker Hill Ave.
Boston, MA 02120
(617) 732-5055

Lakeville Hospital
Asthma Rehabilitation Unit
Main St.
Lakeville, MA 02346
(617) 947-1231

Michigan
University Hospital
1405 E. Ann St.
Ann Arbor, MI 48109
(313) 764-3184

Henry Ford Hospital
2799 West Grand Blvd.
Detroit, MI 48202
(313) 876-2600

Mary Free Bed Hospital and Rehabilitation Center
235 Wealthy St. S.E.
Grand Rapids, MI 49503
(616) 774-6774

Minnesota
University of Minnesota Hospitals and Clinics
516 Delaware St.
Minneapolis, MN 55455
(612) 373-8484

Mayo Clinic and Foundation
200 First St. S.W.
Rochester, MN 55901
(507) 284-2511

Missouri
Children's Mercy Hospital
24th St. and Gillham Rd.
Kansas City, MO 64108
(816) 234-3000

Barnes Hospital-Washington University Medical School
Barnes Hospital Plaza
St. Louis, MO 63110
(314) 454-2000

St. Louis University Medical Center
1402 Grand Blvd.
St. Louis, MO 63104
(314) 664-9800

Nebraska
St. Joseph Hospital
601 N. 30 St.
Omaha, NE 68131
(402) 449-4001

New Jersey
Betty Bacharach Rehabilitation Center
4100 Atlantic Ave.
Pomona, NJ 08240
(609) 652-7000

Children's Seashore House
Jim Leeds Rd.
Atlantic City, NJ 08401
(609) 345-5191

New York
Mount Sinai Medical Center
1 Gustav Levy Place
New York, NY 10029
(212) 650-6500

Children's Hospital of Buffalo
219 Bryant St.
Buffalo, NY 14222
(716) 878-7000

Nassau County Medical Center
2201 Hempstead Turnpike
East Meadow, NY 11554
(516) 542-0123

R. A. Cooke Institute of Allergy-Roosevelt Hospital
428 W. 59th St.
New York, NY 10019
(212) 554-7000

Cornell Medical School-New York Hospital
510 E. 70th St.
New York, NY 10021
(212) 472-5900

New York University Medical Center
552 First Ave.
New York, NY 10016
(212) 340-5241

Strong Memorial Hospital of the University of Rochester
601 Elmwood Ave.
Rochester, NY 14642
(716) 275-2121

St. Mary's Hospital for Children
29-01 216th St.
Bayside, NY 11360
(212) 224-0400

Blythedale Children's Hospital
Bradhurst Ave.
Valhalla, NY 10595
(914) 592-7555

North Carolina
Duke University Medical Center
Durham, NC 27710
(919) 684-8111

Ohio
Children's Hospital Medical Center
Elland and Bethesda Aves.
Cincinnati, OH 45229
(513) 559-4200

Cleveland Clinic Foundation
9500 Euclid Ave.
Cleveland, OH 44106
(216) 444-5780

Ohio State University Hospitals
456 Clinic Dr.
Columbus, OH 43210
(614) 422-4851

Health Hill Hospital for Children
2801 East Blvd.
Cleveland, OH 44104
(216) 721-5400

Oklahoma
Children's Convalescent Center
P.O. Box 888
6800 Northwest 39th Expressway
Bethany, OK 73008
(405) 789-6711

Pennsylvania
Children's Hospital of Pennsylvania
34th St. and Civic Center Blvd.
Philadelphia, PA 19104
(215) 596-9100

Hahnemann Medical College and Hospital
Feinstein Bldg.
216 North Broad St.
Philadelphia, PA 19102
(215) 448-7000

Hospital of University of Pennsylvania
34th and Spruce Sts.
Philadelphia, PA 19104
(215) 662-4000

Thomas Jefferson University Hospital
11th and Walnut Sts.
Philadelphia, PA 19107
(215) 928-6000

Children's Hospital of Pittsburgh
125 De Soto St.
Pittsburgh, PA 15213
(412) 647-2345

Children's Heart Hospital
Conshohocken Rd.
Philadelphia, PA 19131
(215) 877-7708

Rhode Island
Rhode Island Hospital
593 Eddy St.
Providence, RI 02902
(401) 277-4000

Texas
University of Texas Health Sciences Center
7703 Floyd Curl Dr.
San Antonio, TX 78284
(512) 691-6011

University of Texas Medical Branch Hospitals
8th and Mechanic Sts.
Galveston, TX 77550
(713) 765-1011

Texas Children's Hospital-Baylor College of Medicine
6621 Fannin
Houston, TX 77030
(713) 791-4219

University of Texas at Houston
Medical School: Department of Pediatrics
6431 Fannin
Houston, TX 77030
(713) 792-5330

Virginia
University of Virginia Hospitals
Private Clinic Bldg.
Hospital Dr.
Charlottesville, VA 22908
(804) 924-0211

Medical College of Virginia
Hospitals
12th and Marshall Sts.
Richmond, VA 23298
(804) 786-9000

Washington

University Hospital
1959 N.E. Pacific St.
Seattle, WA 98195
(206) 543-3300

Wisconsin

University of Wisconsin Hospital
and Clinics
600 Highland Ave.
Madison, WI 53702
(608) 263-8000

Milwaukee County Medical
Complex
8700 W. Wisconsin Ave.
Milwaukee, WI 53226
(414) 257-5915

15

DAILY DOS AND DON'TS

Knowing how to cope with asthma on a daily basis can transform a mildly successful treatment program into a very successful one. This chapter will provide you with a long list of the dos and don'ts of living with asthma. Over the years I have offered my patients many helpful hints. Some of them I derived by listening to my patients. Some that I present here will be written in "doctorese" and some will be in "patientese," but all will be practical and useful and in conjunction with your physician.

Not all of these dos and don'ts will be relevant for each asthmatic. Use those that apply to your individual situation.

Since this is a list of either dos and don'ts, there's no room for maybes. Speaking in extremes may seem to deny the existence of a middle ground. However, there is one at times. For example, if I say, "Don't have pets," and you have lived with your beloved cat (and your asthma) for ten years, I understand that you may be adamant in your refusal to give the cat away. I will operate with the belief that you will be able to recognize the seriousness of the problem and take other steps to compensate (not allowing the cat in your bed, improving the air quality in your home, immunotherapy, or cromolyn sodium).

In fact, this list is presented with the conviction that you are committed to helping yourself (and your doctor) to reduce or eliminate your asthma symptoms.

Your Environment

1. Don't smoke.
2. Don't allow smoking in your home, especially in the bedroom.
3. Don't be afraid to ask others to stop smoking, with the explanation that you are asthmatic.
4. Don't have pets.
5. Don't spend a long time in places where there are pets (for instance, friends' homes, circuses, zoos, or stables).
6. Don't plan to be around when your house is being painted or even for a few days afterward.
7. Don't expose yourself to too much dust. Arrange for someone else to do the heavy cleaning, dusting, and vacuuming, whenever possible.
8. Don't empty the vacuum cleaner bags.
9. Don't wear perfume or cologne, and avoid fragrant toiletries.
10. Don't buy perfumed tissues.
11. Don't browse in candle shops or perfume departments.
12. Don't allow yourself to be sprayed with free perfume samples. Duck!
13. Don't fill your shelves with dust collectors.
14. Do use a dust mask if you cannot avoid exposure to dust.
15. Do have your mattress vacuumed regularly.
16. Do have your sheets, pillowcases, quilts, and comforters cleaned often.
17. Do have your vents cleaned often (professionally, if possible).
18. Do keep your humidifier and air conditioner filters clean.
19. Do filter or vent cooking odors.
20. Do keep refrigerator drip trays clean to control mold growth.
21. Do keep your windows closed during the height of the allergy season. This applies to car windows too.
22. Do use air-conditioning during the summer months.
23. Do use a damp mop when cleaning floors or walls.
24. Do rake leaves promptly and trim the vegetation near your home.

25. Do ask your companions for the evening not to wear perfumes (even your husband or wife).
26. Do keep your workplace as clean as your home.
27. Do be aware of other potential environmental irritants such as newsprint, room deodorizers, ammonia, and mothballs.

Handling Your Medication

1. Do become familiar with your medication—by name and dosage.
2. Do keep an up-to-date list of your medications with the schedule and doses. Make this list known to some family member or friend, and keep a copy in your wallet.
3. Do use a checklist if you are on a complicated drug regimen. This will make sure that you don't repeat a dose or forget one.
4. Do use a calendar to remember what day (even or odd) to take your cortisone if you are on an every-other-day dose.
5. Do keep a generous supply of your medications. Don't wait until the last minute to refill a prescription.
6. Do keep extra medication in your car's glove compartment in case you've left your pills or sprays in another handbag or attaché case.
7. Do get your morning medications ready the night before, if your mornings are rushed.
8. Do learn exactly how to use your medications. One of the major causes of failure of albuterol (Proventil and Ventolin), beclomethasone (Vanceril and Beclovent), metaproterenol (Metaprel and Alupent), and cromolyn sodium in effectively treating asthma is the patient's failure to use the medications properly.
9. Do clean and cover your spray medications.
10. Do take any medications that cause jitteriness or nausea or headaches about ten minutes after eating.
11. Do tell your family and/or friends where your medications are and how they are to be administered.
12. Do take your cortisone dosage all at once, in the morning.

13. Do try to manipulate your medication schedule so that you are symptom-free at special times; for instance, if you know you have an important job interview at 10:00 A.M., try to insure that your medications are then near peak effectiveness, rather than at their lowest level of effectiveness.
14. Do follow your doctor's instructions carefully: Don't abuse any medications.
15. Do take your allergy shots regularly.
16. Do ask your doctor to prescribe noncolored medications if you are allergic to artificial colorings.
17. Do inform your asthma specialist of any other medications you may add because of nonasthma-related problems you may be having. Don't take any medication (even a sleeping pill) without his permission.
18. Do take cromolyn sodium fifteen mintues to half an hour before exercising if you have exercise-induced asthma.
19. Do ask your doctor about EpiPen, an easy to administer premeasured dose of Adrenalin. Many of my patients carry it with them wherever they go just in case of an emergency.
20. Do teach a family member or friend how to administer Adrenalin.
21. Don't remove the foil wrapping of the cromolyn sodium until you are ready to use it, since cromolyn sodium may absorb moisture from the air and become soggy and unusable.
22. Don't keep your medication on your night table. You might take them when you are too drowsy to know what you are doing.
23. Don't take theophylline with caffeine (coffee, tea, or cola drinks).
24. Don't delay in taking your medication if your symptoms suddenly require them.
25. Don't be embarrassed to take your medications in public. It will be more embarrassing to have a coughing spell and breathing difficulty.
26. Don't alter your medications unless you consult your doctor.

27. Don't take megadoses of vitamins—they may be harmful. A multivitamin is fine.
28. Don't take aspirin or aspirin-containing compounds until you have checked with your physician. (Twenty percent of all asthmatics are sensitive to aspirin.)

Dealing with Foods

1. Do take the time to read the labels on the products you plan to eat.
2. Do call the hostess of your next dinner party to inquire about the menu. You can then make provisions for yourself. On occasions when there will be a set menu, call the caterer.
3. Do take the time to eat before you leave home for extended periods when you are not sure what food will be available to you.
4. Don't be afraid to ask what ingredients are in the foods you order in a restaurant. If the waitress can't help you, ask to see the chef.
5. Don't forget to bring some allowable foods with you when you are going someplace where you cannot control the food offered to you.
6. Don't overeat.
7. Don't eat too fast.
8. Don't talk while you are eating.
9. Don't be afraid to call the manufacturer of a product to find out its ingredients. Consumer service departments are usually very cordial and helpful.
10. Don't drink alcoholic beverages if you are taking a lot of medication. They may trigger an attack. Consult your doctor.

General Health Factors

1. Do avoid people who have colds or other infections.
2. Do make it very clear to others that it is very important that you not get a cold. Even if Aunt Tillie is traveling two hours just to see you, don't let her in if she is ill.

3. Do get a flu shot to prevent influenza. It should be taken in September or October. If you are allergic to eggs (since the flu serum contains an egg base), and cannot eat them without an allergic reaction, or if you have had difficulty in the past with a flu shot, it may not be wise to have a shot.
4. Do discuss with your physician whether you should receive Pneumovax, an injection to prevent pneumococcal pneumonia.
5. Do drink plenty of fluids.
6. Don't forget to cover your mouth in cold weather so that the air you breathe will be warmed, reducing the chance of bronchospasm.
7. Don't avoid exercise, even if you have exercise-induced asthma. Exercise is important. You can engage in activities that do not keep you in action for a prolonged time. Try walking, short sprints, swimming, or baseball. Cromolyn sodium half an hour before exercise can be very helpful.
8. Don't let yourself get too fatigued.
9. Don't forget to eat well and stay in good condition. Pamper yourself.
10. Don't use any stimulant, especially cocaine, at any time.

Emergency Times

1. Do ask your doctor about EpiPen.
2. Do have a friend and family member ready to act in times of emergency.
3. Do have the telephone number of the rescue squad available.
4. Do have the telephone number of the nearest emergency room readily available.
5. Do have your doctor's name and telephone number readily available.
6. Do have any emergency equipment (medications, syringes, nebulizer, or oxygen) in a ready-to-use state.
7. Do wear a Medic-Alert bracelet. This will make available the information needed by the emergency medical team. (See Glossary for address.)

8. Do keep an up-to-date schedule of your medications and doses in your wallet.
9. Do familiarize yourself with relaxation techniques (hypnosis, biofeedback, and progressive relaxation). While you are waiting for medications or other emergency measures to work, these techniques may be very helpful.
10. Don't forget to keep your Adrenalin drugs fresh. Check the expiration date and check for discoloration.

Coping with Asthma in Children

1. Do your best to teach your child about his disease.
2. Do teach your child to declare himself an asthmatic to his teachers, counselors, and friends.
3. Do inform the school nurse of the problem and ask her to keep extra medications in school.
4. Do pay attention to your child's moods after medication. Be understanding.
5. Do avoid wool clothing and stuffed animals.
6. Do be wary of the circus and the zoo, as well as friends and neighbors who have pets. This can be particularly difficult for children. You may have to be imaginative and compensate for this one.
7. Do teach your child what foods he can and cannot have. Be firm. Again, imaginative cooking may be required.
8. Do make sure that someone else is competent to care for your child's asthma if you are not there when he has an attack. Train a family member or friend.
9. Don't give your child a spray medication unless he is clearly mature enough to handle it judiciously.
10. Don't treat your child like an invalid. Allow him to exercise as much as his asthma will safely allow. Suggest swimming.
11. Don't let the teacher seat your child next to the cage with the class pet. If possible, ask the teacher to keep the gerbils in the next room.
12. Do check with your local lung or allergy association and your local "Y" for special physical conditioning programs for asthmatic children.

Vacations

1. Do make sure that you are not allergic to your vacation haven. If you're allergic to horses, don't spend a week at a dude ranch.
2. Do learn the word for *asthma* in the foreign language spoken in the country you are visiting. You might also want to learn the foreign words for your medications.
3. Do get a note from your doctor specifying that you are asthmatic and need special medication. Understandably, some customs officials will be suspicious when they discover vials and syringes, pills, and sprays.
4. Do take your favorite pillows along with you. Many places still use feather pillows and many of my patients find it helpful to sleep with their head elevated by several pillows.
5. Do make sure that you choose a vacation spot where you can get the kinds of foods you need. If you are allergic to rice, don't visit China.
6. Do pay attention to the location of the nearest hospital or doctor when you are in a new city. Then enjoy your vacation.
7. Do ask your doctor if he knows a physician in the area you are planning to visit. In addition, if he does not, usually he can look up the name of a competent physician in one of his reference books.
8. Don't forget to take special precautions with your medications when you travel. If you are going by airplane or train, where your luggage will not be available to you, keep an extra set of medication with you. If you're headed for Minneapolis and your luggage winds up in Omaha, you'll be especially glad you have your drugs with you.
9. Don't forget to take an oversupply of medication. It may not be easily available where you are going.
10. Don't forget to request the nonsmoking section on an airplane. Do this early and request that your seat be as far from the smoking section as possible.
11. Don't go far from your medication. Take it with you to the beach (preferably in a plastic bag) or when you're going on a sailing trip.

Your Attitude

1. Do commit yourself to feeling better. As you can see by this seemingly endless list, there's a great deal of work that must be done. Once you get into the routine, it becomes second nature, but you must be committed.
2. Do know your own limitations and requirements. Tell your child, "No I can't go horseback riding, but I'd love to play Ping-Pong."
3. Do keep yourself knowledgeable about asthma. Reading this book is a fine start. Continue by looking at newspaper articles, listening to TV and radio spots, and talking to other asthmatics.
4. Don't be afraid or embarrassed to declare yourself an asthmatic to others. Saying "Please put out the cigarette because I'm asthmatic" is more effective than saying "Please put out the cigarette because it bothers me."
5. Don't be intimidated by people who think your asthma is caused by emotional weakness. We know better now.
6. Don't be discouraged. The most effective treatment program may take time to develop.

Do discuss these instructions, especially those pertaining to medications or vaccinations with your own physician. He is the best judge of what you should do.

16

THE FUTURE

It is always fascinating to wonder what the future holds for us. Certainly, speculating about the future in asthma treatment arouses a feeling of challenge in the medical profession and hope among millions of asthma sufferers.

One thing we know for sure is that attitudes toward asthma are changing. While some myths still linger, the asthmatic individual and his family and friends no longer have to cope with the prejudice that his problem is emotionally based. The real facts about asthma are beginning to spread to the public through the media and through books like this, as well as through the efforts of the American Lung Association. There is an increasing trend by employers of the larger corporations to acknowledge the impact of asthma and allergic diseases on their workers by using fewer offending substances in the workplace, doing a better job of dusting the office, installing proper ventilation, and even funding immunotherapy. We are all aware of the movement against air pollution and the enforcement of No Smoking regulations. There is a great deal of work being done in laboratories around the world regarding human physiology.

Now that we all know that asthma symptoms result from a malfunctioning in the respiratory physiology, we can look to the laboratories for future breakthroughs. Some advances will be made in the not so distant future (within the next ten years) and others will take longer to be realized. My "spies" in several laboratories keep me well informed, and so I can make good guesses as to what the next ten years or so may have to offer.

The Near Future

1. *Theophylline:* We have seen that theophylline is a very useful and effective medication for asthma. We know when to use it and how it works. The one problem with theophylline is its side effects.

   As you may remember, theophylline inhibits the enzyme phosphodiesterase, which in turn prevents the destruction of CAMP (cyclic AMP). This increases the level of CAMP in the lung and mast cell and makes them less sensitive and less reactive. This, of course, is our goal since it will reduce the asthma symptoms.

   Unfortunately, at present, theophylline works in many organs, increasing their level of CAMP and causing side effects. It may produce nausea and headaches. If the theophylline molecule could be changed through chemical engineering so as to act only on the lungs and not anywhere else, we would have a more perfect medication. We might even be able to ''engineer'' increased effectiveness without any side effects at all. The application of new chemical engineering techniques to improve theophylline lies in the near future.
2. *Sympathomimetic Drugs:* The drugs in this category are Adrenalin, ephedrine, metaproterenol (Metaprel and Alupent), albuterol (Proventil and Ventolin), and terbutaline sulfate (Brethine and Bricanyl). To review, these drugs mimic the sympathetic nervous system (that's why we call them sympathomimetic) to increase the production of CAMP, keeping the lungs functioning well. Here again, as with theophylline, these drugs work well, but have significant side effects. Chemical engineering again makes the future look rosier. Newer drugs that are longer-acting and act more specifically on the lungs are on the horizon and hopefully will be available soon.
3. *Cromolyn Sodium (Intal):* Cromolyn sodium is now available in many forms: nasal sprays, metered-dose inhalers and nebulizer solution for the lungs, and opthalmic sprays.

A promising drug known as Zaditen or ketotifen is now available in Europe. In the near future, it will be used in the United States. It is a pill taken twice a day and appears to be very effective in asthma and in certain allergic diseases, and it does not have many side effects. This drug (and its future offspring) will be very helpful.

4. *Corticosteroids:* Although cortisone has been controlling asthma symptoms for a long time, its side effects are notorious. As I've said many times, this is the last drug to use and the first to eliminate. The recent introduction of the spray form of cortisone has helped to reduce the side effects by reducing the amount of the drug that is absorbed in the body. Probably within the next five years, the spray will be more refined and will have more positive effects and fewer adverse side effects.
5. *Antihistamines:* In the future, molecular maneuvering will alter antihistamines and make them very useful in the treatment of asthma. The pendulum has moved back and forth with regard to the use of antihistamines. At first they were used frequently and then infrequently in treating asthma.
6. *Prostaglandins:* I discussed in Chapter 2 the role of the prostaglandins as mediators that are released following the interaction of IgE and allergens in an allergic reaction. Some prostaglandins are helpful. Prostaglandins E_1 and F_1 are important in controlling the lungs. I feel that as we begin to understand more about the prostaglandins in the future, we will be able to control bronchial asthma. The use of these drugs is probably not far off and we will probably see them being used in Europe within the next five years.
7. *Allergy Testing:* In the past, all allergy testing was done by injecting extracts of allergens into the patient and waiting to see the reaction. Such skin tests are gradually being replaced by testing procedures that do not require injecting any substances into the patient. Techniques have been developed that test a sample of the patient's blood. The RAST, ELISA, and immunoperidoxiase (IP) tests are such procedures. I feel that these *in vitro* (outside the living

body) testing methods will be at least as effective as skin testing in the very immediate future . . . probably better. They will make it much easier to diagnose allergic conditions and to prescribe better treatment. They are also less of a hassle for the patient (especially when children are concerned).

8. *Allergy Shots (Immunotherapy):* Tremendous progress is being made in perfecting the serum used in allergy shots. These new extracts are not yet available in the United States. They have the ability to immunize the patient against his particular allergen, but not provoke the allergic reaction as is now the case. Therefore, we will be able to immunize patients rapidly, perhaps even with only a few injections. It is possible that these substances will be in use before this book is published. These new serums will immunize patients quickly against pollen, dust, mold, and even penicillin, aspirin, and other drugs.
9. *Food and Environmental Factors:* There has been a great deal of confusion about the role of food and environmental variables in the pathogenesis of asthma. Much work is being done in these fields. It is my feeling that within the next few years we will have a much deeper understanding of how the components of foods or the components of our environment interact with our bodies to produce asthma symptoms. With increased skill at identifying and isolating the various triggers will come better dietary and environmental controls. We are moving in this direction now, and the future will surely bring us closer.

The "Far" Future

As we get nearer to the year 2000, there are two major things that I foresee. First, we will come to fully understand the pathogenesis of asthma. Once we figure out the exact nature of the underlying defect in the sympathetic nervous system, it will be easy to manufacture a drug that will fix the problem. At present our medications work around the defect, fixing something in the cycle that allows CAMP to be built up, maintained, or not destroyed. We will eventually be able to create a specific drug that will add CAMP directly without producing any side effects. We will then be able to turn asthma off with very simple medication.

The second thing that I foresee is an increased understanding of how IgE antibodies behave. The "good" IgE cells fight off parasites, worms, and even cancer. The "bad" IgE cells play a significant role in the chain of allergic asthma. I think we will learn how to turn this system on and off in such a way that it will turn off the allergic reactions while keeping on the surveillance systems against infections, parasites, and cancer. Then it will be easy to control allergies with perhaps one injection a year and virtually no side effects.

By the year 2000, with our very detailed understanding of exactly what causes asthma, we will then be able to track down what genes are involved in producing the asthmatic state. Then through genetic engineering, which is making outstanding progress, we will be able to alter the genetic composition of patients with asthma and fix them! Maybe these procedures will begin to be applied by 2010. The only disadvantage I can see to this fabulous prediction is that it will make this book obsolete.

APPENDIX 1

Pollination Time of Trees, Grasses, and Weeds

These tables can be used to find the trees, grasses, and weeds that grow in the area in which you live or plan to visit. The pollination times vary and are always influenced by changing weather patterns, but the information here is detailed enough to let you know what you are going to be exposed to.

I have given the longest pollen season (which always occurs at the lowest altitude and the most southern part of the zone). Therefore, if you live in the northern or cooler part of the zone or in the mountainous part of the zone, the pollen season for your exact area will be proportionately shorter than the span that I've indicated.

REGION I—NORTH ATLANTIC UNITED STATES

States: Connecticut, Massachusetts, New Jersey, Pennsylvania, Vermont, Maine, New Hampshire, New York, and Rhode Island

Trees	***Pollination Time***
Box Elder/Maple	Mar.–May
Birch	Apr.–May
Oak	May–June
Hickory	May

Trees	Pollination Time
Ash	Apr.–May
Sycamore	May
Cottonwood/Poplar	Mar.–May
Elm	Apr.
Grasses	
Redtop	May–July
Orchard Grass	May–July
Fescue	May–July
Timothy	May–July
Bluegrass/June Grass	May–July
Weeds	
Lambs Quarters	Aug.–Oct.
Ragweed (tall and short)	Aug.–Oct.
Cocklebur	Aug.–Oct.
Plantain	May–July
Dock Sorrel	May–July

REGION II—MID-ATLANTIC UNITED STATES

States: Delaware, Maryland, Virginia, District of Columbia, and North Carolina

Trees	Pollination Time
Box Elder/Maple	Feb.–May
Birch	Apr.–May
Cedar/Juniper	Mar.–Apr.
Hickory/Pecan	Apr.–May
Walnut	May
Ash	Mar.–May
Cottonwood/Poplar	Mar.–May
Elm	Feb.–Apr.
Oak	Mar.–May

Grasses	
Redtop	May–June
Vernal Grass	May–June
Bermuda Grass	Apr.–July
Orchard Grass	May–June
Timothy	May–June
Bluegrass/June Grass	May–July
Rye	May–July
Johnsongrass	May–July

Weeds	
Pigweed	Aug.–Oct.
Lambs Quarters	Aug.–Oct.
Ragweed (tall and short)	Aug.–Oct.
Cocklebur	Sept.–Oct.
Plantain	May–July
Dock Sorrel	May–July

REGION III—SOUTH ATLANTIC UNITED STATES

States: Northern Florida (above Orlando), Georgia, and South Carolina

Trees	*Pollination Time*
Box Elder/Maple	Mar.–Apr.
Birch	Apr.
Cedar/Juniper	May
Oak	Mar.–May
Hickory/Pecan	May
Walnut	May
Ash	May
Cottonwood/Poplar	Mar.–Apr.
Elm	Feb.–Apr.

Grasses	
Redtop	May–July
Vernal Grass	May–July
Bermuda Grass	Mar.–Sept.
Ryegrass	May–July
Fescue	May–July
Timothy	May–July
Bluegrass/June Grass	May–July
Johnsongrass	May–July

Weeds	
Lambs Quarters	Aug.–Oct.
Ragweed (tall and short)	Aug.–Oct.
Sagebrush	Aug.–Oct.
Cocklebur	Aug.–Oct.
Plantain	May–July
Dock Sorrel	May–July

REGION IV—THE GREATER OHIO VALLEY

States: Indiana, Ohio, West Virginia, Kentucky, and Tennessee

Trees	*Pollination Time*
Box Elder/Maple	Mar.–Apr.
Birch	Apr.–May
Oak	Apr.–May
Hickory	Apr.–June
Walnut	Mar.–May
Ash	Mar.–May
Sycamore	Apr.–May
Cottonwood/Poplar	Mar.–May
Elm	Feb.–Apr.

Grasses	
Redtop	May–June
Bermuda Grass	Apr.–July
Orchard Grass	May–June
Fescue	May–June
Rye	May–June
Timothy	May–June
Bluegrass/June Grass	May–June
Johnsongrass	May–July

Weeds	
Water Hemp	Aug.–Oct.
Pigweed	Aug.–Oct.
Lambs Quarters	Aug.–Oct.
Ragweed (tall and short)	Aug.–Oct.
Sagebrush	Aug.–Oct.
Cocklebur	Aug.–Oct.
Dock Sorrel	Aug.–Oct.
Plantain	May–July

REGION V—SUBTROPIC FLORIDA

Trees	***Pollination Time***
Box Elder	Feb.–Apr.
Cedar/Juniper	Jan.–Apr.
Oak	Dec.–Apr.
Pecan	Dec.–Apr.
Privet	All year
Palm	Dec.–Apr.
Australian Pine	Dec.–Apr.
Sycamore	Feb.–Apr.
Elm	Feb.–Apr.
Brazilian Pepper	Dec.–Apr.
Bayberry	Dec.–Apr.
Melaleuca	Dec.–Apr.

Grasses	
Redtop	All year
Bermuda Grass	All year
Salt Grass	All year
Bahia	All year
Canary	All year
Bluegrass/June Grass	All year
Johnsongrass	All year

Weeds	
Pigweed	July–Oct.
Lambs Quarters	July–Oct.
Ragweed (tall and short)	June–Nov.
Marsh Elder	June–Nov.
Dock Sorrel	Mar.–July
Plantain	Mar.–June

REGION VI—SOUTH CENTRAL UNITED STATES

States: Alabama, Louisiana, Arkansas, and Mississippi

Trees	*Pollination Time*
Box Elder/Maple	Mar.–Apr.
Cedar/Juniper	Feb.–May
Oak	Apr.–May
Hickory/Pecan	Apr.–May
Walnut	Apr.
Ash	Mar.–May
Sycamore	Apr.–May
Cottonwood/Poplar	Apr.–May
Hackberry	Mar.–May
Elm	Feb.–Mar.

Grasses	
Redtop	Apr.–Sept.
Bermuda Grass	Apr.–Sept.
Orchard Grass	May–Sept.
Ryegrass	May–Sept.
Timothy	May–Sept.
Bluegrass/June Grass	Mar.–Sept.
Johnsongrass	Apr.–Sept.

Weeds	
Carelessweed/Pigweed	Aug.–Oct.
Lambs Quarters	Aug.–Oct.
Ragweed (tall and short)	Aug.–Oct.
Sagebrush	Aug.–Oct.
Marsh Elder/Poverty Weed	Aug.–Oct.
Cocklebur	Aug.–Oct.
Plantain	May–July
Dock Sorrel	May–July

REGION VII—THE NORTHERN MIDWEST

States: Michigan, Wisconsin, and Minnesota

Trees	*Pollination Time*
Box Elder-Maple	Mar.–Apr.
Alder	Mar.–Apr.
Birch	Apr.
Oak	May–June
Hickory	May–June
Walnut	May–June
Ash	May
Sycamore	Apr.–May
Cottonwood/Poplar	Mar.–Apr.
Elm	Mar.–Apr.

Grasses	
Redtop	May–July
Bromegrass	May–July
Orchard Grass	May–July
Fescue	May–June
Ryegrass	May–June
Canary Grass	May–July
Timothy	May–July
Bluegrass/June Grass	May–July

Weeds	
Water Hemp	Aug.–Oct.
Lambs Quarters	Aug.–Oct.
Russian Thistle	Aug.–Oct.
Ragweed (tall and short)	Aug.–Oct.
Marsh Elder/Poverty Weed	Aug.–Oct.
Cocklebur	Sept.–Oct.
Dock Sorrel	May–July
Pigweed	Aug.–Oct.
Plantain	May–July

REGION VIII—THE CENTRAL MIDWEST

States: Illinois, Missouri, and Iowa

Trees	*Pollination Time*
Box Elder/Maple	Mar.–Apr.
Birch	Apr.
Oak	May–June
Hickory	May
Walnut	Mar.–May
Ash	Apr.–May
Sycamore	Apr.–May
Cottonwood/Poplar	Mar.–Apr.
Elm	Feb.–Apr.

Grasses	
Redtop	May–Aug.*
Bermuda Grass	Apr.–July
Orchard Grass	May–Aug.
Ryegrass	May–Aug.
Timothy	May–Aug.
Bluegrass/June Grass	May–Aug.
Johnsongrass	May–July
Corn	May–Aug.

Weeds	
Pigweed	Aug.–Oct.
Lambs Quarters	Aug.–Oct.
Mexican Firebush	Aug.–Oct.
Russian Thistle	Aug.–Oct.
Ragweed (tall and short)	Aug.–Oct.
Marsh Elder/Poverty Weed	Aug.–Oct.
Plantain	May–July
Dock Sorrel	May–July

REGION IX—THE GREAT PLAINS

States: Kansas, North Dakota, Nebraska, and South Dakota

Trees	*Pollination Time*
Box Elder/Maple	Mar.–May
Alder	Mar.–Apr.
Birch	Apr.–May
Oak	May–June
Hickory	May
Walnut	May
Ash	May
Cottonwood/Poplar	Mar.–Apr.
Elm	Mar.–Apr.

Grasses	
Quack Grass/Wheatgrass	May–July
Redtop	May–July
Bromegrass	May–July
Orchard Grass	May–July
Ryegrass	May–July
Fescue	May–July
Timothy	May–July
Bluegrass/June Grass	May–July

Weeds	
Water Hemp	July–Aug.
Pigweed	July–Oct.
Lambs Quarters	July–Oct.
Mexican Firebush	July–Oct.
Russian Thistle	July–Oct.
Ragweed (tall and short)	July–Oct.
Sagebrush	Sept.–Oct.
Marsh Elder/Poverty Weed	Aug.–Oct.
Cocklebur	Sept.–Oct.
Plantain	May–July
Dock Sorrel	May–July

REGION X—SOUTHWESTERN GRASSLANDS

States: Oklahoma and Texas

Trees	*Pollination Time*
Box Elder	Mar.–Apr.
Cedar/Juniper	Dec.–Mar.
Oak	Mar.–June
Mesquite	Feb.–Apr.
Mulberry	Mar.–May
Ash	Feb.–May
Cottonwood/Poplar	Feb.–Apr.
Elm	Feb.–Apr.

Grasses	
Quack Grass	Apr.–Aug.
Redtop	Apr.–Aug.
Bermuda Grass	Apr.–Aug.
Orchard Grass	Apr.–Aug.
Fescue	Apr.–Aug.
Ryegrass	Apr.–Aug.
Timothy	Apr.–Aug.
Bluegrass/June Grass	Apr.–Aug.
Johnsongrass	Apr.–Aug.

Weeds	
Carelessweed/Pigweed	Aug.–Oct.
Lambs Quarters	Aug.–Oct.
Russian Thistle	Aug.–Oct.
Ragweed (tall, short, false, and giant)	Aug.–Oct.
Sagebrush	Sept.
Marsh Elder	Sept.–Oct.
Cocklebur	Sept.–Oct.
Dock Sorrel	May–July
Plantain	May–July

REGION XI—ROCKY MOUNTAIN EMPIRE

States: Arizona (mountainous), Colorado, Idaho (mountainous), Montana, New Mexico, Utah, and Wyoming

Trees	*Pollination Time*
Box Elder	Apr.
Birch	Apr.
Cedar/Juniper	Mar.–May
Oak	May–June
Pine	Feb.–Apr.
Cottonwood/Poplar	Mar.–May
Elm	Feb.–May
Mountain Cedar	Dec.–Mar.

*Grasses**	
Quack Grass	Apr.–Sept.
Redtop	Apr.–Sept.
Bermuda Grass	Apr.–Sept.
Orchard Grass	Apr.–Sept.
Ryegrass	Apr.–Sept.
Timothy	Apr.–Sept.
Fescue	Apr.–Sept.
Bluegrass/June Grass	Apr.–Sept.

Weeds	
Pigweed	July–Oct.
Saltbush/Scale	May–Sept.
Lambs Quarters	July–Oct.
Mexican Firebush	Aug.–Oct.
Russian Thistle	July–Oct.
Ragweed (false, giant, short, and western)	July–Sept.
Sagebrush	July–Oct.
Cocklebur	July–Oct.
Plantain	May–June

REGION XII—THE ARID SOUTHWEST

States: Arizona and Southern California (S.E. Desert)

Trees	*Pollination Time*
Sycamore	Mar.–May
Cypress	Feb.–Apr.
Cedar/Juniper	Apr.
Mesquite	Mar.–June
Ash	Feb.–May
Cottonwood/Poplar	Jan.–Apr.
Elm	Jan.–Mar.
Oak	Mar.–May

*Grasses in Arizona's mountainous region and New Mexico pollinate from Apr. to Aug.; grasses in Colorado and Idaho pollinate from May to Sept.; grasses in Utah and Wyoming pollinate from May to July; and grasses in Montana pollinate from May to Aug.

Grasses	
Bromegrass	Apr.–July
Bermuda Grass	Feb.–Dec.
Ryegrass	Feb.–Dec.
Canary Grass	Mar.–July
Bluegrass/June Grass	Feb.–Dec.

Weeds	
Carelessweed	May–Nov.
Saltbush/Scale	May–Sept.
Lambs Quarters	May–Nov.
Russian Thistle	May–Nov.
Ragweed	Mar.–Apr. and Sept.–Oct.
Sagebrush	Sept.–Oct.

REGION XIII—SOUTHERN COASTAL AND CENTRAL CALIFORNIA

Trees	***Pollination Time***
Mulberry	Mar.–Apr.
Box Elder	Mar.–Apr.
Oak	Feb.–May
Walnut	Apr.–June
Acacia	Feb.–Mar.
Alder	Jan.–Apr.
Ash	Apr.–May
Sycamore	Apr.–June
Elm	Feb.–Mar.
Cottonwood/Poplar	Feb.–Apr.

Grasses	
Oats	Apr.–July
Redtop	June–Aug.
Bromegrass	Mar.–June
Bermuda Grass	Feb.–Nov.
Orchard Grass	Apr.–Sept.
Ryegrass	Apr.–June
Canary Grass	Mar.–July
Timothy	June–Aug.
Johnsongrass	Apr.–Sept.

Weeds	
Carelessweed	June–Oct.
Pigweed	May–Aug.
Saltbush/Scale	May–Sept.
Lambs Quarters	June–Oct.
Russian Thistle	Aug.–Oct.
Ragweed	June–Sept.
Sagebrush	June–Oct.
Cocklebur	Aug.–Oct.
Plantain	Apr.–July
Dock Sorrel	Apr.–June

REGION XIV—INTERMOUNTAIN WEST

States: Idaho (Southern) and Nevada

Trees	*Pollination Time*
Box Elder	Apr.–May
Alder	Mar.–Apr.
Birch	Apr.
Cedar/Juniper	Mar.–May
Ash	Mar.–May
Sycamore	Apr.–May
Cottonwood/Poplar	Feb.–May
Elm	Feb.–Apr.

Grasses	
Quack Grass	May–July
Redtop	May–July
Bromegrass	May–July
Bermuda Grass	May–July
Orchard Grass	May–July
Ryegrass	May–July
Timothy	May–July
Bluegrass/June Grass	May–July

Weeds	
Pigweed	July–Oct.
Saltbush/Scale	May–Sept.
Lambs Quarters	July–Oct.
Mexican Firebush	Aug.–Oct.
Russian Thistle	July–Oct.
Ragweed	July–Oct.
Sagebrush	July–Oct.
Cocklebur	July–Oct.

REGION XV—PACIFIC NORTHWEST

States: California (Northwestern), Oregon, and Washington

Trees	*Pollination Time*
Box Elder	Mar.–Apr.
Alder	Feb.–Apr.
Birch	Feb.–May
Oak	Apr.–June
Walnut	Apr.–June
Cottonwood/Poplar	Feb.–Mar.
Willow	Feb.–Apr.
Hazelnut	Feb.–Mar.
Ash	Mar.–May
Elm	Mar.–June
Acacia	Jan.–Dec.

Grasses	
Redtop	May–Aug.
Bromegrass	May–Aug.
Orchard Grass	May–Aug.
Ryegrass	May–Aug.
Timothy	May–Aug.
Bluegrass/June Grass	May–Aug.
Oatgrass	May–Aug.
Bermuda Grass	May–Aug.

Weeds	
Pigweed	July–Oct.
Lambs Quarters	July–Sept.
Ragweed	June–Sept.
Sagebrush	Sept.–Oct.
Plantain	May–July
Dock Sorrel	May–July

REGION XVI—ALASKA

Trees	*Pollination Time*
Alder	Mar.–June
Aspen	Mar.–June
Birch	Mar.–June
Cedar	Mar.–June
Hemlock	Mar.–June
Pine	Mar.–June
Poplar	Mar.–June
Spruce	Mar.–June
Willow	Mar.–June

REGION XVII—HAWAII

Trees	*Pollination Time*
Acacia Australian Pine Cedar/Juniper Monterey Cypress Date Palm Eucalyptus Mesquite Paper Mulberry Olive Privet	Good data are not available for these plants in the Hawaiian region
Grasses	
Bermuda Grass Corn Finger Johnsongrass Lovegrass Bluegrass/June Grass Redtop Sorghum	
Weeds	
Cocklebur Plantain Kochia Pigweed Ragweed (slender) Sagebrush Scale (saltbush)	

GLOSSARY

Adenyl Cyclase. The enzyme that produces CAMP. The action of adenyl cyclase is partially blocked in the asthmatic patient. *See* Chapter 5 for further details. *See* CAMP.

Adrenalin (epinephrine). A sympathomimetic drug that is given by injection to help control asthma attacks.

Aero-allergen. Any substance, such as pollen, dust, dander, or mold, carried in the air that can induce an allergic reaction.

Alveoli. The tiny air sacs found at the termination of the bronchioles. The thin lining of the alveolus is in contact with the capillary membrane. It is in this area that the blood takes on oxygen and loses carbon dioxide.

Anaphylaxis. The most severe form of allergic reaction. It is manifested by generalized swelling, hives, wheezing, and choking (in its most severe form, death ensues).

Antibody. Any substance found in the blood or body fluids that may exist naturally, but is usually produced in response to a stimulus from any foreign substance (antigen). Usually, an antibody is composed of proteins that are similar in structure and are called immunoglobins. The immunoglobins are capable of reacting with foreign substances and inducing reactions that destroy these substances. When they react with bacteria, fungi, and parasites, they usually destroy them. This process is called immune defense. When antibodies attack pollen or other harmless substances such as dust and mold, they also damage or destroy these substances. This is characterized as an allergic or hypersensitivity response. In both the immune defense process and in the hypersensitivity reactions, some tissue damage occurs. *See* Immunoglobins.

Antihistamine. A drug that blocks the action of histamine. This drug is very useful in ameliorating symptoms of hay fever and itching. It is occasionally useful in asthma.

Autohypnosis. The process by which an individual induces the hypnotic state in himself.

Autonomic Nervous System. Regulates the lungs, heart, blood vessels, visceral smooth muscles (stomach and intestine), and many exocrine (mucus and salivary) glands. Its functioning is not under voluntary control.

Biofeedback. The use of instrumentation that can measure biological functions and their variations of which an individual would normally not be aware. These measurements are fed back to the individual, informing him of variations in his biological functions so that he can learn to control them. For example, a device is placed on the tip of a patient's finger that can measure his temperature. The patient's temperature is recorded on a screen so that the patient can read it and be taught techniques to regulate it.

Bronchi. They start as two large air tubes that branch out from the trachea. They continue to branch forming smaller bronchi until the diameter of the air tubes is only 0.5 millimeters (1/50 inch); they are then called bronchioles. *See* Figure 1 on page 234. All of these airways convey air to and from the lungs.

Bronchioles. Smaller air tubes leading into the alveoli.

Bronchiolitis. An inflammation of the smallest bronchioles and caused by a virus. It usually occurs in infants and small children. Symptoms include coughing, wheezing, fever, and in severe cases, difficulty in breathing. Bronchiolitis is often confused with asthma. Bronchiolitis usually occurs once whereas asthma is a recurrent illness.

Capillaries. Very small blood vessels with very thin walls allowing oxygen and other nutrients to be exchanged across the walls of these vessels.

Cardiologist. A physician who specializes in diseases of the heart.

Cataract. An opacity in the lens of the eye. As it increases in size it impairs vision.

Chronic Bronchitis. An inflammation of the bronchial airway resulting in coughing and excessive mucus secretion. It is a disease that can produce wheezing and is often mistaken for asthma. There is chronic damage to the bronchi (air tubes) that causes marked irritation and results in the production of a large amount of mucus. Many patients with this disease have a long history of smoking. There is less likelihood of reversibility than there is in asthma.

Corticosteroids. Drugs such as cortisone, Prednisone, and Decadron used to treat severe bronchial asthma. *See* Chapter 5 for further details.

Cromolyn Sodium (Intal). A drug used to treat bronchial asthma. It is inhaled with a metered-dose inhaler and is also available as a liquid that can be nebulized. It is not effective when swallowed.

Croup. An illness caused by inflammation of the larynx and trachea. It is usually caused by a virus and only affects infants and small children. Symptoms include hoarseness, fever, a barking cough, and a sore throat. In severe cases the airways can close off and produce severe difficulty in breathing.

CAMP (Cyclic adenosine 3^1, 5^1-monophosphate). A substance that is diminished in asthmatics. When CAMP is diminished the mast cell more readily releases mediators and the bronchi more readily constricts, causing allergic reactions, than if CAMP were present in normal levels.

Cystic Fibrosis. A disease that in early life sometimes resembles asthma. It is a much more serious disease and produces severe damage to the lungs. It is differentiated from asthma by a sweat test. *See* Sweat Test.

Dehumidifier. Any device to remove moisture from the air.

Dyspnea. Shortness of breath or difficulty in breathing usually induced by diseases of the heart or lungs or by alterations in metabolism. There is a feeling of not being able to get enough air into the lungs.

Electrocardiograph (ECG or EKG). An instrument that measures the electric potential associated with the electric currents traversing the heart. It can help to determine the presence of certain forms of heart disease.

Electrostatic Air Cleaner. Works by electrically charging the particles that pass through it. On one side of the system the particles are given a positive charge and on the other side they are given a negative charge. The particles then clump together and are filtered out of the air. This system can filter out any particles 0.1 micron or greater in size. This device is best for a forced air system.

Emphysema. A disease characterized by distention of the air sacs. An asthmatic patient may experience acute emphysema during an asthma attack. When the asthma attack is over, the air sacs return to normal. In chronic emphysema the air sacs remain permanently distended. Unless asthma is absolutely uncontrolled, it does not usually lead to chronic emphysema. Emphysema can be mistaken for severe asthma because wheezing occurs in both.

Epiglottis. The elastic cartilage cap over the larynx that prevents the swallowing of food and liquid into our respiratory system.

Extrinsic Asthma. A term of convenience for a form of asthma in which the cause is known. Cat dander, which may induce asthma, is an example of extrinsic asthma.

FEV_1 (One Second Forced Expiratory Volume). That portion of the Forced Vital Capacity that one can exhale in one second. Normally 82 percent of the forced vital capacity may be exhaled in one second. Patients whose disease is characterized by bronchospasm (asthma, emphysema, and chronic bronchitis) tend to have an FEV_1 that is less than 82 percent. The FEV_1 is inversely proportional to the amount of bronchospasm.

Forced Vital Capacity. The amount of air that one can exhale after a deep inhalation, exhaling as hard and as fast as one can.

Fungi. Plants without chlorophyll that lack definite root, stem, and leaf structure. Fungi reproduce by expelling spores into the air. The spores are allergens. If you are allergic to fungi, you may develop allergic symptoms when you inhale the spores.

HEPA Filter (High Efficiency Particulate Air). A filter made of tightly meshed material that can filter particulate matter (pollen, dust, or mold) of 0.013 micron or greater in diameter out of the air. This type of filter functions best in an enclosed room. Its disadvantage is that it cannot work as the filtering device for a forced air system.

Humidifier. Any device to add moisture to the air.

Hyperventilation Syndrome. The patient breathes too rapidly. This syndrome is produced by anxiety. The symptoms (rapid breathing, dyspnea, and chest pain) may be confused with asthma.

Hypnotic State. A trance state (hypnosis) in which one is awake and has lost peripheral awareness, but possesses central awareness and is therefore capable of intense concentration. A person in this state is highly susceptible to suggestion and may be able to gain some control over his autonomic functions.

Hypnotism. The procedure whereby a hypnotic state is induced either naturally (by circumstances) or artificially by deliberate intervention of another person.

Hypnotist. One who induces hypnosis in others.

Hypoxemia. That state in which the level of oxygen in the blood is below normal.

Immunoglobin E (IgE). An immunoglobin present in very small quantities in the bloodstream of humans. The exact functions of this immunoglobin are unknown. However, it is known to be the major antibody involved in the allergic reaction.

Immunoglobins. Structurally related proteins in the blood separated into five major classes: IgG, IgA, IgM, IgD, and IgE. These proteins are important in certain phases of defense against viruses, bacteria, and parasites. They also help mediate some allergic reactions.

Immunoglobulin Test. A test to measure the level of Immunoglobulin in the blood.

Immunotherapy. Immunotherapy, desensitization, hyposensitization, and allergy shots are terms used to describe the treatment process of sequentially injecting a patient with substances to which he is allergic to induce in him a tolerance or immunity to those substances. This treatment is most effective in patients with allergies to pollen, dust, mites, mold, and danders. It is not effective in treating food allergy. *See* Chapter 4 for further details.

Intradermal Skin Test. A test in which small quantities of an allergen are injected, using a syringe, into the superficial layers of the skin (the dermis). The intradermal test is more sensitive than the scratch or puncture tests, but there is more risk of a generalized reaction (very uncommon). Intradermal skin tests may be too sensitive and falsely label a nonallergic person allergic.

Intravenous. Within the vein.

Intrinsic Asthma. A term of convenience for a form of asthma for which no known cause has been determined.

In Vitro Test. A test or procedure done in the test tubes; for instance, a RAST or PRIST test.

In Vivo Test. A test done in the living body; for instance, a skin test.

Ion. An atom or group of atoms that have a positive or negative charge.

Ionization. The process of producing ions.

Larynx. The upper part of the respiratory tract extending from the pharynx to the trachea. It contains the vocal cords that are important in the production of speech and sounds.

Leukotriene LTE 4. A mediator that is very important in bronchial asthma.

Liter. 1.06 quarts or slightly more than a quart, which is 0.967 liters.

Mast Cell. Cells distributed throughout the body, which are more concentrated in any area of the body that comes in contact with the external environment. Thus, they are found in greater quantities in the mouth, trachea, bronchi, skin, and gastrointestinal tract. Histamine exists in a preformed state within the granules of the mast cell. The mast cells produce SRS-A, and most of the other mediators that are involved in allergic reaction. Pairs of IgE molecules are situated on receptor sites on the outer membrane of the mast cell. When the appropriate antigen combines with the paired IgE molecules a reaction occurs, the end result of which is a biochemical signal to the mast cell to release its contents into the surrounding body fluids. The release of mediators into the surrounding body fluids causes the allergic reaction.

Medic-Alert Bracelet. Can be obtained by sending away to Medic-Alert, P.O. Box 1009, Turlock, CA 95381-1009.

This device is a distinctive bracelet that can be worn around the wrist. It indicates what drugs you are allergic to, whether you have asthma or take steroids, and any other important medical information. In addition, information is kept concerning your medical background in a central computer. In an emergency the doctor taking care of you can call this computer number and receive information concerning your medical background. If you have any significant disease, allergy, or asthma, it is a very good idea to get this bracelet. If you are unconscious it may save your life.

Mediator. Any chemical substance that can activate some aspect of the immune system. Histamine, SRS-A, and prostaglandins are mediators.

Mite (Human); *Dermatophagoides Farinae*. An insect that is thirty microns in diameter. It is barely visible to the naked eye. The human mite lives on human dander. It does not bite. However, when it dies, it decomposes and becomes part of the house dust. Mite is the major antigen in house dust.

Mitral Valve Prolapse. A slight loosening of the support of the mitral valve in the heart. This process may cause chest pain.

Mold. Same as fungus.

Multiphasic Blood Scan. A test that measures various components of the blood such as sugar, calcium phosphorous, and various enzymes that relate to the functioning of organs such as the liver, kidneys, heart, and pancreas. It is a sensitive indicator of various disease states. It is an automated test that is done as part of a general medical workup.

Nebulizer. An apparatus that can vaporize a liquid.

Oxygenation. The addition of oxygen to any physical or chemical system. For example, the blood is oxygenated when it passes through the lungs.

Peak Flow Meter. A device that measures the peak flow of air expelled at the beginning of forced expiration. This measurement is very important for asthma patients because a reduced expiratory flow rate may be an early warning of an impending asthma attack.

Pharynx. A muscular and membranous cavity leading from the mouth and nasal passages to the larynx and esophagus.

Phosphodiesterase. An enzyme that breaks down CAMP. This enzyme is blocked by theophylline. Since CAMP prevents asthma, administering theophylline to prevent the breakdown of CAMP by phosphodiesterase will reduce the severity of asthma.

Physical Therapy. The use of physical (nonmedicinal) forces such as massage, relaxation techniques, postural drainage, and therapeutic exercise to compensate for a deficit induced by disease.

Pneumonia. An inflammation of the lungs. The most common forms of pneumonia are caused by bacteria and viruses. Symptoms include chest pain (especially on deep inspiration), fever, cough, and in severe cases, shortness of breath.

Pollen. The male fertilizing element of a plant. It is a grain usually 15–50 microns in diameter (3–10 × the diameter of a red blood cell). Pollen may be wind-borne, which causes problems for people with allergies or it may be insect-borne, which is not a problem unless you make an effort to smell the plant. (The flower ragweed is an example of the wind-borne type. Roses are examples of the insect-borne type.)

Postural Drainage. A method of treatment whereby the patient is placed in an anatomic position that will allow gravity to favor the expulsion of excess mucus when the use of mechanical force (cupping of the hands and percussion over the appropriate area of the lung) or electronic energy (ultrasound) is utilized. This method is more useful in the treatment of emphysema, cystic fibrosis, and chronic bronchitis than it is in the treatment of asthma. *See* Chapter 8 for full details of this procedure.

PRIST (Paper Radioimmunosorbent Test). A test to measure the IgE level in the bloodstream.

Progressive Relaxation. A method of inducing relaxation developed by Edmund Jacobson. The subject is trained to progressively tense and relax groups of muscles starting in the extremities and proceeding to the torso and head and neck. When this method is used a state of deep relaxation is induced in most individuals. Jacobson Progressive Relaxation is very similar to hypnosis, yoga, and meditation.

Prostaglandins. Substances with similar chemical structure that are mediators. They are involved in many body functions and are also important in some phases of bronchial asthma.

Psychosomatic. Any physical disease state that is induced by any mental process. Psychosomatic disease states are currently believed to be physical states that can be aggravated by mental processes such as stress and tension.

Pulmonary Function Test. A test to measure the health, strength, capacity, and functioning of the lungs. The test is performed with an instrument that measures the patient's ability to breathe (sometimes a series of tests is used).

Pulmonologist. A physician who specializes in diseases of the chest.

Puncture (Prick) Test. A test in which a drop of the substance to which the patient is thought to be allergic is placed on the patient's skin. The skin is then pricked with a needle at this site. This test is slightly more sensitive than the scratch test and is less sensitive than the intradermal test. There is virtually no danger of a systemic reaction with the puncture test.

RAST (Radioallergosorbent Test). A blood test developed in 1967 to measure the amount of specific IgE in the blood against various substances to which a patient may be allergic; for instance, ragweed, grass, eggs, milk, or penicillin. RAST is easier to perform than skin testing and it is more specific and accurate than skin testing. Skin testing is more sensitive than a RAST, and in certain ambiguous cases, a skin test may have to be performed to ascertain the presence of an allergy.

Residual Volume. The amount of air that is left in the lungs when you exhale as hard and as fast as you can. An increase in residual volume makes it mechanically harder to breathe. In asthma, there may be an increase in residual volume because the alveoli are slightly stretched. In emphysema, there is a marked increase in residual volume.

Retraction. Occurs when the excessory muscles of respiration are used and cause the ribs to appear to be sucked in when the patient inhales. Retraction occurs when one is having difficulty breathing.

Scratch Test. A test in which a drop of the substance to which the patient is thought to be allergic is placed on the patient's skin at the site where a superficial scratch has been made. The substance being tested enters the top layer (epidermis) of the skin. A wheal will develop if the patient is allergic to the substance. It is the least sensitive of all skin tests.

Spirometer. An apparatus that measures the ability to breathe, and the general function of the lungs. *See* Chapter 3 for further details.

Sweat Test. A test to measure the amount of sodium ions and chloride ions in sweat. It is important in establishing the diagnosis of cystic fibrosis. It is performed by sending a very weak electric current through the skin producing sweat. The presence of 60 mEq/L or greater of sodium ions or chloride ions in the sweat is considered diagnostic of cystic fibrosis.

Sympathomimetic. Mimics the effects of the sympathetic nervous system. Adrenalin, Isuprel, metaproterenol (Metaprel and Alupent), and albuterol (Proventil and Ventolin) are sympathomimetic agents.

Theophylline Blood Level. The level of theophylline in the blood. A level of 10–20 milligrams is considered effective.

Theophyllinization. The process of titrating the amount of theophylline that a patient takes until a therapeutic level of theophylline is achieved in the bloodstream. *See* Chapter 8 for further details.

Therapeutic Level. That level of a medication in the bloodstream that is effective in producing the desired therapeutic blood level.

Trachea. The largest air tube that extends from the larynx to a point high in the chest where it divides into the two large air tubes that are the bronchi. See bronchi.

Vital Capacity. The total amount of air that one can exhale after a deep inhalation.

Wheal. An acute transitory circumscribed area of edema (swelling) in the superficial layers of the skin. The most common examples of wheals are mosquito bites and hives. A wheal is also produced by allergy skin tests.

Wheezing. A sound that is made as air passes through narrowed bronchi, usually occurring during an asthma attack; difficult and noisy breathing, often with a whistling sound.

A special thank-you to my wife, Marcia, who labored many hours to help compile this glossary.

Index

A
Absenteeism, 1, 280
Achromycin, 254
Acute attacks, 285–303
  adrenalin, 295–296
  children, 277–278
  emergency room, 297–301
  hospitalization, 301–302
  mild asthmatic, 289
  moderate asthmatic, 290–292
  nebulizers, 294–295
  planning ahead, 287–288
  pregnancy, 259
  self-monitoring, peak flow meter, 286
  severe asthmatic, 292–294
  situations for immediate attention, 287
  sporadic asthmatic, 288–289
Adenosine monophosphate, 144–145
Adenosine triphosphate, 144–146
Adenyl cyclase, 144, 145, 168
Adrenal glands, 173, 305
Adrenalin, 139, 141, 145, 295–296
  and anaphylactic reaction, 69, 74
  body weight and dose, 295
  children, 278
  for emergency treatment, 155
  long-acting brand, 296
  training for injection of, 295
Aero-allergens
  nature of, 41–42
  types of, 41–50
  See also Environmental stimuli.
AeroBid, 168, 172, 180
Aerochamber, 274
Aero-irritants, 10, 42, 50, 57
  pollution, 51–52
  smoke, 49–50
  as trigger, 10
  types of, 50
  weather, 51–52
Aerosol sprays, 50
Afrin, 257
Age factors, food allergies, 69–70
Air-conditioning, 60
Air filters, 60–61
  electrostatic air purifiers, 60
  HEPA (High Efficiency Particulate Air), 60–61
Air pollution. *See* Pollution.
Air ventilation system of home, as environmental control, 60–61
Albuterol, 160, 254, 255, 256, 275
  brand names, 155
  nebulized liquid, 157–158
  side effects, 156, 159
  spacers, 157
  spray, 156–157
  syrup, 159
  tablets, 158–159
Alcohol, 12
  sensitivity to, 104
Allergens
  definition of, 38
  elimination of, 38–39
  types of, 38–39
  See also Allergies; Environmental stimuli.
Allergic reaction
  inflammatory response, 165–166
  late phase response, 166
  mechanisms in, 165–166
Allergic shiners, 208
Allergies, 6
  aero-allergens, 41–50
  aero-irritants, 50–52
  chemical mediators and, 8, 40
  elimination diets, 77–103
  environmental stimuli, 38–66
  extrinsic asthma, 7–8
  food reactions, 67–134
  as trigger, 7–9
  See also specific topics.
Allergists, 23, 54, 139
Allergy shots. *See* Immunotherapy.
Allergy tests, 134–137
  ELISA, 30, 329
  future view, 329
  PRIST, 30–31
  RAST (Radioallergosorbent Test), 136–137, 141
  skin tests, 29–30, 135
Alpha one antitrypsin defect, misdiagnosed as asthma, 19
Alupent, 159, 160, 180, 254, 255, 258, 260, 275, 291
American Academy of Allergy and Immunology, 31
Aminophylline, 146, 147, 181
Anaphylactic reaction, 69, 72, 74–75
  adrenalin, 69, 74
  emergency treatment, 74–75
  planning guidelines, 69, 74–75

Anesthesia
  dental surgery, 307
  pregnancy, 261
Animal dander, 9, 48, 206–207
Antibiotics
  and pregnancy, 256
  TAO, 175
Antibodies
  actions of, 8
  immunoglobulin-E (IgE), 8
  role in asthma, 8
Anticholinergic agents, 12
Antihistamines, 139, 141, 167, 329
Antitrypsin deficit, 19
Arachidonic acid, 8
Aristocort, 168, 169, 174
Artificial coloring and flavoring, 70, 83, 103
Aspartame, 105
Aspirin, 9, 70, 105, 208
Asthma
  acute attacks, 285–303
  attack, features of, 3–4
  CAMP (cyclic adenosine 3'5'-monophosphate) deficit, 144–146
  centers/clinics for, 309–317
  in children, 265–284
  daily routines, guidelines, 318–326
  differential diagnosis, 19
  doctors, 20–36
  environmental stimuli, 38–66
  extrinsic asthma, 7–8
  food reactions, 67–134
  future advances, 327–331
  gender and, 1
  genetic factors, 248–250
  immunotherapy and, 141–142
  impact of, 1–2
  intrinsic asthma, 8
  late phase response, 166
  lifestyle changes, xiii, 3, 26
  Lung-Line, 36–37
  mechanical respiratory problems created by, 232–234
  medications, 142–201
  myths related to, 5–6
  physical exam/diagnostic tests, 26–32
  physical therapy approach, 235–247
  in pregnancy, 248–264
  psychological aspects, 219–231
  respiratory system and, 6–7, 12, 41
  sporadic asthma, 205–206, 210
  and surgery, 304–308
  symptoms of, 2, 14–17
  syndromes mimicking asthma, 18–19
  triggers, 6–13
  See also specific topics.
Atarax, 254
ATP (adenosine triphosphate), 144–146
Atrovent, 12, 174–175, 177, 182
  children, 276–277
Auto fumes, 39
Autonomic nervous system, 7, 38
Azmacort, 168, 172, 173, 182, 255

B
Barometric pressure, 52
Baseball, 9
Basement/attic/crawl spaces, environmental control, 59
Basophil chemotatic factor of anaphylaxis (BCF-A), 8
Bathroom, environmental control, 59
Beclomethasone, 168
Beclovent, 168, 172, 173, 183, 255, 256
Beconase, 255, 257
Bedroom, environmental control, 56–58
Benadryl, 75
Benzoates, 84
Beta-2 action, 156
Biofeedback, stress reduction, 225–226
Blood levels, theophylline, 151–152, 290
Blood test, 27
Breast-feeding, 263–264
Breathing dynamics, pulmonary function tests, 28–29
Breathing exercises, 235–239
  abdominal breathing, 236
  effects of, 236
  exercise/positions, 237–239
  pursed-lip breathing, 236–237
  weights, use in, 237
Brethaire, 183, 255, 258, 260
Brethine, 161, 183, 254, 291
Bricanyl, 161, 184, 254, 291
Bronchi, 3, 40
Bronchial spasm, 3
Bronchioles, 3
Bronchiolitis, in differential diagnosis of children, 268
Bronchodilator, 28
Bronkodyl, 146, 147
Bronkosol, 68
Bronkotabs, 163

C
Caffeine, 12
Calcium, 165
Calcium channel blockers, 112
CAMP (cyclic adenosine 3'5'-monophosphate) deficit, in asthma, 144–146, 168, 328, 331
Camps, asthma camps, listing of, 282–284
Candida, 80
Car, environmental control, 62–63
Carpeting, 57
Celestone, 168, 169, 174
Chemical mediators, and allergies, 8, 40
Chest X-ray, 27
Children, 265–284
  compared to adults, 266, 267
  asthma camps, listing of, 282–284
  corticosteroids, 170
  cromolyn sodium, 166
  daily routines, guidelines, 324
  differential diagnosis, 267–271
    bronchiolitis, 268
    congenital abnormalities, 270
    croup, 268–269

Children (*continued*)
cystic fibrosis, 270
epiglottitis, 269
foreign-body obstruction, 269
heart disease, 270
hyperventilation syndrome, 270
mitral valve prolapse, 271
pneumonia, 269
discipline and, 281
doctor, choosing, 22, 23, 272–273
elimination diets, 273–274
emergency situations, 277–278
environmental control, 273
food allergies, 69–70
common sensitivities, 83–84
multiple elimination diet, 82–103, 107, 109–110
immunotherapy, 278–279
infections, 278
medication, 274–278
for mild to moderate asthma, 275–277
nebulizers, 274–275
for severe asthma, 277–278
spacers, 274
metaproterenol, 160–161
National Jewish program, 310–311
nebulizers, 158
physical fitness, 246
psychological aspects, 281–282
school factors, 280–281
spacers, advantages of, 157
sports, 279–280
statistical information, 265–266
symptoms, 266–267
team approach and asthma, 266, 279, 280
terbutaline sulfate, 161, 162
theophylline, 148–149, 152–153
Chinese food, MSG, 68, 71, 84, 105
Chloride ions, 27
Chlor-Trimeton, 75
Chocolate, 12
Choledyl, 146, 184
Chronic bronchitis, 2
Cigarette smoke. *See* Smoke
Cimetidine (Tagamet), 12, 153
Citrus fruits, 12
Clinics/centers
listing of, 312–317
National Jewish Center, 309–311
Coffee, 12
Colds, 209
antihistamines, 167
children, 278
Congenital abnormalities, in differential diagnosis of children, 270
Constant-T, 147, 185
Cooking odors, 59
Corticosteroids, 145–146, 167–174, 178
and acute attack, 293–294
brand names, 168
"burst" technique, 292
children, 170, 277
future view, 329
long-acting, 168
long-term use, 169–170
mechanism of action, 168, 173
and pregnancy, 256
short-acting, 168
short-term use, 168
side effects, 170–172
spray, 168, 172–173
steroid dependency, 174, 305
stopping dosage, 173
surgery/dental treatment precautions, 173–174
Cottonseed, 9, 48–49
Coughing, 2
in asthma attack, 4
as symptom, 17
types of cough, 17
Cromolyn sodium, 72, 164–166, 177
and acute attack, 291
children, 166, 275, 276, 280
future view, 328
improvements to, 165
mechanism of action, 165–166
nebulized liquid, 165
old usage, 164
and pregnancy, 256
spacer, 165
spray, 165
therapeutic level, time span, 166
therapeutic uses, 164, 166
Croup, 18
in differential diagnosis of children, 268–269
Cystic fibrosis, in differential diagnosis of children, 2, 27, 270
Cytotoxic test, 32

D

Daily routines, guidelines, 318–326
children, 324
emergencies, preparedness for, 323–324
environmental control, 319–320
foods/eating, 322
general health factors, 322–323
medication, 320–322
mental attitude, 326
vacations, 325
Death
anaphylactic reaction, 69, 74–75
from asthma, 2
Decadron, 168, 169, 173
Decadron Turbinaire, 255
Dehumidifier, 61
Delayed food reactions, 69
tests for, 75
Dental procedures, precautions in, 173–174, 307
DeVilbiss, 158
Diabetes, 27
Diaphragm, 233–234
Diets. *See* Elimination diets.
Differential diagnosis, 19, 27
See also Children, differential diagnosis.
Doctors
for children, 22–23, 272–273

Doctors (*continued*)
communication about medications, 179
first visit, 23–35
guidelines for patients, 32–35
history, taking, 24–26
patient procrastination and, 20–21
patient's bill of rights, 35–36
physical examination, 26–32
pregnancy, 22
signs for need of, 20–22
types of, 22–23
Downy mildew, 45
Dry rot, 45
Dust, 9, 10, 46–47
as allergen transport system, 47
Dust mites, 9
Dyspnea. *See* Shortness of breath.

E
Egg-free diet
foods to avoid, 119–120
sample menus, 121–122
Electrocardiogram (EKG), 28
Electrostatic air purifiers, 60
Elimination diets, 77–103, 213–214
children, 273–274
corn-free diet, 116–119
egg-free diet, 119–122
eliminating one food, 77–78
eliminating two foods, 78–79
milk-free diet, 111–113
multiple elimination diet, 82–103
adding foods back, 101–103
for adults, 93–101
basics of, 82–83
for children, 83–93
sample menus, 84–87, 96–101
rotation diet, 110
salicylate-free diet, 122–125
survival guide, 107–110
vitamins and, 105
wheat-free diet, 113–116
yeast-free diet, 80–82, 125–128
ELISA (Enzyme-linked Immuno-Assay), 30, 329
Elixophyllin, 146, 147, 185, 289
Elixophyllin-S.R., 147
Emergencies
adrenalin, 69, 74, 155
anaphylactic reactions, 74–75
children and, 277–278
emergency surgery, 307–308
information needed in, 302–303
See also Acute attacks.
Emergency room, 297–301
leaving emergency room, 300–301
procedure in, 297–299
Emotions, as trigger, 11
Emphysema, 2, 27
Environmental control, 53–64
air pollution alerts, guidelines for asthmatics, 65–66
air ventilation system of home, 60–61
away from home, 63–64
basement/attic/crawl spaces, 59
bathroom, 59
bedroom, 56–58
car, 62–63
children, 273
kitchen, 59
moderation in, 54, 56
property outside house, 62
situations for action, 53–54
smoke, avoiding, 64
and tight building syndrome, 61–62
Environmental stimuli
aero-irritants, 42, 50
animal dander, 48
cottonseed, 48–49
dust, 46–47
feathers, 48
flaxseed, 49
fungus, 45–46
kapok, 48
mites, 47
pollen, 42–44
pollution, 51–52
pyrethrum, 49
smoke, 49–50
weather, 51–52
Eosinophil chemotatic factor of anaphylaxis (ECF-A), 8
Ephedrine, 255
Epidermis, animals, 48
Epiglottitis, 20
in differential diagnosis of children, 269
Epinephrine. *See* Adrenalin.
EpiPen, 69, 74, 278, 296
EpiPen Jr., 278
Exercise, recommendations, 246
Exercise-induced asthma, 9, 176, 204–205, 271, 279
cromolyn sodium, 164, 166
hypnosis, 231
Exhalation, 232
in asthma attack, 4
Eyes, allergic shiners, 208

F
Family history, 21
FAST, 30
Fatty foods, 12
Feathers, 9, 48
Fibrosis, 11
Flaxseed, 49
Flunisolide, 168, 172
Food additives, 9, 70, 83, 103
Food allergens, 39
Food families, listing of, 72–74
Food reactions, 31
alcohol, 104
allergic food reactions, 67
anaphylactic reactions, 69, 72, 74–75
changes over time, 69–70
delayed reactions, 69, 75
drugs for prevention of, 72
elimination diets, 77–103
and food families, 71–74

Food reactions (*continued*)
food intolerances, 68
and form of food, 70, 71
hidden food allergies, 75–76
immediate reactions, 68–69, 71
most notorious substances, 105–106
tests for food allergies, 70, 75
treatment, 71
See also Elimination diets.
Foods, fungus in, 46
Forced expiration volume, 28
Foreign-body obstruction, in differential diagnosis of children, 27, 269
Formaldehyde, 50, 53
Fungal overgrowth, 157
Fungus, 45–46
in foods, 46
indoor sources, 45
nature of, 45
outdoor sources, 45
seasons for, 46
Future advances, 327–331
for allergy testing, 329–330
for environmental factors, 330
for immunotherapy, 330
for medications, 328–329, 330–331

G
Gastroesophageal reflex, 215
actions of, 11
reducing, 12
as trigger, 11–12
Genetic factors, 7
asthma, 248–250
Geographic areas, 6
fungi seasons, 46
pollination seasons, 43–44, 332–348 (regional tables)
GI (gastrointestinal) series, 12
Glottis dysfunction, misdiagnosed as asthma, 18–19
Gold, 175
Golf, 9
Grass pollens, 42, 43
Group therapy, 223

H
Hair analysis, 31
Heartburn, 11
Heart disease, in differential diagnosis of children, 270
Heart failure, 2, 20, 21
Heating system, 60
HEPA (High Efficiency Particulate Air), 60–61
Hiatus hernia, 11
Histamine, 8, 40
History, doctor's visit, 24–26
Hoarseness, 157
Hospitalization, 301–302
Humidifiers, guidelines for use, 61
Humidity, 39
Hydroxyzine hydrochloride, 163, 254
Hyperventilation syndrome, in differential diagnosis of children, 270
Hypnosis
Hypnotic Induction Profile, 229
stress reduction, 228–231
Hyposensitization. *See* Immunotherapy.

I
Immediate food reactions, 68–69
anaphylactic emergencies, 74–75
treatment, 71
Immunoglobulin-E (IgE), 8, 39–40, 41
Immunoglobulin test, 27
Immunoperidoxiase (IP) tests, 329
Immunotherapy
allergy testing, 134–137
appropriateness of, 137
asthma and, 141–142
children, 278–279
effectiveness factors, 137, 141
future view, 330
injections, administration of, 139
perennial approach, 138
and pregnancy, 256–257
reactions, 140–141
results, 141–142
schedule for, 139–140
seasonal approach, 138
serum in, 138
stopping therapy, 211–212
theory in, 134
Inderal (propranolol), 153
Infants, wheezing, 20
Infections
children, 278
indications of, 287, 292
treatment regime, 176, 209
as trigger, 10, 287
Inflammatory response, allergic reaction, 165–166
Inhalation, 232
in asthma attack, 4
Insect particles, 9
Inspirease, 157, 274
Intal, 255
capsules, 186
nebulized liquid, 186
spray, 186
See also Cromolyn sodium.
Internists, 22
Intradermal test, 30
Iodides, 167
side effects, 167
Ionization of atmosphere, 52
Ipratropium bromide, 174–175
Isoproterenol, 12

J
Jacobson, Dr. Edmund, 226
Job setting, environmental control, 63

K
Kapok, 9, 48
Ketoconazole, 80

Ketotifen (Zaditen), 72, 329
Kirschman spirals, 17
Kitchen, environmental control, 59
Klorvess, 171
K-Lyte/C1, 171

L
Late phase response, allergic reaction, 166
Leukotriene (LTE_4), 8, 40
Lifestyle changes, xiii, 3, 26
Linguet, 162
Lithium, 154
Locked-lung syndrome, 156, 289
Lung cancer, 2
LUNG LINE, 36–37, 311

M
Marax, 163, 187, 254
Mast cell-IgE complex, 8, 9, 40, 41
Mast cells, 30, 165
Mecholyl challenge test, 19
Medic-Alert bracelet, 174, 307
Medications, 54, 143–201
  adrenalin, 155
  albuterol, 155–159
  antihistamines, 167
  atrovent, 174–175
  corticosteroids, 167–174
  cromolyn sodium, 164–166
  ephedrine, 162
  gold, 175
  iodides, 167
  isoproterenol, 162
  metaproterenol, 159–161
  methotrexate, 175
  most commonly used (chart), 181–200
  natural medications, 104
  over-the-counter drugs, 103
  pregnancy, 253–257
  sample regimens, 175–178
    for mild asthma, 175–176
    for moderate asthma, 177–178
    for severe asthma, 178
  TAO (troleandomycin), 175
  terbutaline sulfate, 161–162
  theophylline, 146–154
  theophylline-sympathomimetic combinations, 163
  See also specific types of medications.
Medihaler-Iso, 162
Medrol, 168, 169, 173, 175
Mental attitude, guidelines, 326
Meperidine, 12
Metabisulfites, 68, 84, 108
  listing of foods containing, 106
Metaprel, 159, 160, 187, 254, 255, 258, 291
Metaproterenol, 160, 254, 255, 256, 291
  brand names, 159
  children, 160–161
  nebulized liquid, 160
  side effects, 161
  spray, 159–160
  syrup, 160–161
  tablets, 160–161
Methotrexate, 175
Milk allergy, 208
Milk-free diet
  foods to avoid, 111–112
  sample menus, 112–113
Milk products, pure forms, 101–102
Mistometer, 162
Mites, 47, 58
  nature of, 47
Mitral valve prolapse, in differential diagnosis of children, 271
Mold, 9, 45
  home, areas for, 59
  pamphlet on, 59
Monaghan Aerochamber, 157
Monosodium glutamate (MSG), 68, 71, 84, 105
Morphine, 12
Mucus
  in asthma attack, 3, 4, 10
  excess, as symptom, 17
  excessive, postural drainage, 235, 240–245
  excessive production, 233
  mucus plugs, 17
Multiphasic blood scan, 27
Mycostatin, 80

N
Nasal congestion, 208, 212
Nasalcrom, 255, 257
National Jewish Center for Immunology and Respiratory Medicine, 36, 37
  activities of, 309–311
Nebulizers
  Albuterol, 157–158
  children, 158, 274–275
  cromolyn sodium, 165
  equipment, 158
  metaproterenol, 160
  training in use of, 295
Neocalglucon, 208
Nicotine, 12
Nitrogen dioxide, 50, 53, 59
Nitrous oxide, 307
Nonsteroidal anti-inflammatory drugs (NSAID), 106
Nutrasweet, 105
Nystatin, 80

O
Osteoporosis, and steroid use, 171
Over-the-counter drugs, 103–104
  and pregnancy, 256

P
Paint odors, 50
Peak flow, 29
Peak flow meter, 286
Pediatricians, 22
Peppermint, 12
Perfumes, 10, 50, 63
Phethysmography, 29
Phosphodiesterase, 144–145

Physical examination/diagnostic tests, 26–32
  blood test, 27
  chest X-ray, 27
  cytotoxic test, 32
  electrocardiogram (EKG), 28
  ELISA (Enzyme-linked Immuno-Assay), 30
  forced expiration volume, 28
  hair analysis, 31
  immunoglobulin test, 27
  peak flow, 29
  phethysmography, 29
  PRIST (Paper Radioimmunosorbent Test), 30–31
  provocative neutralization challenges, 32
  pulmonary function test (spirometry), 28
  RAST (Radioallergosorbent test), 30
  sinus X-ray, 27
  skin tests, 29–30
  sweat test, 27
  vitamin screening panels, 31–32
Physical therapy approach, 235–247
  breathing exercises, 235–239
  exercise, 246
  patient candidacy for, 235–236
  postural drainage, 235, 240–245
  relaxation exercises, 245
Platelet-aggregating factor of anaphylaxis (PAF-A), 8
Pneumonia, 11
  in differential diagnosis of children, 269
Pollen, 9, 42–44
  grass pollens, 42, 43
  pollen counts, 44
  ragweed, 42, 43, 44
  seasons of pollination, 43–44
    regional tables, 332–348
  tree pollens, 42, 43
  weather conditions and, 43
Pollution, 10, 51–52
  air pollution alerts, guidelines for asthmatics, 65–66
  indoor pollution, 53
  outdoor pollution, 52–53
Postural drainage, 235, 240–245
  "clapping" chest/back, 240, 241
  effects of, 240
  liquid intake in, 240
  positioning, 241–245
Posture, of asthmatics, 233–234
Potassium iodide (SSKI), 167, 254
Potassium loss, and steroid use, 171
Prednisone, 168, 169, 173, 174, 175, 178, 209, 277, 292, 294
Pregnancy, 248–264
  acute attack, 259
  breast-feeding, 263–264
  cesarean section, 262
  delivery, 259–263
    anesthesia, 261
    medications during labor, 261
    natural childbirth, 260–261
    postdelivery period, 262–263
  major concerns, 248
  medication, 253–257
    acceptable drugs, 161, 255–257
    drugs to avoid, 254
  rhinitis, 257
  and risk to mother, 250–251
  and risk to newborn, 250
  treatment plan, 251–253, 258, 260
Preservatives. *See* Metabisulfites.
PRIDE Program (Progressive Rehabilitation through Individual Development and Education), 310
Primatene, 188
Primatene "P" Formula, 163
PRIST (Paper Radioimmunosorbent Test), 30–31
Progesterone, 12
Progressive relaxation, stress reduction, 226–228
Property outside house, environmental control, 62
Prostaglandins, 8, 40
  future view, 329
Proventil, 155, 156, 159, 189, 210, 212, 254, 255, 275, 277, 288, 291
Provocative neutralization challenges, 32
Psychological aspects/treatment approaches, 219–231
  children, 281–282
  group therapy, 223
  misconceptions about, 220
  problem-oriented psychological therapy, 222–224
  psychological interpretation of asthma, 219–220
  psychological support services, 222
  "psychosomatic" asthma case, 5–6
  stress and asthma, 220–221, 224–228
Pulmonary function test (spirometry), 28
Pulmonologists, 23
Puncture test, 29–30
Pyrethrum, 49
Pyribenzamine, 257

Q
Quibron, 147
Quibron-S.R., 147
Quibron-T, 192
Quibron-TSR, 193

R
Rackermann, Francis, 7
Ragweed, 42, 43, 44
Rainy conditions, 52
Ranitidine (Zantac), 12, 153
RAST (Radioallergosorbent test), 30, 70, 136–137, 141, 329
Recipes, 128–133
Reflux. *See* Gastroesophageal reflex.
Relaxation techniques. *See* Stress reduction.
Respiratory system
  of asthmatics, 6–7, 12, 41
  mechanical problems, asthma induced, 232–234
Reversibility, 28
Rhinitis, 207
  pregnancy, 257

S
Salicylate-free diet
  foods to avoid, 125–126
  sample menus, 123–125
Salicylates, 83
Saline spray, 257
Saliva, animals, 48
Scratch test, 29, 135
Self-monitoring, peak flow meter, 286
Serum, in allergy shots, 138
Shortness of breath, 204–205, 271
  as symptom, 15–16
Sinus X-ray, 27
Skin tests, 29–30, 135, 329
  intradermal skin tests, 135
  intradermal test, 30
  puncture test, 29–30, 135
  scratch test, 29, 135
Sleep, 19
Slo-Bid, 146, 147–148, 176, 193, 276
Slo-Phyllin, 146, 147, 194, 289
Slo-Phyllin-S.R., 147
Slow-K, 171
Smog, 39
Smoke, 10, 39, 49–50
  avoiding, 64
  passive, effects of, 50
  respiratory effects, 49–50
Sodium ions, 27
Somophyllin, 146, 195
Somophyllin-T, 147, 289
Spacers
  advantages of, 157
  albuterol, 157
  children, 274
  cromolyn sodium, 165
Spiegel, Herbert, 229
Spirometry. *See* Pulmonary Function Test.
Sporadic asthma, 205, 205–206, 210
Sprays
  albuterol, 156–157
  corticosteroids, 168, 172–173
  cromolyn sodium, 165
  dosage, 156, 159–160
  locked lung syndrome, 156, 289
  overuse problem, 156, 255
  and pregnancy, 255
  terbutaline sulfate, 161
  usage guidelines, 156–157
Spectrophotometer Phadezym, 30
SR Gyrocaps, 194
Steroids. *See* Corticosteroids.
Stress and asthma, 5, 11
  asthma as stress trigger, 221
  cyclical nature, 224–225
Stress reduction
  biofeedback, 225–226
  hypnosis, 228–231
  progressive relaxation, 226–228
Surgery, 304–308
  elective surgery, 304
  emergency surgery, 307–308
  information needed about asthmatic, 304–306
  and steroid dependency, 173–174, 305
SusPhrine, 196, 296
Sweat test, 27
Swimming, 9, 246, 279
Sympathetic nervous system, 330
Sympathomimetic drugs, 145
  and acute attack, 291–292, 293
  adrenalin, 155
  albuterol, 155–159
  brand names, 155, 157, 159, 161
  children, 158, 159, 160, 160–161, 162, 275
  ephedrine, 162
  future view, 328
  isoproterenol, 162
  metaproterenol, 159–161
  nebulized liquid, 157–158, 160
  and pregnancy, 255–256
  pregnant women, 161
  side effects, 156, 159, 161
  spacers, 157
  spray form, 156–157, 159–160, 161
  syrup, 159, 160–161
  tablets, 159, 160–161
  terbutaline sulfate, 161–162
  theophylline-sympathomimetic combinations, 163
  See also specific drugs.
Symptoms, 2
  asthma attack, 3–4
  coughing, 17
  excess mucus, 17
  shortness of breath, 15–16
  situations related to discomfort, 14–15
  wheezing, 16–17

T
Tachypnea, 18
TAO (troleandomycin), 175
Tedral, 163, 197
Telephone services, LUNG LINE, 36–37
Tennis, 9
Terbutaline sulfate, 254, 255, 291
  brand names, 161
  children, 161, 162
  dosage, 161–162
  pregnant women, 161
  side effects, 161
  spray, 161
Terramycin, 254
Theo-24, 146, 147, 150, 152, 153, 198
Theobid, 198
Theo-Dur, 146, 147, 148, 176, 199, 211, 212
Theolair, 146, 199
Theolair-S.R., 147
Theophyl, 146
Theophyl-S.R., 147
Theophylline, 12, 145, 146–154, 177, 213, 255
  and acute attack, 290–291, 292–293
  blood levels, 151–152, 290
  brand names, 146, 147
  children, 148–149, 152–153, 275–276
  dosage, 148–151
  future view, 328

Theophylline (*continued*)
  intermediate-acting, 146–147, 149, 151–152
  long-acting, 147, 148, 149, 152, 276
  metabolism of, affecting factors, 152–154
  for mild asthma, 147
  for moderate asthma, 147
  and pregnancy, 255
  for severe asthma, 147–148
  short-acting, 146, 147, 148, 149, 151, 276
  side effects, 149, 154, 328
Theophylline-S.R., 147
Theophyllinization, 290
Thunderstorms, 52
Tight building syndrome, 61–62
Tiredness, 21
Tomato, 12
Treatment approaches
  case examples, 202–218
  steps in, 217–218
  See also Elimination diets; Environmental control; Immunotherapy; Medications; Physical therapy approach; Psychological aspects/treatment approaches; Stress reduction.
Tree pollens, 42, 43
Triamcinolone Acetonide, 168, 172
Triamcinolone clathrate, 172
Triggers, 6–13
  airborne irritants, 10
  allergies, 7–9
  chain of events related to, 39–41
  emotions, 11
  exercise, 9
  gastroesophageal reflex, 11–12
  infections, 10

U
Uniphyl, 146, 147, 150–151, 152, 153, 200

V
Vacations, 110
  environmental control, 64
  guidelines, 325
Vancenase, 255, 257
Vanceril, 168, 172, 173, 201, 213, 255, 256
Ventolin, 155, 156, 201, 254, 255, 275, 288, 291, 292
Vibramycin, 254
Vistaril, 254
Vitamins, 171
  supplemental dose, 105
Vitamin screening panels, 31–32
Vocal cords, glottis dysfunction, 18–19

W
Weather, 51–52
  components of, 51
  ionization of atmosphere, 52
  and pollination season, 43–44
  trends related to asthma, 51–52
Weather and Air Pollution Committee, 65
Wheal, 29, 30, 140
Wheat-free diet
  foods to avoid, 114
  sample menus, 118–119
Wheezing, 2
  in asthma attack, 3
  infants, 20
  other causes of, 16–17
  as symptom, 16–17
  treatment regimen, 176
Wind, 52
Wood smoke, 53, 59

Y
Yeast, 76
Yeast-free diet, 79, 80–82
  foods to avoid, 125–126
  sample menus, 126–128
Yellow dye #5, 84, 108

Z
Zaditen, 329

ABOUT THE AUTHORS

■■■■■

DR. STUART H. YOUNG

Dr. Stuart H. Young graduated from Colgate University and received his medical degree from the State University of New York-Downstate Medical Center. He completed a fellowship in allergy, immunology, and asthma at the National Jewish Hospital and Asthma Research Center and the University of Colorado, in Denver, Colorado.

In addition to his private practice, he is also the Chief of Allergy Clinics in both the Department of Medicine and the Department of Pediatrics at the Mount Sinai Medical Center. He is a clinical associate professor of medicine and a clinical associate professor of pediatrics at the Mount Sinai Medical School.

Dr. Young is board-certified in pediatrics, pediatric allergy, and allergy and clinical immunology (a conjoint board of The American Board of Internal Medicine and The American Board of Pediatrics). In addition, he is a fellow of the following national medical societies which are instrumental in the diagnosis and treatment of allergic disease: The American Academy of Pediatrics (Allergy Section), The American College of Allergy, The American Academy of Allergy and Clinical Immunology, and The American College of Chest Physicians.

Dr. Young has lectured extensively and published numerous papers in his field. In addition, he is the coeditor of two medical textbooks: *The Psychobiological Aspects of Allergic Disease,* and *Practical Points in Allergy*. He is currently engaged in research on many aspects of allergy and asthma and is active in several societies to help control bronchial asthma. He resides in New York City with his wife, Marcia.

SUSAN A. SHULMAN

After suffering with asthma for many years, Mrs. Shulman was referred to Dr. Stuart Young who has helped her significantly. She has tried many of the treatment approaches available to the asthmatic patient and has developed her own "bag of tricks" and long list of helpful hints. Her dedication to understanding her own problem and to helping others who have asthma have compelled her to join with Dr. Young in writing this book.

Mrs. Shulman is a graduate of Brooklyn College with a B.A. in mathematics and an M.A. in math education from the University of Minnesota. Mrs. Shulman currently serves as an assistant professor in the Department of Mathematics at Middlesex County College and teaches at the Real Estate School of Central New Jersey.

She is the author of *Mathematics Review for the Real Estate Licensing Examination*. At present she resides in East Brunswick, New Jersey, with her husband, Martin, and her two sons, Lawrence and Andrew.

MARTIN D. SHULMAN, PH.D.

Martin D. Shulman, Ph.D. is a speech-language pathologist and coordinator of the Speech and Hearing Programs at Kean College of New Jersey, Union, New Jersey, where he serves as associate professor in the Department of Special Education and Individualized Services. He has been appointed by Governor Thomas Kean to serve the state of New Jersey on the Advisory Committee for Audiologists and Speech-Language Pathologists.

Dr. Shulman has written and presented many scientific papers in his field and is an associate editor for *Language, Speech, and Hearing Services in Schools,* a journal published by the American Speech-Language-Hearing Association. He brings his writing experience to this book as well as his familiarity with asthma stemming from nineteen years of marriage to Susan. By living through the ups and downs of Susan's asthma, Dr. Shulman has suffered and compensated in his own way, bringing yet another perspective on asthma to this book.